Pregnancy and Birth

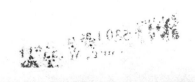

Pregnancy and Birth

A Guide to Making
Decisions That Are Right for
You and Your Baby

Teresa Pitman
and Joyce Barrett, M.D.

KEY PORTER BOOKS

For our families: John, Liza and Pam Hambley, Adam Mabee, and
my granddaughter Emma, whose birth illuminates my life
To Matthew, Lisa, Daniel, Jeremy, Esmaralda, Sebastian, and Callista Pitman.

Library and Archives Canada Cataloguing in Publication

Barrett, Joyce, 1944–
Pregnancy and birth : a guide to making decisions that are right for you and your baby / Joyce Barrett, Teresa Pitman. —
2nd ed.

Includes index.
ISBN-13: 978-1-55263-791-3, ISBN-10: 1-55263-791-3

1. Pregnancy—Popular works.   2. Prenatal care.   3. Childbirth.   I. Pitman, Teresa   II. Title.

RG525.B37 2007   618.2'4   C2006-906434-2

The publisher gratefully acknowledges the support of the Canada Council for the Arts and the Ontario Arts Council for
its publishing program. We acknowledge the support of the Government of Ontario through the Ontario Media
Development Corporation's Ontario Book Initiative.

We acknowledge the financial support of the Government of Canada through the Book Publishing Industry Development
Program (BPIDP) for our publishing activities.

Key Porter Books Limited
Six Adelaide Street East, Tenth Floor
Toronto, Ontario
Canada M5C 1H6
www.keyporter.com

Every reasonable effort has been made to trace ownership of copyright materials. All line drawings by Karen Visser. Photo by John-Mark
Romans/istockphoto page 19. Photo by Kateryna Govorushchenko/istockphoto page 49. Photo by TCL/Masterfile pages 75 and 91. Photo
by John Carleton/istockphoto page 103. Photos by Adrienne Leong pages 119, 149, 171, 211, and 255. Photo by Tom Skudra page 186.
Photos by Reg Vertolli pages 235, 238, and 239. Photo by Nastasha Nicholson pages 292, and 293.

Text design: Marijke Friesen
Electronic formatting: Jean Lightfoot Peters

Printed and bound in Canada

07 08 09 10 11 5 4 3 2 1

CONTENTS

ACKNOWLEDGEMENTS   7

INTRODUCTION
Why Should I Read This Book?   8
The Basics of Birth   14

IN THE BEGINNING:
THE FIRST MONTH   19
1   Choosing a Caregiver   20
2   Calculating Your Due Date   30
3   Lifestyle Risks   32
4   Where Will Your Baby Be Born?   37
5   "High-risk" Pregnancy   46

TWO MONTHS:
FIVE TO EIGHT WEEKS   49
6   Nutrition and Supplementation   50
7   Ultrasound   56
8   The Discomforts of Early Pregnancy   62
9   Sex during Early Pregnancy   66
10 Rubella (German Measles)   68
11 Toxoplasmosis   70
12 Rh-negative Mother   71

THREE MONTHS:
NINE TO TWELVE WEEKS   75
13 What Happens at a Prenatal Checkup?   76
14 Weight Gain in Pregnancy   78

15 Miscarriage and Tubal (Ectopic) Pregnancy   83
16 Tests to Assess the Baby during Pregnancy   91

FOUR MONTHS:
THIRTEEN TO SEVENTEEN WEEKS   103
17 Prenatal Classes   104
18 Preparing to Breastfeed   109
19 More Than One Baby   111
20 Urinary Tract Infections   115

FIVE MONTHS:
EIGHTEEN TO TWENTY-ONE WEEKS   119
21 Your Developing Baby   120
22 Preparing for Baby   122
23 Caesarean Birth   125
24 Vaginal Birth after Caesarean
    Section (VBAC)   134
25 Sexually Transmitted Diseases   141

SIX MONTHS:
TWENTY-TWO TO TWENTY-FIVE WEEKS   149
26 The Discomforts of Late Pregnancy   150
27 Hospital Routines   153
28 Do You Want a Doula?   157
29 Gestational Diabetes   159
30 Bleeding in the Third Trimester of
    Pregnancy   164
31 Group B Streptococcus   166

SEVEN MONTHS:
TWENTY-SIX TO TWENTY-NINE WEEKS   171
32 Your Baby's Position in the Uterus   172
33 Hypertension (High Blood Pressure)
     and Pre-eclampsia   180
34 Premature Labour and Birth   186
35 Sex during Late Pregnancy   196

EIGHT MONTHS:
THIRTY TO THIRTY-THREE WEEKS   199
36 Labour and Its Variations   200
37 Problems with the Amniotic Fluid   208
38 Coping with Pain in Labour   211
39 Assessing the Baby during Labour   227

NINE MONTHS:
THIRTY-FOUR TO THIRTY-EIGHT WEEKS   235
40 Supporting Your Partner through Labour 236
41 Induction of Labour   241
42 Pre-labour Rupture of the Membranes   251
43 Here Comes the Baby!   254
44 Delivery of the Placenta   265

TEN MONTHS:
BIRTH AND BEYOND   271
45 "Overdue"   272
46 You and Your Newborn Baby   276
47 Postpartum Depression   281
48 Getting Started with Breastfeeding   285

CONCLUSION
Making Decisions   299

APPENDICES
Northern Babies   305
Understanding Research Methods   308
How to Deliver a Baby   312
Resources   314
Index   316

Acknowledgements

We are pleased to bring you this revised edition that includes the most recent research on important issues for women having babies, and hope you will find the new month-by-month format useful.

Many thanks to the midwives, doctors, and parents who told us they found our first edition helpful and to those who made suggestions for new items to include.

Thank you to Holly Bennett who did her usual outstanding editing work and who is always a pleasure to work with, and to Key Porter Books' editor Carol Harrison who helped us stay on track.

And thank you to all the families who have shared their stories and experiences with us, and who have invited us to be a part, even in a small way, of this special time in their lives.

-Introduction-
Why Should I Read This Book?

In the years since the first edition of this book was published, the landscape of birth in North America has seen many changes. From one perspective, it looks now as though there are two hills, one much higher than the other, with a shallow valley in between.

One hill—the larger one—represents an approach that has been described as "medicalized." Typically, this involves conducting a number of routine tests during pregnancy; often labour is induced or augmented, and pain medication is given beginning when the mother arrives at the hospital, early in labour. There may be a "cascade of interventions" where one intervention leads to or increases the risk of the need for a second intervention, which leads to a third and so on. The baby may be delivered with forceps or a vacuum extractor or, increasingly often, by Caesarean section. Caesarean births may be planned in advance, on the doctor's recommendation, or even by request of the mother. The baby may then be removed to a hospital nursery, at least for a period of time, or kept in a small plastic bed in the mother's room.

The smaller hill is perhaps bigger than it used to be, especially in Canada where midwifery and home births are paid for by some provincial health insurance plans, but still includes only a small percentage of women. The mothers on this hill often choose to have fewer prenatal tests and make plans to give birth at home with minimal intervention and no pain medication in labour. The baby usually stays with the mother, often sharing her bed, after the birth.

Some women are in the valley. A mother may plan a hospital birth with minimal medication, for example, or a mother who had planned a home birth may find herself needing to use some of the interventions from the "bigger hill" and so crosses the valley towards it, while bringing her doula and midwife to provide support.

The experience of being pregnant and giving birth is clearly quite different, depending on where you stand and the choices you make.

These changes in childbirth practices only reinforce the importance of the premise of this book: with this range of options available, it is more important than ever for women to have the information they need to make the decisions that are right for them, their families, and their babies.

What Can We Learn from Research?

Trish has been waiting all morning to share her news. As the other women from her aerobics class gather for their traditional early morning snack and chat, she grabs the opportunity to make her announcement.

"Guess what? I'm pregnant!"

"Congratulations!" There is a chorus of excited comments.

Then Rita says, "Have you found an obstetrician yet? Mine was excellent, if you want his name."

Shelley jumps in. "Don't go to an obstetrician! Get a midwife. I had one and she was wonderful—they give you so much support."

Rita shakes her head. "No, you need an obstetrician just in case something goes wrong. They're the experts."

Alana adds, "Well, I wouldn't go with a midwife but I stayed with my family doctor and he was pretty good. I had a huge episiotomy, though, and it still bothers me."

"Sure," says Gwen, "but think about what would have happened if you didn't have the episiotomy. You'd probably have a bad tear instead, and everyone knows that's worse."

Shelley disagrees. "My midwife said that isn't true. Most women don't need episiotomies and she's good at delivering babies without tearing."

Jane turns to Trish and asks, "Are you having an amnio? When's your first ultrasound scheduled?"

Trish shrugs her shoulders. She doesn't even know what an amnio is and thought ultrasound was something used to detect fish swimming under a boat.

Shelley says, "I didn't have any ultrasounds."

"I had seven," Gwen counters. "But of course, I had gestational diabetes so I was high risk."

Rita says, "And make sure you get the epidural as early as possible."

Trish heads off to work with her head full of new questions and concerns. She hadn't known that being pregnant meant making so many decisions.

In the years since the first edition of this book was published, we've talked to many women about their pregnancies and births. If anything, it has become more rather than less complicated to navigate your way through a long list of tests, interventions, medications, and procedures.

As a pregnant woman, your conversations with other mothers are guaranteed to reveal different opinions about almost every aspect of pregnancy and childbirth. Every woman you talk to will have a different birth story—and that's understandable, because every pregnancy and every birth is unique. (Yours will be, too!) But you may find yourself feeling very confused by the dramatically different ideas you're hearing about everything from prenatal tests to how to take care of a newborn.

It often seems that what should be a natural, normal part of life has become a very medical process. When you are pregnant, you will be offered a whole range of tests, visit your doctor or midwife on a regular basis, and in most cases plan to give birth in a hospital. But even within those medical parameters, some normal pregnancies and births seem to be much more "high-tech" than others. That's what Trish discovered as she listened to her friends discussing their birth experiences.

It doesn't seem possible that these very different approaches can all be right. Is an episiotomy beneficial to the mother and baby or not? Should you be concerned about developing gestational diabetes, or should you decide not to be tested for it? Does using a monitor to continuously listen to the baby's heartbeat in labour keep the baby safer? Should you have your labour induced if you are "overdue"?

Hasn't anyone researched all of this?

Yes, someone has!

In fact, since the 1950s, literally thousands of studies have been conducted in countries all over the world, researching the risks and benefits of various tests, treatments, and approaches to different parts of pregnancy and childbirth.

This is a lot of research for even the most dedicated doctor or midwife to keep up with. To help people sort this out, the Cochrane Collaboration—a group of physicians and researchers—evaluate the methods that have been used to do the research and decide which studies are properly done and significant. These studies are then analyzed—if several small studies have been done on the same topic, their results are compared. The authors then make recommendations based on what the research studies showed. New material is constantly being reviewed and added to an updated database, available at www.cochrane.org. The information is also published quarterly on a CD-ROM.

Although the reports on the studies in the Cochrane database include a "plain language" summary, they are not always easy for people without a medical background to follow. The goal of *Pregnancy and Birth: A Guide to Making Decisions That Are Right for You and Your Baby* is to make this valuable information available to pregnant women and their partners.

What Is Effective Care?

What do we mean by **effective care** during pregnancy? Ideally, effective care would result in a healthy mother and a healthy baby. It sounds simple, but in the real world decisions about effective care can be complicated.

One of the reasons there are so many (and often conflicting) approaches to pregnancy and birth is that this is a process that has evolved to work very well, most of the time. If you never had a single prenatal visit or test and gave birth at home alone, in the majority of cases you and your baby would be just fine. That doesn't mean we'd recommend that approach, because there are situations where things go wrong, and a knowledgeable caregiver can make a big difference, but it does tell you something about how normal pregnancy and birth usually is.

A normal pregnant woman is healthy, not ill. While pregnancies are usually monitored by doctors or midwives to make sure things are proceeding as expected, that doesn't mean something is likely to go wrong.

Because most births are normal without any intervention, it's important to consider all the risks and benefits of any intervention carefully. Remember that there are at least two people involved in every pregnancy and birth! Some procedures may only minimally improve the baby's chances of being healthy, but greatly increase the mother's risk of complications. Some medications can reduce the pain of labour for the mother, but increase the risk of the baby having breathing problems after birth. Interventions can also affect the emotional experience of pregnancy and birth, and can affect how parents feel about themselves and their babies.

In examining the research done about pregnancy and childbirth, there are three important questions:

1. What kinds of interventions during pregnancy and childbirth will actually improve the outcome for women and babies? An **intervention** is anything a doctor, midwife, or other caregiver might do, like giving advice on nutrition, recommending a test, or performing surgery. The **outcome** is the measurable results of that intervention for the mother and the baby. Outcomes can include effects such as: more or fewer fevers, infections, or injuries to the mother; more or fewer illnesses, breathing problems, or need for special-care treatment in babies. An improved or positive outcome means healthier mothers and babies.
2. Are there routinely used interventions that make outcomes worse for mothers or babies?
3. Are there questions for which we don't have answers yet?

With some issues, research makes the choice fairly clear. Some interventions are clearly beneficial; others are clearly ineffective or even harmful.

However, there are also plenty of grey areas: issues where the research doesn't come down strongly one way or another and where there are both pluses and minuses to be considered. And there are a surprising number of situations where no good research has been done to determine whether "the way we have always done it" is effective care.

In every situation, you are the one who should assess the evidence available and make the decisions. Research just gives you guidelines; it doesn't make decisions for you. You are the one who will live with the consequences and who knows best what your priorities are. You are the one who must decide what will be effective care for you.

Taking on this responsibility can be frightening—especially in those situations where there are no clear answers. But it is important to realize that if you simply let your caregiver make all the decisions, you are making a conscious decision to do that.

But Shouldn't My Doctor Know All This?

If all this research is available and known, why are there still routines and policies in place that clearly ignore it? This discrepancy between research-based evidence and practice happens not just in pregnancy and childbirth, but in all areas of medicine.

One reason is that practice (what doctors and hospitals actually do) sometimes lags behind the research. Doctors tend to keep on doing what they were taught in medical school, even if those procedures have since been demonstrated to be not beneficial or even potentially harmful. It is time-consuming and often difficult to keep up with reading and evaluating all the studies that are done.

In some situations, practice leaps *ahead* of the research—as happened when electronic fetal monitors were introduced. These machines that track the baby's heartbeat during labour seemed, in theory, like a good idea. By the time research showed they weren't, the use of monitors was firmly established in many hospitals.

Once medical procedures are established, they are very difficult to discontinue. "The way we usually do it" becomes what is called the standard of care in the community, even if it is not supported by research. The standard of care becomes the way in which care is measured—women expect it, and doctors expect all other doctors to do it. New techniques of unproven benefit are often introduced quickly, but when it comes to abandoning tests and procedures that have been shown not to be helpful, inertia sets in. It's hard to admit that something you've been doing for years was not helpful or was even harmful.

Also, our ability to diagnose conditions is ahead of our ability to treat them. Pregnancy diabetes (or **gestational diabetes**) may be a real condition that can be diagnosed by special blood tests; and the babies of women who have gestational diabetes probably do have a slightly higher complication rate. But the research shows that knowing this does not mean we can do anything about it—none of the treatments for gestational diabetes have improved the complication rate at all.

Finally, medical training tends to emphasize the importance of "doing something," and so, rightly or wrongly, this has also become the usual approach to pregnancy. Even when interventions aren't likely to be helpful, "doing something" makes the caregiver (and sometimes the parents) feel better.

Physicians also have a sense that they are less likely to be sued over a complication if they have "done everything." A doctor feels more protected when a complication occurs if he has done a lot of tests and a Caesarean section rather than if he has sat and patiently waited for the baby to be born—even if none of those interventions could have prevented the complication.

One of the ways that standard medical practices change, though—especially in the area of pregnancy and childbirth—is under pressure from women who have read the research and made their own informed decisions. Your discussions with your caregiver will contribute to the ongoing improvement of prenatal care.

What This Book Can Do for You

Pregnancy and Birth will give you factual information to help you make decisions that are right for you, your baby, and your family. It summarizes and explains the research, giving plenty of examples from the experiences of other women. It will also discuss how to negotiate these choices with your caregiver.

Both authors have been involved in childbirth for many years—Dr. Joyce Barrett, now retired, was a family physician with a large pregnancy practice, and Teresa Pitman has worked as a childbirth educator, doula (providing support for women in labour), and writer. Teresa is currently the executive director of La Leche League Canada. To the research described in the Cochrane database, we have added our own experiences, and those of women we have worked with or who have written to us about their births.

Let's imagine that right after work, Trish drops into a bookstore and buys a copy of this book. She finds out what an ultrasound is, and decides to discuss with her husband whether or not they want to have this done. Since midwifery care is covered in her provincial health plan, she thinks she'll call to set up an appointment and see if this is a good choice for her.

She still has lots of questions and lots of decisions to make, but now she feels she can make them based on solid information.

This book can't answer all your questions—some of them don't have answers. It can't make your decisions for you. It *can* give you a foundation of knowledge that will enable you to make your own decisions. That's a foundation that can make you feel more confident and prepared throughout your pregnancy, labour, and birth, and help your experience be as positive as possible.

The Basics of Birth

As we explain the research that has been done, we will be using many pregnancy-related medical terms. If you are already familiar with most of these, feel free to skip ahead. If not, you may find this section helpful.

The Anatomy of Pregnancy

A new baby is conceived when the sperm and egg (or **ovum**) meet and fuse into a single cell, and that cell rapidly divides to form a cluster of cells. This living cluster floats down from its point of origin in the **Fallopian tubes** (tubes inside the mother's abdomen that lead from the **ovaries**, where the eggs are made, to the **uterus**, or womb). Once inside the uterus, the **embryo** (a term for the developing baby early in pregnancy) will settle into the lining of the uterus. (This lining is what comes away through the vagina during a woman's monthly menstrual period. This month the lining will stay in place, providing nourishment for the embryo, and the woman will "miss her period"—her first clue that she is pregnant.)

Some of the cells in this cluster begin to form a **placenta**, which will transmit oxygen and nutrients from the mother's bloodstream to the baby's. At first, the placenta consists of **chorionic villae**, small protrusions of cells along the wall of the uterus. When it's fully formed, the placenta will look like a large slab of beef liver with a slick and shiny membrane on one side. Out of this side emerges the **umbilical cord**, which attaches at the other end to the baby's abdomen. (When it dries up and falls off after the baby is born, the place where the cord was attached becomes the baby's navel.)

Pregnancy is divided into three **trimesters**: the first trimester is the first three months, the second trimester is the next three months, and the third goes from the end of the sixth month to the day the baby's born. The number of weeks from the mother's last menstrual period is the baby's **gestational age**.

Within the mother's uterus, the baby (called a **fetus** as it continues to develop) is floating in liquid called the **amniotic fluid**. (It's mostly water.) This fluid is contained by amniotic membranes (or just "membranes") that make up the amniotic sac, or bag of waters. At the bottom of the uterus is the **cervix**, leading into the **vagina**. During pregnancy, the cervix is thick and the opening in the centre of it is plugged with mucous. When the cervix begins to open and the mucous plug comes out through the vagina, it is often streaked with a little blood and is called a **bloody show**.

How Labour Works

The whole purpose of labour is to thin out the cervix (the thinning-out process is called **efface-ment**) and pull it open (called **dilation**) wide enough for the baby to come through it, into the vagina, and then out into the world. Most babies are born at **full term**. This means that it has been about 40 weeks since the mother's last menstrual period, give or take two weeks. A baby born earlier than 37 weeks is called **pre-term** or **premature**. When the pregnancy goes on longer than 41 or 42 weeks, it is called **post-term** or **prolonged pregnancy**.

When labour starts, the uterus contracts and this pulls against the cervix, which first thins out and then gradually opens. The whole time that the contractions are working to open the cervix is called the **first stage of labour**; it can be divided into early labour, active labour, and tran-sition. Once the cervix is completely open, the baby can move down into the vagina; this is called the **second stage of labour** or the "push-ing stage." As the baby emerges, it stretches the skin around the vagina called the **perineum**. Once the baby is born, the **third stage of labour** begins as the uterus contracts again to push the placenta out through the vagina.

When the baby is born, the midwives or nurses attending will examine it and give it an **Apgar score** (out of 10) at one minute and five minutes after birth. This simple score was devel-oped to give a quick indication of the baby's health. To determine the score, the baby is given zero, one, or two points in each of five cate-gories: colour, muscle tone, breathing, crying, and response to reflex stimulation. A low score means your baby probably needs extra help with breathing and coping with life outside the womb; a high score tells you the baby is doing well.

The Birth of Your Baby

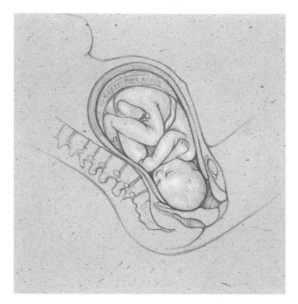

Once the cervix is fully open, the baby is ready to move out of the uterus.

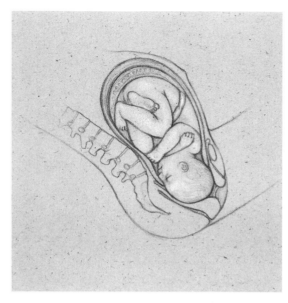

As the baby slips through the open cervix, the baby turns to face her mother's back.

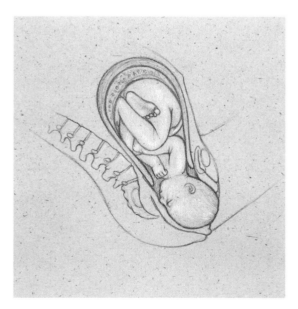

The baby moves through the vagina by gradually lifting her head away from her chest.

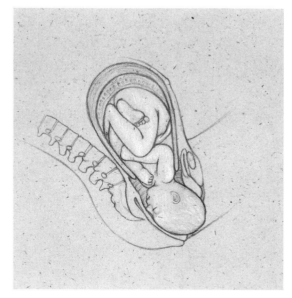

The muscles of the uterus gather behind the baby, helping to ease her down and out into the world.

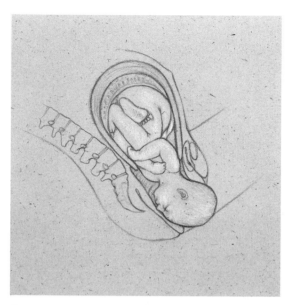

The baby's head crowns. As the outer vaginal tissues are stretched, the mother may experience a burning or tingling sensation.

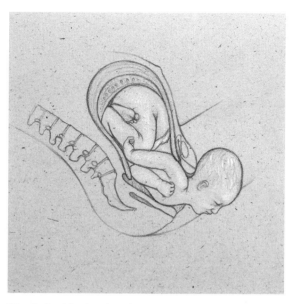

The baby lifts her head completely away from her chest.

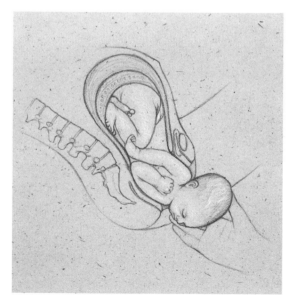

The baby moves her head to the side.

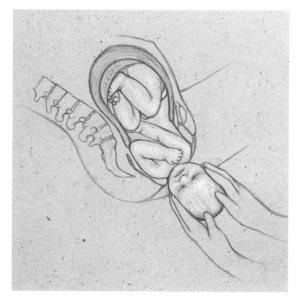

This brings the baby's shoulders into position, ready to be born.

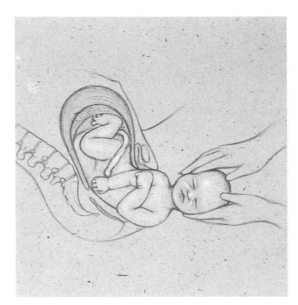

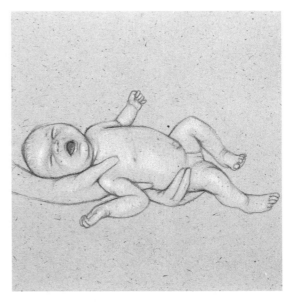

Once the baby's shoulders are born, the rest of the body will slip out quickly.

In a matter of hours, nine months of waiting and planning are fulfilled.

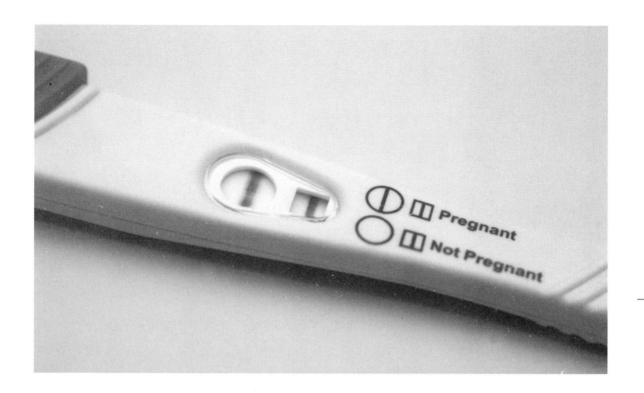

In the Beginning
❧ *The First Month* ❧

Congratulations! You're pregnant! Whether this was a surprise or whether you've been trying for months, you probably feel both excited and a little scared. Having a baby will change your life—and the changes are already starting.

And while you might still be adjusting to the whole idea of being pregnant, you have some important decisions to make. We're here to help with information about your choices in caregiver and place of birth and research about how alcohol and other lifestyle issues can affect your baby.

-1-

Choosing a Caregiver

One of the first and most important decisions you will have to make is choosing who will provide your medical care during your pregnancy and the birth of your baby.

You should expect your caregiver to treat you with respect, to explain any procedures, tests, or concerns about your pregnancy, and to be skilled and competent. Caregivers should be familiar with current research and standards. You want to have your caregiver available when you need him or her, and to have suitable arrangements made for backup care for you when not on call.

Those are the basics. Beyond that there is no one caregiver who will be perfect for everybody. You need to think about the kind of care you want, and then seek out the person who will provide it. Some women prefer a formal approach, while some like the camaraderie of a friendship. Some women like to discuss issues and expect to have their ideas and feelings taken seriously; other women expect to ask questions and get answers. Some women expect their caregiver to make recommendations, other women want to have options outlined, from which they will choose the one that suits them best. Some

women expect emotional and psychological support from their primary caregiver, others expect to get this from their family and friends, or to be referred to another professional if they need extra help.

Susan remembers: "I knew I had found the right person when I asked if I should take vitamins, and 15 minutes later we were still talking about vitamin supplements and general nutrition." But Ruth's first appointment with the same doctor was also her last: "Everything I asked her, she would say, 'Well, that depends.' I wanted advice and she never really told me what to do." Both of these women were very happy with their choices: Susan stayed with this caregiver, and Ruth found someone else with whom she was more comfortable.

How Do You Choose a Caregiver Who Will Meet Your Needs?

There are three different kinds of caregivers currently practising obstetrics in North America: obstetricians, family doctors, and midwives. Each group has different training and often a different approach to pregnancy and birth. (In addition, doulas or labour support people may also be available in your community. Doulas do not provide medical care or catch the baby; rather, they provide support, encouragement, information, and specific techniques for labouring women and their partners. (See Chapter 28) As a pregnant woman, you need to determine which kind of care will best meet your emotional and physical needs.

OBSTETRICIANS

Obstetricians are medical doctors who have specialized in the care of pregnant women. Their medical training focuses on dealing with problems and complications; obstetricians are surgeons who are trained to perform **Caesarean sections** and difficult forceps deliveries. Some obstetricians do **primary care obstetrics**, which means they will care for healthy women throughout their pregnancies. Others have a referral practice for complicated pregnancies only.

As specialists, obstetricians are very familiar with the technology used in pregnancy and birth (which has become quite complex). The routines and policies governing the care of pregnant and labouring women in hospitals are increasingly designed by obstetricians. Even though you may not go to an obstetrician for your care, it is usually obstetricians who set up the rules that must be followed by family doctors and midwives in the hospital.

For several reasons, a policy of having obstetricians care for women with normal, uncomplicated pregnancies is not ideal.

Obstetricians have to keep up their expertise and skills in dealing with complications, and for that reason they should spend most of their time caring for "problem pregnancies." However, the vast majority of pregnancies are normal. The small percentage of complicated births in any community may not provide enough work for a full-time obstetrician. For that reason, most obstetricians also attend normal births. Unfortunately, the interventions appropriate for the complicated pregnancy may sometimes end up being used routinely for their normal births.

There are times when an obstetrician is the best choice as your primary caregiver. If, for example, you have a health problem such as diabetes or high blood pressure before you get pregnant, an obstetrician may be the best physician to care for you during pregnancy—possibly in conjunction with another specialist. Or perhaps you discover that you are expecting triplets—again, an obstetrician may be the best person to help you with this unexpected challenge.

Pregnant women sometimes choose an obstetrician because they see these specialists as being "most qualified." The obstetrician's expertise, training, and specific interest is generally in the area of managing pregnancy complications or problems, not in providing care for normal pregnancies. However, some individual obstetricians are very interested in working with women without any complications and in helping them have the birth they want.

Lee-Anne says, "My family doctor doesn't do births, so he referred me to an obstetrician. He very much supported my desire to have a natural, unmedicated birth. When I arrived at the hospital in early labour, he stopped by to see how

I was doing, and he was very encouraging. After he examined me, he said, 'Just go out and walk—go outside if you want.' So I put on my robe and my husband and I walked for hours, until the baby was almost ready to be born. That wasn't the kind of advice I expected from an obstetrician, but it worked and it suited me just fine."

FAMILY DOCTORS

General practitioners or family doctors sometimes care for pregnant women with normal pregnancies as part of their larger practice (a few family doctors choose to specialize in providing pregnancy care only). A family doctor who has cared for a woman and her family before the pregnancy is likely to have more knowledge of their particular circumstances. As Tracey comments, "Both my husband and I already knew and felt comfortable with our doctor even before I got pregnant. He knew about the problems I'd been through with the recent death of my father, and he had treated me for an earlier miscarriage that was followed by a depression. I appreciated his support and his understanding of my sometimes conflicting emotions."

The care that a family doctor can give to the majority of women whose pregnancies are not affected by any major illness or serious complication will often be more responsive to their needs than that given by specialist obstetricians. Your family doctor will handle all your health needs during the pregnancy—if you sprain your ankle or get stomach flu, these events will be handled by the same doctor with the pregnancy always in mind.

However, the number of family doctors who attend births has been declining sharply in recent years. The reasons for this include increased responsibility and risk of liability, poor pay for pregnancy care, and more hours spent on call. In some communities, this shortage of family doctors willing to attend births has become a serious problem. Family doctors who don't do obstetrics may refer the pregnant women in their practices to either another family doctor who does attend births, or to an obstetrician.

Pregnant women are sometimes concerned that their family doctor may be uninformed about pregnancy and birth, since it is only a small part of the doctor's overall practice. Now that more family doctors are eliminating obstetrics from their practice, those who continue to attend births are generally interested in pregnancy and childbirth and make a point of keeping up to date. If problems develop that need an obstetrician's expertise, your family doctor will be able to refer you.

MIDWIVES

Midwives are specialists in normal pregnancy and birth. If you are seeing a midwife and complications develop with your pregnancy that the midwife does not handle, she will refer you to an obstetrician.

In some provinces and states, midwives have full hospital privileges, so the woman attended by a midwife can choose either a hospital or home birth. In these communities, the midwife will provide all the prenatal care as well, and the mother does not need to see a doctor for prenatal care. In other places, midwives can attend

MIDWIFERY STATUS ACROSS CANADA (AS OF AUGUST 2006)

British Columbia
Self-regulated profession
Both home and hospital births
    Fully funded

Alberta
Registered and regulated under
    Health Disciplines Act
Both home and hospital
    Not funded

Saskatchewan
Midwifery Act was passed, but
    not declared
Home births only
    Not funded

Manitoba
Salaried employees of Regional
Health Authorities
Both home and hospital
    Fully funded

Ontario
Regulated
Both home and hospital
    Fully funded

Quebec
Regulated
Home, hospital, and birthing
    centres
    Fully funded

New Brunswick
Not regulated
Home births only
    Not funded

Nova Scotia
Not regulated
Home births only
    Not funded

Prince Edward Island
Not regulated
Home births only
    Not funded. Women must
    usually purchase midwifery
    services from outside the
    province

Newfoundland
Not regulated
Home births only
    Not funded

Yukon
Not regulated
Home births only; birthing centre
in Whitehorse has closed
    Not funded

Northwest Territories
Registered under Health and
Social Services Authority
Home and hospital
    Fully funded

Nunavut
Two midwives employed by
    provincial government
Legislation is being drafted and
    training of Inuit midwives has
    begun
Home, hospital, birthing centre
    Fully funded

Note: In most cases, where a midwife does not have hospital privileges, she will go with a mother who needs to be transferred to a hospital, and continue to provide support.

For information about midwifery in the United States, please see Midwives' Alliance of North America (www.mana.org) and the American College of Nurse-Midwives (www.acnm.org).

births at home, but if the woman chooses a hospital birth, a doctor must be involved as well. The midwife will generally come to the mother's home for early labour, help her decide when to go to the hospital, and continue to provide support while they are at the hospital. The doctor will then arrive and attend the birth. In that situation, the doctor may also see the mother for prenatal visits. Not all doctors are comfortable working with midwives, but your midwife will be able to give you names of doctors with whom she has worked in the past.

Midwives usually schedule lengthy prenatal visits. Different midwifery practices schedule the midwives in different ways. You may have one primary midwife and expect that she will be at your birth; usually she will have a backup midwife in case she is not able to attend, and will make sure you meet this person during the pregnancy. Most midwives will have another midwife with them at the birth. In some practices, the midwives work on a rotating schedule so you will be cared for by whichever midwife is on duty when you go into labour. With this approach, prenatal visits are usually rotated as well so that you have the opportunity to meet all the midwives.

Midwives are not covered by all health plans, so you will have to determine what the situation is where you live, and whether hiring a midwife is within your budget (most midwives have a sliding fee scale for low-income families).

Heather was living in Alberta when she became pregnant with her first child, and saw her family doctor for the first five months. Then she moved to Ottawa, Ontario, and sought out a midwife. She was very pleased with the care her midwife provided. "Visits lasted at least an hour, were personal, comfortable, and enjoyable. My midwives became like sisters or friends to my husband and me."

Research comparing midwifery care (with appropriate medical backup) to traditional obstetrical care found that midwifery is associated with improved outcomes for both mother and baby. Some of these improved outcomes were **psychosocial**—women felt more supported during their pregnancies and more confident about their ability to have and care for a baby. This isn't surprising, as midwives take more time to be responsive to the emotional needs of the mother and family.

Midwifery care also led to better physical outcomes—fewer **episiotomies** (incisions made in the skin at the opening of the vagina at the time of the baby's birth—see Chapter 43), fewer forceps and vacuum deliveries, and fewer **epidurals** (a type of anaesthetic often used in labour—see Chapter 38, page 220). This is an important benefit for both mothers and babies.

Your Options

Your choice of caregiver will definitely be influenced by geography.

If you live in a large city, you can probably choose between a midwife, a family doctor, or an obstetrician. You may base your choice on whether the practitioner attends births at home, in a birthing centre, or in a teaching hospital.

Women consistently prefer to see the same person during pregnancy and at the birth, or to work with a small group of caregivers and get to know all of them. This is standard practice for midwives, but is not always the case with family doctors and obstetricians. It can be stressful for women to have appointments with one doctor during pregnancy, to discuss concerns and issues, and to make plans with that doctor, but to know that whoever is "on call" will show up when they go into labour.

Research supports the importance of keeping the same caregivers for pregnancy, labour, and birth. Controlled studies show that continuity of care leads to less drug use in labour, shorter labours, and babies less likely to need resuscitation at birth. Parents also feel more satisfied with the care they have received.

Group practices of obstetricians or family doctors can let you know ahead of time how likely it is that your own practitioner will actually be there for your birth. Many groups arrange for you to meet all the practitioners in the group during your pregnancy, so that you will not meet a stranger when you are in labour.

Not always, though. When Margot asked her doctor if she could meet the others who shared his practice, he said that wasn't something they did. "He said that by the time I was in hard labour and the doctor showed up, I wouldn't care who it was. I knew that wasn't true! Knowing I might meet a stranger at my birth confirmed my decision to hire a labour support person (**doula**) to be with me and my husband throughout the whole process."

If you live in a small town or more remote area, your choices will be much more limited. There may not be midwives in your area. Only some of the family doctors may do obstetrics, and often the obstetricians will see only women with complicated pregnancies on the referral of their family doctor. The nearest hospital that has a labour and delivery department may be miles away, as the trend for small hospitals to close their obstetrics wards continues. It may be that you will see your family doctor in your own town for your pregnancy care, then be referred to a doctor who attends deliveries in the community with the hospital two or three hours' travel away.

If you have pre-existing health problems it may be useful for your care to be shared by your pregnancy caregiver and your other practitioner. Christy, for example, who has been diabetic since age 10, saw both her obstetrician and her **endocrinologist** (diabetes specialist) during her pregnancy.

Preparing a Birth Plan

Some couples prepare a formal birth plan. This can include all the things that are important to you around your labour and birth, and what you hope your birth will be like. Some are several pages long, to cover all the possible situations.

On the other hand, your birth plan might just cover one or two points that are important to you. Jacky says, "I wrote a one-line note that said, 'DON'T CALL ME DEAR!!!'." (Some women have also asked the nurses not to call them "Mom.") Some women write very general thoughts about their philosophy of birth; other women are very specific: "Please do not ask me at any time if I want an epidural or other painkiller. If I want it, I will ask for it."

Sometimes writing a birth plan can be a start in gathering information. Sara remembers, "I'm kind of anti-doctor, and I took this birth plan to my first appointment. It was really dogmatic—'I won't have an epidural, I won't have an episiotomy, I won't have a Caesarean section.' My doctor took me seriously and spent a lot of time talking to me about it. He pointed out a few reasonable 'what ifs'—what if I had a placenta previa, what if my baby's heartbeat was really low and none of the things we tried improved it—situations that made me think. I revised my plan to allow for the possibility of problems and made a point of reading more about what can happen at birth."

WHO'S BEST FOR YOU?

How can you choose the best caregiver for you? Some factors you might consider:

1. **Where do you want to give birth?** If you have a choice of hospitals in your area, you may want to choose the hospital first and then look for a doctor or midwife who practises there. Dolores, for example, decided she wanted to have her baby at the family birthing centre in a hospital not far from her home community. She says, "I chose the birthing centre because of their approach to birth and the support they provide for families. When I went for a tour, I knew for sure that it was the right place for me." She was referred to the team of nurse-midwives who provide care for pregnant women and attend births at the centre and was very positive about the care she received.

   If you are planning a home birth, you will need to look for a midwife or a doctor who attends home births, and you may not have many choices. (You can call your provincial or state midwives association; the local La Leche League may also know which doctors are attending home births.) (See also Chapter 4)

2. **Are there any special concerns you have?** Some survivors of sexual abuse, for example, feel strongly that they want to be cared for by women during pregnancy and birth, and need to choose a female caregiver who will attend their birth. For these women, a group practice where there is the possibility of being met by a male physician during labour is probably not a good option.

3. **Are there pre-existing health problems (diabetes, high blood pressure, or other conditions), or past pregnancy complications (a history of premature births) that might require care by a specialist?** You might also develop complications during the pregnancy (such as discovering that you are pregnant with triplets!) that could mean you would want to switch to a specialist.

4. **Talk to other people.** Ask everyone you know who has a baby about their experience and their caregiver. Remember that unless someone has had a really dreadful experience, most people will be positive about their doctors or midwives. Be as specific as you can in your questioning: "Did you discuss episiotomy during your pregnancy? What happened at the birth?" "My husband is concerned that a midwife will be providing all my emotional support in labour, so he won't have a role to play. How did your husband find working with your midwife?" Ask about the issues that most concern you, and try to talk to as many people as possible.

5. **With whom do you feel most comfortable?** Make interview appointments (clearly designated as such when you make the booking) with all your possible choices, to see how comfortable you feel with them. Discuss your concerns with them all and see what kind of reaction you get. (Your gut feelings are probably right!) If you are told over the phone that the practitioner doesn't do "that kind of appointment" it sends a pretty good signal that he or she is not used to being questioned.

Mary decided her plan would be the story of her ideal birth, the one she hoped to have. She says, "Before I wrote my plan, I had a doctor and knew what hospital I was having the baby in. When I started writing, I could picture things going as I wanted up until I left for the hospital, then I couldn't imagine it after that. In my mind, I kept leaving for the hospital closer and closer to the birth. Finally, I realized that I really wanted to have my baby at home. It took a lot of doing, but I got a midwife, convinced my husband, and had Samantha in my bed at home."

Birth plans can be helpful if your caregiver is in a group practice and may not be present for your birth. A copy of your birth plan can be sent to the hospital ahead of time with your pre-registration form, or you can take it in with you in labour and give it to the nurse who is admitting you. This avoids having to discuss issues with a stranger when you are in hard labour. Make sure the birth plan gets onto your chart; then it is part of the written record. Usually nurses and doctors are quite respectful of patients' written preferences; caregivers also realize that your ideas can change during labour and that your plan is not engraved in stone.

Writing a birth plan and going over it with your caregiver can sometimes be an eye-opener. Janice and Bob found that "just about everything on our birth plan our doctor said either he didn't do it that way or the hospital wouldn't allow it." Janice remembers holding Bob's hand during the discussion and feeling miserable. "The things we had written were very important to us."

Bob explains, "We wanted the baby to stay with us all the time and I was quite willing to pay for a private room so I could stay, too. Also, we didn't want our baby to have the eye drops.

Neither of us have ever had any other sexual partners so I knew our baby didn't need them. Our doctor was very pleasant but inflexible; he said that it just couldn't be as we wanted. Janice and I talked about it for hours, then changed doctors and hospitals—driving an hour farther to do it—but were able to get agreement about everything we wanted. And it was worth it."

Your birth plan can include whatever is important to you. Sheila and Marc had requested that their own baby blankets be used to dry off the new baby, as they wanted to take these blankets home to familiarize their two dogs with the baby's smell. Sheila says, "Labour was a lot harder and more painful than I had expected. By the time the baby was actually being born, the dogs were the last thing on my mind. But the nurse had read our plan, and she had our blankets ready and a plastic bag to put them in. Afterwards, I was so pleased that they had cared enough to remember what we wanted."

There is no blank birth plan form to fill out that will suit everybody. Not everybody even wants to have one. But writing out a birth plan can help you clarify your own priorities, reveal areas you want to learn more about, and help to make sure that your feelings and desires are understood and respected—even when labour gets too intense for discussing issues.

Being Assertive with Your Caregiver

The teacher of the prenatal class Vijay and Jamill were attending had just finished explaining why episiotomies were rarely needed or helpful. Vijay raised his hand: "But my doctor says that almost

FINDING MY CAREGIVER: ONE MOTHER'S STORY

"We had just moved to a new community when I found out I was pregnant with my third child. I really didn't know anyone when I came here so it was difficult. I started my search for the doctor I wanted right away, and these are the steps I took:

- I called my old doctor to see if she happened to know anyone in this area she could recommend. No luck.
- I asked a neighbour who worked as a nurse in labour and delivery at the local hospital. She gave me a couple of names of the doctors she thought were the best. I made appointments to go interview them.
- I called the childbirth educator who taught the course at the hospital and asked which doctors she would recommend. She said she didn't make recommendations.
- I went to a parent drop-in group at the parent-child centre and asked about doctors. From the mothers' birth stories, I added a couple more names to my list. Some I could tell right away

from the stories were wrong for me—although the mothers I talked to loved them.

- I called the local La Leche League (LLL) leader and asked who her doctor was. She told me, but said he wasn't taking new patients. I wrote down his name anyway.
- I went for interview appointments with two doctors who were on my list and taking new patients, but didn't feel comfortable with either of them.
- I called the doctor the LLL leader used, and found out that he wasn't taking new patients but a new doctor had just joined their group and she would be happy to see me. I set up an appointment to meet her.
- I had a great interview and decided to have this doctor provide my care.

I didn't try to do this all in one week—it took a little time—but it was worth it. I'm very pleased with our new family doctor and the way she's approaching my pregnancy."

all first-time mothers need episiotomies. Are we supposed to argue with our doctor?"

"Yes, I've been wondering about that too," says Gina, one of the pregnant women. "My doctor said I have to get the **glucose tolerance** test done, but you said the research doesn't support that. How can I disagree with a doctor?"

How can you become more assertive with your caregiver? This is often easier with midwives, who typically invite their clients to participate in decision making and who want them to make fully informed choices. They are often more flexible about how various aspects of pregnancy and birth will be handled.

Some family doctors and obstetricians, on the other hand, have developed set routines, and expect that people will follow them. Most of their patients do. They may be surprised if you disagree with something they suggest, but many doctors are happy to discuss issues and concerns with you, and will respect your choices.

"My heart was pounding when I went into my doctor's office," says Marva. "I was afraid she'd be really upset when I told her I didn't want an **ultrasound**. But she just said, 'Yes, you were pretty sure about your dates, weren't you?' and crossed it off on the form. It was much easier than I'd expected!"

> ### *The Evidence About...*
> ## Choosing a Caregiver
>
> Finding the right caregiver is an important, but very personal decision. Your choices may be limited by what is available in your community. For normal pregnancies, a family physician or midwife will probably be the first choice; obstetricians focus more on complicated or problem pregnancies.

It's true, unfortunately, that some caregivers are not very open to discussing options or to sharing decision making. In a worst-case scenario, you may decide to change to a more receptive caregiver.

Calculating Your Due Date

Your period is late. Maybe you picked up a pregnancy test kit from the drugstore and it confirmed what you already suspected—a baby is on the way. But when will that baby's birth day be? There are three ways to calculate when the baby is likely to arrive.

1. Take the first day of your last menstrual period, subtract three months, and add seven days. So, if your last period started on September 15, three months earlier would be June 15, and when you add seven days you get June 22.
2. Take the first day of your last menstrual period and add 280 days. (There are calculators on the Internet that can do this for you, and most doctors and midwives will have a chart or wheel to show the dates.)

Both of these methods assume a regular menstrual cycle of about 28 days with ovulation and conception taking place on day 14 of your cycle. If you know that your menstrual cycles are normally shorter or longer than this, you should add or subtract days accordingly. For example, if you had a due date of June 22 based on the first method, but you know that your cycles are normally about 33 days, not 28, you would add five days and have an estimated birth date of June 27.

3. If you have been tracking ovulation by taking your basal temperature or observing cervical mucous, and you know when you ovulated and conceived, you can add 266 days to that date. This is more accurate than relying on your last menstrual cycle.

What if you don't know the date of your last period, or if your cycles are very irregular? You might be able to estimate these, or your caregiver might make an estimate based on other things, such as the size of your uterus. Your caregiver may also recommend an ultrasound, which will show how big your baby is at this point. Ultrasounds to estimate due dates are more accurate if they are done early in the pregnancy rather than later.

What does this date mean? Only about 5 per cent of women actually give birth on their "due dates." A baby is considered to be full term if he or she is born within three weeks before that date, and a week or so after that date. If the pregnancy continues more than a week past the date given, it is generally described as **post-term** and many caregivers will recommend inducing labour.

Lifestyle Risks: Smoking, Drinking, and Drugs

When a Manitoba woman, pregnant with her fourth child, was brought to court by the child welfare system to force her to get treatment for her solvent-sniffing addiction, the country's attention was drawn in a very dramatic way to the issue of drugs during pregnancy. This mother's previous three children were already in the care of the Children's Aid Society and showed clear evidence of damage due to their mother's drug use during her pregnancies. In the commentary on this case, it was pointed out that many women smoke cigarettes or consume alcohol in amounts that put their babies at increased risk. Should these women, as well, be forced into treatment programs?

The Manitoba court decided that the pregnant woman could not be legally required to have treatment for her addiction. The Supreme Court of Canada upheld this opinion: "Nobody has the legal right to interfere with a pregnant woman whose behaviour threatens her fetus." This judgment supports women's right to make their own decisions, including harmful ones. It does nothing to settle society's responsibility to that fetus. Another statement from the Supreme Court's decision rings very true from the medical point of view: "The mother and her fetus are one."

Tobacco, Alcohol, and Illegal Drugs

The research in some areas is quite clear. "Recreational" drugs—including tobacco, alcohol, and illegal drugs from glue-sniffing to crack cocaine—put the developing fetus at risk.

SMOKING

Smoking is known to lead to a slightly increased risk of miscarriage, increased risk of accidental separation of the placenta, reduced birth weight, and an increased risk of SIDS (**sudden infant death syndrome**—sometimes called "crib death") after the baby is born. Babies born to mothers who smoke have more problems with their lungs and are more prone to respiratory problems. In later life, babies who were exposed to the toxins of tobacco smoke in utero seem to have more behaviour problems—they are more likely to be arrested for crimes or to have problems with substance abuse.

There is also some evidence that exposure to second-hand smoke during pregnancy also increases these risks for babies.

What isn't clear is how to best help pregnant women who are addicted to cigarettes. Simply telling women to stop smoking does not help them with their addiction, and hearing lectures about the dangers of smoking during pregnancy can make women feel guilty and inadequate. We do not know if feeling stressed and anxious harms pregnancies or affects the mother's subsequent relationship with her baby. But the stress of knowing she is potentially causing problems for her baby may actually increase the tobacco-addicted woman's desire to smoke—10 per cent of women who smoke actually smoke *more* when they are pregnant.

The ideal situation would be to give up tobacco before the baby is conceived, but this isn't always possible. For pregnant smokers, smoking cessation courses can be useful. Their specific behavioural strategies and support are much more likely to help you stop smoking than trying to do it on your own, even if you have to check out a couple before you find one that suits you. There are a variety of programs currently available for those who want to stop smoking. Having your partner quit with you not only gives you some support while you quit, but has other benefits—a non-smoking household is healthier for the baby after birth (having parents who smoke is a significant risk factor in SIDS, in lung infections, and asthma in infants).

If the mother can't quit smoking altogether, it is useful to cut down. The harm from cigarettes seems to be "dose-related," and although research has not determined a safe lower level, it appears that the less smoked the better.

For other women, pregnancy can provide the motivation they've been looking for to stop smoking. Kim says, "I'd been talking about quitting for years. When I got pregnant, I decided this was the time. One of my worries had been that I would gain weight if I quit smoking, so pregnancy was a good time to quit—I was gaining weight anyway!"

ALCOHOL

Alcohol is the most commonly used recreational drug in the world.

Fetal alcohol syndrome is a condition seen in some babies whose mothers have been steady drinkers throughout pregnancy (averaging two drinks per day or more), although some affected babies have been born to mothers who did not drink all the time but binged heavily on a few occasions. Babies with FAS usually have small, abnormally shaped heads and are developmentally delayed. Large amounts of alcohol during early pregnancy seem to be most likely to cause problems for the fetus—and this is a concern, because about 50 per cent of pregnancies are unplanned and many women don't realize they are pregnant in the early weeks. However, those two glasses of wine you had when your period was just a couple of days overdue are not something to be concerned about.

Fetal alcohol effect is a less obvious complication of alcohol exposure during pregnancy. The infant has no physical signs at birth, but has developmental problems during

OTHER POSSIBLE HAZARDS

Other substances and behaviours have been shown in some studies to potentially increase the risk of miscarriage or birth defects. These include:

- **Sitting in hot tubs or saunas** heated over 38°C (100°F) for longer than 15 minutes. Either of these can raise the mother's body temperature enough to increase her risk of miscarrying the baby.
- **Exposure to X-rays.** X-rays can cause problems prior to pregnancy (they can cause mutations in the mother's egg cells). If the mother is exposed to X-rays in early pregnancy, the baby may be at a higher risk of developing cancer after it is born. Because this is well known, women of child-bearing age will be given lead aprons to protect them if they need X-rays.
- **Pesticides and other toxic chemicals.** Many pesticides and chemicals have been linked to birth defects. This can be a concern for women whose jobs require them to work with these chemicals. It may be possible, in some workplaces, to ask for a transfer to another area with less exposure to the chemicals.
- **Caffeine.** Caffeine is in many common drinks (coffee, tea, colas, etc.) and some foods as well. Women who consume the equivalent of more than three cups of coffee daily have an increased risk of miscarriage.
- **Fish containing mercury.** Due to pollution, most fish and shellfish contain at least small amounts of mercury, and the developing fetus is quite sensitive to this element. Pregnant women are advised to avoid shark, swordfish, king mackerel, and tilefish, as these are all high in mercury. Eating up to 12 ounces a week of low-mercury fish such as shrimp, canned light tuna, salmon, pollock, and catfish is considered safe. Albacore or white tuna is higher in mercury than light tuna.
- **Soft cheeses.** Some meats and cheeses may contain listeria bacteria, which can cause miscarriages, premature births, and fetal death when consumed by pregnant women. This is a rare problem, but the risk can be reduced by avoiding mould-ripened cheeses (such as brie and feta), blue-veined cheeses (such as roquefort and camembert) and unpasteurized raw-milk cheese. Hard cheeses, cream cheese, cottage cheese, and other pasteurized cheeses are safe. Processed meats such as hot dogs, packaged meat pâtés, and deli meats can also harbour listeria bacteria and should be heated thoroughly before eating.

childhood that continue on into the teen years and adulthood.

Recently, researchers have been looking at the effects of lower levels of alcohol during pregnancy. One study found that when women drank consistent but low levels of alcohol during pregnancy, their children were more likely to be aggressive, anxious, and depressed at age six, and more likely to demonstrate problem behaviours at home and school.

Like addiction to cigarettes, alcohol addiction is a complicated and difficult-to-treat disease. The information available about fetal alcohol syndrome tends to worry women who are light or infrequent drinkers during pregnancy, even though their babies are not likely to be at risk.

On the other hand, simply being told that heavy drinking may affect the baby isn't likely to help a woman who is addicted to alcohol.

ILLEGAL DRUGS

The effect of illegal drugs depends on the amount and frequency of drug use and the particular drugs involved. Babies born to mothers who are addicted to heroin or cocaine are also born addicted to the drug from the exposure in the uterus. The babies go through withdrawal symptoms after birth, and many have developmental delays and health problems as they grow up. As with cigarettes and alcohol, information about the risks seems to have minimal effect on drug usage during pregnancy in women who are already using drugs.

Prescription and Over-the-Counter Drugs

The rule with any medication you might take during pregnancy is caution.

Some prescription drugs have been studied and are felt to be safe during pregnancy—some antibiotics, high blood pressure medicine, pills to stop vomiting, and painkillers.

Many drugs have not been specifically researched for safety for the developing baby; they might be safe, we just don't know for sure. They are usually labelled, "Safety in pregnancy not established; weigh the potential benefits against the possible hazards to the fetus." This is good advice—if you can manage without them, don't take them.

Some drugs are thought to be dangerous for the developing fetus, usually because animal studies have demonstrated **teratogenicity** (this means the drug causes fetal abnormalities). Tragically, some drugs are known to be teratogenic to humans (like **thalidomide**) because they were given to pregnant women before the danger was known.

Whenever you are given a prescription, remind the doctor that you are pregnant. If you have forgotten to mention it to the doctor, you can ask the pharmacist to check the drug's safety for you before you get the prescription filled.

Most diseases have more than one possible treatment. If one drug is not safe during pregnancy, another may be.

Filomena developed pneumonia during her second pregnancy. "I was really sick, I felt terrible. But it wasn't easy to find the right medication, because I was allergic to one antibiotic and the other the doctor recommended wasn't safe during pregnancy. The one we ended up with was probably the least effective. I needed to stay in bed and rest much longer than I might have with a different antibiotic, but eventually the pneumonia cleared up, and I felt my baby was safe."

Caution is also recommended if you are considering herbal remedies. The fact that these are from natural sources does not mean they are safe for the baby. Check with your midwife, naturopath, or physician before taking any herbs, including herbal teas.

Drugs are a very common part of our lives, and many of us consume tobacco, alcohol, aspirin, allergy pills, and more without thinking about possible risks. The rapidly growing fetus is very sensitive to many of the chemicals we take

The Evidence About...
Smoking, Drinking, and Drugs During Pregnancy

Smoking, drinking, and drugs (recreational and prescription) have the potential to harm the fetus.

We have to use this knowledge to develop helpful strategies for addicted women; simple advice to stop smoking or drinking is not useful. Women who are concerned about their use of these drugs are encouraged to seek out treatment programs that will give them practical strategies and ongoing support for quitting.

Knowledge about the harmful effects of alcohol has raised unnecessary fear in women who have had the occasional drink in early pregnancy.

in, and pregnant women need to be aware and cautious.

For more information about specific drugs and their safety during pregnancy, you can check the Motherisk website at www.motherisk.org or contact the Motherisk phone line at the Hospital for Sick Children in Toronto at 416-813-6780. Pauline says, "Please tell mothers about the Motherisk number. The person who spoke to me was so helpful, and I felt very reassured that the medication my doctor was recommending was safe."

-4-
Where Will Your Baby Be Born?

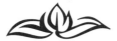

As you prepare to give birth, you will decide not only who you want with you to give you support, but where you want to have your baby.

How do you visualize your ideal birth? Imagine yourself in labour and create a picture of the perfect setting. What do you see?

Elaine: "I see myself walking along the beach near our home, my feet sinking into the sand and the waves rolling in. The contractions get stronger, and we go back into the house. My midwife is there, waiting. The sunlight is coming in through the bedroom window. I get in the shower and let the water run down my back until the contractions get so strong that I want to get onto the bed."

Vicki: "I'm rocking in the rocking chair in the birthing suite at the hospital. The curtains are drawn, the lights are dim, and my tape is playing. My sister is there, talking quietly to me, and Mike is rubbing my feet between contractions. My doctor sits on the edge of the bed, reassuring me that everything is going well. I feel safe."

Some common elements that women often describe in their ideal birth settings:

- a calm, peaceful atmosphere, quiet and dimly lit
- privacy—not being alone, but not feeling exposed or watched by others
- feeling able to moan or cry out as needed
- freedom to walk around or find a comfortable position
- familiar, caring support people who will stay with her
- a tub, shower, or whirlpool available

Keep your imagined ideal birth in mind as you make decisions about where you want to give birth.

Hospital Births

Most North American women assume that they will have their baby in the hospital, just as their own mothers did.

It's hard to generalize about hospital births. Many hospitals have instituted a policy of family-centred maternity care in their birthing suites, and are striving to achieve a warm, home-like approach. They try to be more flexible about routines than the rest of the hospital, and to respond to the mother's needs and wishes. On the other hand, a few hospitals still have routines that have been shown in research studies to be undesirable: giving all women **IV**s in labour or taking the baby to the nursery shortly after birth rather than keeping mother and baby together, for example.

Jennifer says, "When I was in labour with my first baby, I really wanted to have my sister with me for support as well as my husband. The hospital said no way, you get one support person and that is it. I felt like my husband should be there, but I know having my sister too would have helped a lot. But it wasn't allowed."

Three years later, when Jennifer was pregnant again, she found a hospital where the policies were different. "When I called to ask about bringing my sister, the nurse who answered the phone told me I could bring whoever I wanted. It was up to me. I ended up bringing not only my sister, but my daughter Chelsea and my mother-in-law to look after Chelsea. It was a real family birth experience!"

Even with a family-centred approach, though, most women feel as though a hospital birth is a more medical experience. You are given wristbands to wear just as if you were coming in for surgery; high-tech equipment is all around you; nurses you've never met before come in and out of the room where you are labouring.

In a hospital, you are also more likely to experience various interventions—and every intervention has some risk to it. If you are noisy in labour, for example—moaning or crying out— you will probably be offered medication for pain. While some women appreciate this, other women use crying or groaning to help them manage painful contractions. Other interventions, too— from fetal monitors to separation of mother and baby—are all more common in hospital births.

In some metropolitan areas, you may be able to choose between several hospitals or birthing centres. In other communities, your choice may be limited to the one hospital there. In small towns, you may have to leave your community altogether to travel to the closest city that has a hospital with a labour and delivery ward.

If you have some options, go for a tour of each labour and delivery unit or birthing centre. It's important to ask questions about routines and any specific concerns you have, but it's also important to think about how this place makes you feel. Anne burst into tears when she saw the chilly delivery room in her local hospital, with the bright overhead light, gleaming tiles, and the walls lined with shiny stainless-steel equipment. She felt so unhappy at the thought of giving birth in that room that she decided to investigate home births instead.

WHY WOMEN CHOOSE HOSPITAL BIRTHS

You might feel more comfortable in a hospital setting. Liz, for example, already has toddler twins at home, and enjoyed the clean, efficient atmosphere of the hospital when they were born. This time, she plans to leave for the hospital with her first contractions, feeling that in the hospital things will be quieter and less stressful than in her busy, active home, where her small children are likely to want her attention when she needs to be focused on labouring. She chose the local hospital both for its proxim-

WHERE DO YOU WANT YOUR BABY TO BE BORN?
SOME POINTS TO CONSIDER

Birth at Home
- Your familiar things around you
- Feel free to walk, make noises, or do whatever else helps
- Can have any support people you choose
- Consistent, one-to-one care from caregiver
- No separation from baby
- Reduced risk of infection
- Unnecessary interventions are less likely
- Birth can be messy, and you'll need help with cleaning up
- May have to move to hospital for pain medication or if complications arise

Birthing Centre
- Philosophy supports unmedicated births and minimal intervention
- Often have Jacuzzis, birthing chairs, and other special equipment
- Usually one-to-one nursing care
- Emergency equipment is readily available, if needed
- No separation from baby
- May have strict guidelines about which mothers can use the centre; may have to move to regular hospital maternity ward if complications arise

Hospital Birth
- May be only option available in your community
- Pain relief medication is usually quickly available (epidurals not always available at smaller hospitals)
- Emergency equipment, including operating rooms for Caesareans, is readily available
- Policies may not be the same as mother's choices (but this varies, so ask)
- Higher risk of infection
- Higher risk of interventions
- Cared for by strangers
- May feel inhibited about moaning or walking around

ity to her home and the peaceful setting it offered for labour.

If you have a complicated pregnancy, or a medical condition, a hospital birth will be the obvious choice for you. As governments re-evaluate the organization and funding of hospitals, they have created different levels of maternal-infant care at different hospitals. So if you do have a medical problem, you may need to travel out of your home community to give birth at a hospital with the facilities you need.

Remember, too, that you can often negotiate with your hospital if some of their routines and policies are a problem for you. It may be something as simple as wearing your own nightgown instead of a hospital gown, or wrapping your baby in the blanket you bring from home instead of one stamped with the hospital's name that helps you feel happier about your birth experience.

Anna says, "I was quite happy with Callie's birth except for one thing—while I was in labour the nurses kept offering me drugs. I thought I was doing okay until one said, 'Now let me know when you want something for the pain.' I hadn't even been thinking about it until then. When the shift changed, the next nurse was even more

HOME OR HOSPITAL?
MARTHA'S STORY

Your plans about where your baby will be born may change during pregnancy or even while you are in labour, depending on many things.

When Martha became pregnant with her third baby, she expected her labour would be short and intense: "My first labour took three hours start to finish. We live on a farm about 20 minutes from town. My labour just started out of the blue fast and furious, and I could barely manage to get Curtis from the barn so we could leave for the hospital, the pains were so bad. I was only in the hospital an hour when the baby was born.

"With my next baby, the labour only took an hour. It was the same thing—it just started with long, really painful contractions right away. This time we only made it to the parking lot of the hospital. Curtis flew in to the emergency entrance yelling that I was having a baby in the car. The next thing I knew, I was on a stretcher with a crying baby on my tummy and everybody cheering."

During Martha's third pregnancy, the local hospital closed its labour and delivery department, and Martha was told she'd need to drive an hour and a half to the hospital in the nearest city when her labour began. "Based on my past history," she says, "I knew I'd probably give birth in the car, and I didn't want that."

Martha and her husband sought out a local physician who attended home births. The more she thought about it, the more the idea of birth at home appealed to her.

Curtis, however, wasn't so sure. "The two times I had to drive Martha to the hospital in labour were the most scary times of my life. Martha was groaning and crying and I didn't know what I'd do if the baby started coming before we got to the hospital. When she had Joshua in the parking lot, there was blood all over her legs, and I was afraid she might bleed to death before I could get help. It was terrible."

While a planned home birth would avoid the drive, Curtis was afraid the doctor might not make it in time. "It would take the doctor an hour to get out here at least. And what if she was busy and we couldn't get a hold of her right away when labour started? Then it would just be me and Martha, and I was not prepared to deal with that."

Two weeks before Martha's due date, she and Curtis met with the doctor again and talked about the possibility of inducing labour in the hospital. Martha says, "I would have preferred to give birth at home, even if it meant being alone. But Curtis was dreading it, and I needed him to feel confident about what we were doing. We decided I'd go into the hospital when I hit 40 weeks and be induced."

When Martha arrived at the hospital, the doctor found her cervix already soft and starting to dilate, although Martha hadn't felt any contractions. The doctor broke the water, and within half an hour Martha was in very active labour. One hour after her induction, Martha pushed out a 7-pound (3,175-g) baby girl.

Martha says, "It was a bit strange to go from a planned home birth to an induced labour in hospital, but it worked out well. Our situation was difficult, because my labours are so fast and we live so far from the hospital. I don't think there's any one right answer in these situations, but for us, this seemed to be the best solution."

insistent. Every time she checked the baby's heart rate, she'd ask me if I wanted anything yet. When I said no, she'd kind of shake her head, as if she thought I was making a big mistake."

When Anna arrived at the hospital to have her second baby, she told the nurse who admitted her that she did not intend to have any medication and did not want to be asked about it. "If I want drugs, I'll let you know," she told her nurse. "The care was perfect. When the labour got hard and I really started to moan, the nurse just came in and brought my husband some cream to use to rub my back so my skin wouldn't get raw. When I started shivering, another nurse appeared with hot blankets to wrap around me. Finally, when I gave a real yell—I was starting to push—the nurse came in with baby blankets and put them under the warmer in the birthing room. She said to my husband, 'That sounds like we are going to see a baby soon.' That positive support was so helpful, so much more than any offer of drugs would have been."

Birthing Centres

Birthing centres, either free-standing or as part of a larger hospital, can offer a good atmosphere and setting for birth.

Birthing centre staff is usually very respectful of the wishes of the family, and try to avoid any protocols around admission, labour, or birth. They try not to disturb the labouring woman unnecessarily, and try to offer encouragement rather than telling the woman "how to do it." They often have a stated goal: an unmedicated birth with minimal intervention. The room is usually warm and softly lit with a selection of comfortable chairs, stools, and an ordinary low bed. A large heater to put over the bed and keep the mother and newborn warm after the birth is a nice touch, but not essential. Typically, the family goes home within a few hours after the birth.

Kellie says, "People thought I was crazy to go the birthing centre route as the centre's philosophy is to go as naturally as possible (translated to 'no drugs!'). It was great. My first child was about a five-hour labour from start to finish, with the wonderful support of the midwifery staff and, of course, my ever-supportive husband. I thoroughly enjoyed the experience and was home in four hours eating Chinese food with my new family."

Tracy also had a wonderful experience in a family birthing centre. She says, "I can't say enough about the benefits of the centre and the impact it had on my birth experience. The centre has two suites, which consist of a bedroom decorated with lovely linens and curtains and wallpaper, a bathroom with bidet and whirlpool tub, and a sitting room with kitchen facilities, a television and a pullout bed where my husband was able to sleep overnight."

It wasn't just the attractive setting that appealed to Tracy, though; she feels the birthing centre's philosophy was even more important. "I received constant one-on-one care from a nurse trained in midwifery throughout my stay. My baby's birth was attended by my family doctor. I wore my own comfortable clothes. Once my baby was born, he did not leave my side—really my stomach or breast—at all. He was cleaned and weighed only when I was ready to let him go for a few minutes."

Birthing centres vary widely in their policies about which pregnant women can use the centre, and about drug use during the labour. Some have a clear stand—no drugs—and any decision to use pain-killing medication or drugs to speed up the labour means transfer from the birthing centre to the regular labour and delivery unit of the nearby or attached hospital. Other birthing centres use **injectable drugs** for pain relief (for example, **Demerol**), but not **epidurals**. If you are considering using a birthing centre, ask for information about their policies.

Birth at Home

THE QUESTION OF SAFETY

Most women in North America believe that birth in a hospital is safer for their baby than birth at home. Many women who would like to deliver at home eventually dismiss the idea because of their belief that it is not as safe. Women often say, "I would never forgive myself if anything went wrong."

The belief that home birth is not safe is deeply ingrained in our North American culture. Since 1900, the usual place of birth has changed from home to hospital. During this time period, birth has also become safer—death rates for mothers and babies have decreased steadily. These two events have often been seen as being related but it is not a cause-and effect relationship. The shift from home to hospital birth has not *caused* the overall improvement in infant survival.

Why do fewer mothers and babies die today than in 1900? The drop in mortality rates for *babies* has been gradual, and is almost entirely due to improved living standards, better nutrition, and better overall health. Giving birth became safer for *mothers* beginning around the 1930s, and this was because of the introduction of antibiotics, safer blood transfusions and Caesarean sections for certain complications, and other medical advances. These twentieth-century advances have increased the safety of *both* hospital and home births.

When properly gathered statistics are carefully analyzed, they consistently point to the same conclusion: women with specific pregnancy complications greatly benefit from hospital obstetric care and interventions. There is no evidence that a policy of *all* women delivering in hospital has resulted in general benefit. *The research consistently shows that birth at home for mothers with uncomplicated pregnancies attended by a skilled caregiver is as safe for mother and baby as birth in a hospital.*

This has not been an easy area to research. A randomized controlled trial (the most reliable design for a research study, as explained in "Understanding Research Methods" on page 308 of the Appendix) is not possible, as women feel strongly about where they want to give birth and are not willing to be randomly assigned.

The most useful studies have compared groups of women similar in all other respects except for place of birth. These studies have compared outcomes for planned home-birth women, including those who planned to deliver at home but were transferred to hospital during labour, with a similar group of low-risk women with planned hospital births. Complicated pregnancies were excluded from both groups by screening during pregnancy. Unplanned and unattended home births were also excluded.

SIBLINGS AT THE BIRTH

Whether you are at home or in the hospital, you may want to have your older child or children present for the arrival of the newest family member. If you are considering this option, here are a few points to keep in mind:

- How does your child feel about the idea? Some children are eager to be part of the experience; others are equally firm about not being around for the birth. These feelings should be respected.
- If you are giving birth in a hospital, what are the policies about siblings being present? You may need to meet with administrative staff or even change your planned place of birth if siblings are not permitted.
- You will want to have an adult present who is responsible only for the child or children, and who is not intent on being at the birth. Even an older child who doesn't need a babysitter will need someone to be there for him and to explain things if any problems arise.
- Movies of births can help prepare a child for the sounds and surprises of birth. You can discuss what you see on the screen and mention that you also might moan, yell, or cry out, and that there might be a lot of blood. Encourage your child to discuss any concerns or fears about being at the birth.

Be aware that children often change their minds at the last minute. The child who definitely wanted to be there might leave the room; the child who was disinterested in the whole idea might end up at his mother's side, completely enthralled as his baby sister emerges.

The conclusions: the same, very small number of babies die in hospital as at home. The hospital groups had higher incidence of reported fetal distress, babies who needed resuscitation at birth, babies who needed admission to the neonatal intensive care unit, and higher rates of **postpartum hemorrhage** (bleeding by the mother after birth) than the home birth group. The incidence of interventions during labour was much lower in the home birth than in the hospital groups: fewer inductions, fewer artificial rupture of membranes, fewer pain-killing drugs, fewer episiotomies, and fewer forceps or vacuum deliveries.

Having a baby has risks whether the birth takes place at home or in a hospital. The goal of obstetric care is to reduce those risks as much as possible. Having a baby at home may involve choosing to accept situations that could potentially be more quickly handled in the hospital. However, choosing to have a baby in a hospital also involves accepting risks—risks of unnecessary intervention and infection, which do not exist at home.

WHY WOMEN CHOOSE HOME BIRTH

The numbers of women giving birth at home remains small, but it is increasing, especially in areas where midwives are licensed and paid by health plans to attend home births.

Most women who have experienced a planned home birth become advocates. For

WHAT DO YOU NEED FOR A HOME BIRTH?

Your midwife or doctor will be able to provide you with a specific list of birth supplies, but you will typically need:

- waterproof disposable pads (for you to sit on)
- plastic garbage bags for throwing out soiled items
- laundry hamper lined with a plastic garbage bag (most of your laundry will be wet)
- washcloths, towels, and a bowl for washing blood and fluid off you before and after the birth
- a basin for the placenta
- a portable lamp, a space heater if the room is cool, and a heating pad for warming up receiving blankets
- lots of receiving blankets for the baby

- diapers and clothes in which to dress the baby
- large-sized sanitary pads (to use during labour if you are leaking fluid as well as after the birth)
- waterproof sheet for the bed (Usually you make up the bed with a clean fitted sheet on the bottom, the waterproof sheet next, and an older sheet on top. Once the baby is born, the top two layers can be stripped off, leaving a fresh clean sheet underneath for mother and baby to sleep on.)
- comfortable pajama tops, short nightgowns, or an oversized T-shirt to wear during labour
- a nursing nightgown to change into once the baby is born
- a full tank of gas in the car and emergency phone numbers handy, just in case

example, Diane's first baby was born in the hospital, her second at home. She says, "I want you to know that there was nothing particularly disturbing about our eldest son's hospital birth. That is, at least, until we experienced the peacefulness of birth at home."

Wendi's first two children were born in the hospital and her last one was born at home. "I have fast, violent, painful labours. With my first birth, within two hours of my admission to hospital, I was crying and screaming with the contractions. The nurse was very nice, but she kept offering me drugs because I was being so noisy. Finally, I had a shot of painkiller; it made me throw up and feel really groggy. In no time at all I was feeling the urge to push anyway. I don't think anyone had expected my labour to be that fast."

With her next in-hospital labour, Wendi remembers trying not to make any noise because she felt it had been so disturbing to the staff during her first labour. "I buried my face in the pillow with every contraction and just held my breath. I think it made it hurt a lot worse because I felt I couldn't give in to it."

Her home birth for her third baby was "the best." "By seven-thirty, when my husband was putting Shannon to sleep, I was moaning loudly. From seven-thirty to eight-thirty my contractions were two to three minutes apart and I was moaning with them. At this point, I decided to get into the Jacuzzi and sit up while pouring hot water over my belly. I was moaning and screaming. After two hours, I got up to use the toilet and I felt my water break. I sat down on a mattress on the floor with my back against the couch. After a few pushes, my daughter was born. Every time I think of her birth, I remember that wonderful feeling as she came out. I had her on my chest and I checked her sex even before my midwife wiped her off."

What happens when the home birth becomes a hospital birth? Sherry's planned home birth with her first baby ended up as a hospital delivery when labour progressed very slowly. Contractions had been intense from the beginning, and after more than 28 hours, Sherry was very tired. "It was my decision to change our plans and go to the hospital. My midwives really helped by supporting my decision and pointing out how reasonable it was." An IV and epidural for the pain helped her get through the last part of the labour. Her second stage was slow because the epidural freezing muffled her pushing urge, but with patience she had a spontaneous delivery of a healthy baby. "I feel really happy with all the decisions I made, even though it wasn't the birth I had dreamed of. The midwives really helped through the whole thing, both at home and in the hospital. I'll definitely plan on a home birth again next time, and just hope my labour goes differently."

These stories illustrate some of the differences in giving birth at home. Not having to

> ### The Evidence About…
> ### Place of Birth
>
> For low-risk mothers, giving birth at home, in a birthing centre, or in a hospital are all good options.
>
> Where there are specific medical concerns, a hospital with appropriate facilities can reduce the risk of complication to mother and baby.

leave home avoids disrupting the flow of labour. Spontaneously moving around your own house is natural and easy—there is no impediment to doing things your own way. At home, Wendi felt reassured that she could yell all she wanted and her midwife wouldn't mind.

For some women, giving birth at home helps remind them that it is a normal, natural process, not a medical one. Kimberley describes the birth of her daughter Skye this way: "There were no special circumstances. It was just a quiet day in our apartment with the loving support of my husband, my doula, my midwife, and her partner. I laboured, I pushed, I reached down and pulled out my baby, began to nurse her, and then I cried. It was simple. I did what my body told me to do and what nature intended."

-5-
"High-Risk" Pregnancy

Is your pregnancy "low" or "high" risk?

Before considering the factors that may lead you to be classified as one or the other, it's important to look at what high risk means.

Jennifer says, "I thought being high risk meant the baby had a high probability of developing problems. And to me that means definitely more than a 50 per cent chance, maybe more than an 80 per cent chance. I was shocked when I discovered that being high risk for **beta strep infection**, for example, means about a 2 per cent chance of the baby having it. Or that being high risk for **Down's syndrome** is still less than 1 per cent."

Because of this very common misunderstanding about what high risk means, it is often better to think of "higher than average risk" or some other less worrying phrase.

The decision about your risk level matters because it will affect the kind of care you receive and the options you have. If you are low risk, you may be able to give birth at home or in a birthing centre, with a midwife or family physician. If you are considered to be high risk, you may be referred to an obstetrician and advised to go to a larger hospital for your baby's birth.

But knowing your relative risk level is only helpful if it means you and your baby are likely to do better as a result. The current methods of determining which mothers are considered at risk—usually just scoring the answers to a list of questions based on the mother's past medical history—are not very helpful.

Depending on the criteria used, somewhere between 10 and 30 per cent of the mothers labelled "high risk" will actually have any of the problems the risk screening process is supposed to highlight. A significant number (between 20 and 50 per cent, again depending on the criteria used) of the babies who have problems (specifically prematurity or low birth weight) will be born to mothers who were rated low risk. In other words, the factors used to divide women into low- or high-risk groups are not very reliable.

Judith and her husband had not been able to conceive after two years of trying, so they saw a fertility specialist who diagnosed the problem as a low sperm count and irregular ovulation. After several months of treatments, Judith still wasn't pregnant, so they decided to "take a break" from trying to conceive. To their delight, Judith discovered she was pregnant three months later.

"I called the fertility specialist to let him know we were pregnant and wouldn't be coming back, and said I was planning to return to my family doctor for my prenatal care and the birth of the baby. The doctor called me back and said that because I had fertility problems I was high risk and needed to be cared for by an obstetrician," says Judith.

Judith and her husband discussed the situation, and decided to return to their family doctor. As Judith says, "We'd had trouble conceiving, but I couldn't see why this made me a high risk. And in the end, we'd gotten pregnant on our own, without the treatments. This was just a normal pregnancy." Judith eventually gave birth to a 9-pound (4,080 g) baby boy in the birthing centre connected to her hospital.

Even if you have been accurately described as "high risk"—meaning you and your baby *are* actually at a higher risk for certain problems— knowing this is not very helpful if nothing can be done about it. Many of the factors can't be changed, and there are not always interventions that will improve the outcome.

In fact, in many studies, being labelled "high risk" meant that mothers were subjected to a number of additional interventions, and often these were not helpful, according to the research. Since all interventions carry some risk to them, it would make more sense to minimize interventions as much as possible for high-risk pregnancies.

Being told you are high risk also means added stress for the parents.

Often women are classified as high risk simply because they are part of a group. If you are a teenager, or a woman over 40, you might be told you are high risk because of your age, even though it has little to do with you as an individual. Or you might be described as high risk because of the number of children you have, as Cally discovered.

When Cally became pregnant with her seventh child, her family doctor, who had delivered her previous six babies, told her she was now high risk and should see an obstetrician. This didn't make sense to Cally. "I had no problems at all with the previous six pregnancies and births," she says. "I keep fit, I'm healthy, and I couldn't see any reason why the last pregnancy would be low risk and suddenly this one high risk." She persuaded her family doctor to continue providing her prenatal care and to attend the birth.

There are also plenty of grey areas, where women are not actually at any higher risk of problems but may be close enough to whatever definition of "high risk" is being used to cause comment. When Keshia was pregnant, her doctor was concerned that Keshia's blood pressure was "borderline." At each prenatal appointment, the doctor would discuss the interventions that would be suggested if her blood pressure went any higher. Keshia found this very stressful, especially when her doctor talked about inducing labour.

Finally, she asked the doctor to put the discussion of possible treatments on hold until her blood pressure actually changed. It never did.

What if you do fall into the category of higher-than-average risk? You may be in this category because you have a medical problem, such as Type 1 or Type 2 diabetes, or because you have high blood pressure. You may have a complicated pregnancy—perhaps you are expecting triplets, or the baby is growing more slowly than expected. You may simply be older than the average mother, which places you at greater risk for having a baby with Down's syndrome or by Caesarean section.

The high-risk label is not very helpful unless it improves the outcome for you and your baby. As a high-risk mother, what do you need?

1. Information about what aspects of this pregnancy are considered high risk and what (if anything) can be done to lower the risk, including minimizing interventions.
2. Information about how you can prepare for possible complications (for example, a premature baby).
3. This may be the most important part: extra emotional support during pregnancy and birth.

Often women who are considered to be high risk find that in labour they are surrounded by medical personnel—most of them strangers—rather than their partners, friends, and others who can provide comfort and emotional support. While there may be a need for extra technology, this doesn't diminish the need for emotional support. In fact, it may increase it—research is very clear that stress increases the risk of all kinds of health problems and complications, and research is equally clear that support during labour and birth reduces stress and leads to more positive outcomes. It may be helpful to hire a doula to be with you at this time, or to make arrangements with your hospital and doctor to bring extra support people with you.

WHO IS AT HIGHER RISK?

Early in your pregnancy, you may be asked questions such as these to determine your risk level:

- How old are you? (oldest and youngest ages are higher risk)
- How much do you weigh? (obese women are at higher risk)
- Do you have any medical problems such as diabetes, epilepsy, high blood pressure, HIV-positive status, heart disease, blood clotting disorders, etc.?
- Have you had any complications during your previous pregnancies? (some of these may recur, such as high blood pressure, postpartum hemorrhage, premature birth)

During your pregnancy, things may happen that place you in the higher than average risk group:

- vaginal bleeding
- developing high blood pressure or diabetes
- premature leaking of the amniotic fluid
- premature labour
- smaller or larger than usual weight gain or fetal size
- being diagnosed with an infection
- carrying more than one baby

Remember: identifying a risk factor does not necessarily mean that anything can be done to reduce that risk.

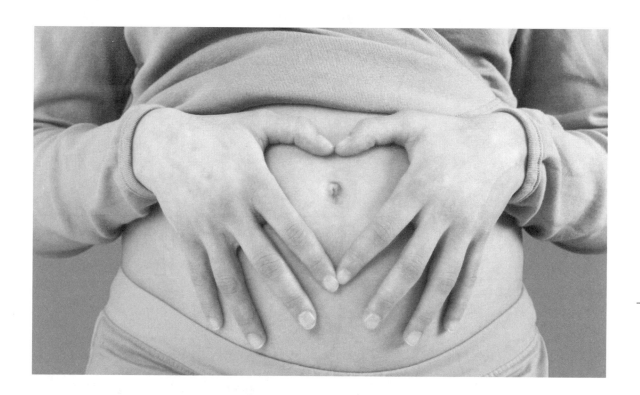

Two Months
∞ *Five to Eight Weeks* ∞

By now, you really feel pregnant. Nobody can tell by looking, but you may be experiencing morning sickness or pressure on your bladder. And you're already beginning to wonder about what the baby you're carrying will be like, how to know if he or she is healthy, and what you can do to give your baby the best chance. This section shares what research has told us about these questions.

-6-
Nutrition and Supplementation

Tara is just out of her teens, single—which in her case means she doesn't have much money—and pregnant. For the past few years, because she's very concerned about staying slim, she's been alternately dieting (eating nothing but celery and carrot sticks for a week) and bingeing on french fries and burgers when her willpower gives out. Now she's pregnant, and her main concern is not gaining too much weight so she'll still fit into her jeans after the baby is born. She does, though, want her baby to be healthy.

Selene is also pregnant. She's been a vegetarian for most of her life, enjoys planning and preparing meals, and is very interested in nutrition. She also takes a number of herbal supplements and vitamins, and wonders if these are safe during pregnancy.

Marta doesn't think much about food. Her husband jokes that the oven in their apartment has never been turned on! Because he and Marta are both very busy at work, they eat almost all their meals out—and because they're usually in a hurry, it's often at fast-food restaurants. Marta doesn't see that changing much now she's preg-

nant, but she's worried about how this diet will affect the baby.

Connie's expecting her fifth child and her oldest is not yet 10. She feels more tired this time than during her previous pregnancies, but doesn't have much time, energy, or money to worry about nutrition. Her focus is on preparing meals her children will eat and that she can afford, so she tends to serve a lot of pasta, rice, and potatoes. She wonders whether this is good enough to grow a healthy baby.

Four pregnant women, each with very different nutritional histories, different lifestyles and incomes, and different concerns about nutrition during pregnancy. In fact, every pregnant woman's nutritional status will be unique, and that's what makes it impossible to say that there is one ideal diet for every pregnant woman.

What do we know about nutrition during pregnancy? The truth is, not a lot. We do know that good nutrition is very important to everyone's health, and that when women who are significantly malnourished become pregnant, their babies are at greater risk. Eating well before you conceive is known to be important. Can you improve the outcome for your baby by changing your diet during pregnancy? There are so many possible variables that this is a very challenging area to research. Most of the studies that have been done focus on supplementation of the diet because this is easier to measure than what people actually eat.

Pregnancy Supplements: The Daily Dose of Vitamins and Minerals

Although multivitamin supplements for pregnant women have been recommended by doctors for years, the actual required amounts of each vitamin or mineral have not been determined by research in most cases.

Folic acid. The supplement that research has found to be most helpful during pregnancy is folic acid. Taking 0.8 milligrams per day of folic acid, beginning *before* pregnancy occurs and continuing through the first trimester, reduces the risk of the baby having **neural tube defects**, either **anencephaly** or **spina bifida**.

Anencephaly means the baby develops without a brain; these babies are either stillborn or die shortly after birth. Spina bifida is an abnormality of the spinal cord which can cause paralysis of the legs and lack of bladder and bowel control. The overall risk of a woman having a baby with neural tube defect is 1 to 2 per 1,000. Although this is rare, because the disease is so severe, the reduction in risk with folic acid is important.

Women who have already had a baby with a neural tube defect have a higher risk of having another one in a subsequent pregnancy. They can reduce this risk by two-thirds by taking a higher dose (4 milligrams per day) of folic acid from before pregnancy until the end of the first trimester.

It's easy to take folic acid supplements during pregnancy, but half of pregnancies are unplanned, and getting sufficient folic acid before conception and in the very early days of pregnancy is at least as important as the folic acid level after pregnancy has been confirmed. However, it is quite possible to get the recommended amount of folic acid in your diet. Folic acid is in many foods, including meat, milk, orange vegetables and fruits, dark green vegetables, and legumes.

Iron. Although the multivitamin supplements for pregnant women all contain iron, the research does not support giving iron supplements routinely to pregnant women.

It is normal for the amount of iron in a woman's blood to drop during pregnancy, but this does not mean it is a problem that needs to be corrected. In fact, the lower iron levels indicate that the mother now has a higher blood volume, something that is normal and desirable in pregnancy.

Iron supplements have been routinely given to pregnant women for many years, but there have been no detected benefits. The supplements do raise the measured level of iron in the mother's blood, but this does not improve the overall outcomes for either the mother or the baby. None of the studies indicate improvement in incidence of low–birth weight babies, incidence of high blood pressure in pregnancy, excessive bleeding after delivery, or stillbirth. This means that routine iron supplementation is certainly wasteful, and can give a woman the

THE PREGNANT WOMAN AND THE FOOD POLICE

Throughout history and around the world, women have always been warned about the foods they must eat or should not eat during pregnancy.

English mothers were warned not to eat strawberries or the baby would be born with a strawberry birthmark.

Mothers in Malta were told that if they craved a certain food they must eat it, or the baby would be born with a handicap. At family gatherings, pregnant women always chose their food first and were encouraged to choose the foods they craved.

Mothers in Siberia were advised not to eat eggs during pregnancy or their babies would be born deaf.

Pregnant Thai women were told not to eat hot chili peppers, which would give their babies a "hot temper," but instead to eat cool foods like bananas to create calm babies.

In Northern India, mothers are traditionally given yak's milk to drink during pregnancy to make the baby strong and fortunate. In other parts of India, honey and butter are eaten during pregnancy to ensure the baby's well-being.

European Gypsy women believed that eating crayfish during pregnancy would cause a more painful and difficult labour.

Women in the East Indies believed they needed to eat a special seafood soup in the days after delivery to have a good supply of breast milk.

Not much different, perhaps, from the warnings North American women were given in recent years to avoid salt or eat large amounts of protein during pregnancy.

mistaken impression that her nutrition is not adequate or that her body is not working properly.

Women do not feel better for having their **hemoglobin** (the measure of iron-containing red cells in the blood) made higher with iron supplements. In fact, iron supplements frequently contribute to constipation. Of more concern, two recent studies found that iron supplementation resulted in an increase in the number of babies born prematurely or with low birth weight.

Women who were **anemic** because of iron deficiency before they became pregnant *should* receive iron supplements. However, iron supplements for all pregnant women are not recommended.

Vitamin D is primarily obtained by being absorbed from the sun and from certain foods that have been fortified (such as milk). Women who don't drink milk or eat cheese and who have little exposure to the sun may become vitamin D deficient and may benefit from supplements during pregnancy, although the benefits appear to be small. Getting sufficient vitamin D during pregnancy is important, though, as the baby stores vitamin D for the first few months after birth in case he or she doesn't get enough exposure to sunlight.

Vitamin B6 supplements may protect mothers against dental decay when given during pregnancy, but no other benefits have been demonstrated.

Magnesium supplements were found in some studies to reduce the number of premature births and the number of low–birth weight babies, but these studies were too small and poorly done to allow any conclusions.

The amounts that should be taken of each of these vitamins and minerals, other than folic acid, have not been established. If you feel that your diet needs to be supplemented (for example, you are exposed to very little sunlight and are concerned about your levels of vitamin D), you could consult with a dietician or nutritionist about the amounts of particular nutrients that would be appropriate for your situation. Some research has suggested, for example, that the levels of vitamin D needed for pregnant and breastfeeding women who are deficient are considerably higher than was thought in the past.

Diets to Prevent Allergies

Enza came from a family with a history of allergies. She herself suffered from hay fever, asthma, and allergies to seafood and strawberries. Her first baby also had eczema and asthma, and was allergic to milk.

When Enza became pregnant again, she decided to try avoiding potentially allergenic foods to see if this would prevent allergies in her new baby. "I didn't drink milk or have any dairy products," she says, "and I stayed away from some of the other things I had been told are often allergenic—citrus fruits and nuts."

When people asked Enza about getting enough calcium, she pointed out that in many parts of the world most of the adults do not drink milk or eat dairy products. Despite this, they continue to have healthy babies. Calcium is present in many foods, including green leafy vegetables, canned salmon (with bones included),

and almonds. Calcium supplements are also available for those who worry that their diet is not adequate.

This baby, however, also had some allergies— but not to milk. "I can't really tell if the special diet made a difference," Enza says, "but I think it may have prevented the milk allergy."

Did it? The research is not clear. Studies suggest that even on these special diets, women with a family history of allergies are still more likely to have babies with allergies. More research needs to be done. It can be difficult and unreasonably expensive to plan nutritious meals when entire food groups are excluded or many foods are eliminated, especially when the evidence for doing so is lacking.

Herbal Supplements: All-Natural Doesn't Always Mean Safe

Caution is recommended in taking herbal supplements. Some herbs can be dangerous during pregnancy, even though they are "natural." The labelling on herbal supplements is sometimes incomplete, so you may not know exactly what you are taking. Make sure you know all the ingredients of any herbal teas or other natural supplements you are considering, and check with your midwife or doctor before taking any herbal supplements while you are pregnant.

Nutritional Attempts to Prevent Pre-eclampsia

We've already pointed out how folic acid supplements can contribute significantly to reducing

---

The Evidence About…
Nutrition during Pregnancy

Folic acid supplements taken before conception and during the first trimester can reduce the risk of neural tube defects in the baby.

Iron supplements for all pregnant women are not recommended.

Vitamin D may be helpful in a few situations, and calcium and magnesium supplements need further research.

Nutrition during pregnancy has not been widely researched. Women with specific concerns or problems should consult with a dietician or nutritionist. Attempts to reduce outcomes such as premature or low–birth weight babies by improving women's nutrition during pregnancy have not been successful; the mother's nutritional status before she conceives seems to be an important factor.

---

spina bifida, a serious birth defect. Researchers and doctors have searched for similar nutritional approaches to other pregnancy complications—in particular, **pre-eclampsia** (formerly called **toxemia**).

Pre-eclampsia (see Chapter 33) is a disease in which the mother's blood pressure goes up, protein is found in her urine, and she becomes swollen from retained fluids. This is a serious condition for both mother and baby.

So far, we have not discovered any modifications of diet and nutrition that will prevent pre-eclampsia. One study has suggested that women who take multivitamins at least once a week during the three months prior to conception and the first month of pregnancy are less likely to develop pre-eclampsia. This

seemed to be more effective in women who were not overweight.

So What Should I Eat?

If you've wondered why your caregiver tends to respond to this question with a muttered, "just eat a balanced diet," now you know. Nutrition during pregnancy has not been widely researched even though it is of considerable concern and interest to most pregnant women.

Some of the research done on nutrition is a little discouraging. Supplementing the diet of malnourished women with extra protein alone actually resulted in a higher incidence of small babies. When researchers tried to supplement the diets of malnourished women with more calories balanced in fat, carbohydrate, and protein, they found that the babies born were still very small. This suggests that it takes more than nine months to repair the effects of many years of malnutrition. It may be that the good food you eat *before* you conceive is as important as the food you eat during pregnancy.

However, good nutrition is known to make an important contribution to overall health, and it seems reasonable to suppose that it plays a role in healthy pregnancy, too. A diet that includes plenty of whole grains, fruits and vegetables, and moderate amounts of dairy products and meats or other protein foods seems likely to be the best approach, as it is for non-pregnant women. Including a wide variety of foods within each food group, and eating foods with minimal processing, will help ensure that you are getting all the important nutrients. A vegetarian diet with adequate protein is perfectly good nutrition during pregnancy. Women with lactose intolerance who avoid milk can continue to avoid dairy products in their diet during pregnancy, but should include adequate amounts of other foods containing calcium.

If you are concerned about eating appropriately during pregnancy, especially if you have a past history of eating disorders or other nutritional problems, ask your caregiver to refer you to a dietician or nutritionist who can evaluate your nutrition, height and weight, and lifestyle, and help you find an affordable and healthy eating plan.

-7-
Ultrasound: Sound-wave Images

If you have friends or relatives with babies, you've probably been treated to a showing of their **ultrasound** pictures. The grainy blurred picture may not have looked much like a baby to you, even after the proud parents pointed out various body parts. Some parents have a whole series of ultrasound pictures to show off, at different stages of the pregnancy.

What is an ultrasound, and when is it useful during pregnancy?

Pregnancy ultrasound was first introduced in the 1970s, and quickly became widely available and frequently used. Improvement in ultrasound imaging equipment has been rapid—the earliest ultrasound images were not very clear, but now even subtle details of the fetus can be seen.

A pregnant woman having an ultrasound will first be asked to drink plenty of water so that her bladder is full; this isn't comfortable for the mother, but it is easiest to see the uterus through the full bladder. She lies down, and warm cream is spread on her abdomen to reduce the friction of the flat paddle-like instrument the technician runs across her abdomen. This instrument bounces ultra high-frequency sound waves off the mother and produces an image of the fetus, placenta, and uterus on a TV-like monitor beside her.

If the ultrasound is being done in early pregnancy when the uterus is still very small, a special instrument can be slipped gently into the vagina to obtain the most detailed pictures. Prints (which look like photographic negatives), can be made from the image on the monitor—these are what parents show off so proudly and have pasted into the front of their "baby book."

The usefulness of ultrasound to answer specific questions about a pregnancy is very clear. What is not clear is whether it is helpful for *every* pregnant woman to have an ultrasound.

Ultrasound to Answer Specific Questions

The selective ultrasound examination is done to answer a specific question. Depending on the question, the ultrasound might be done by a technician and just take a couple of minutes—such as an ultrasound done to check for twins. Another ultrasound might be done by a radiologist and take over an hour—such as an ultrasound done to create a biophysical profile of the baby (see Chapter 16).

There are many different questions that can be answered by doing an ultrasound.

IS THE BABY ALIVE?

Ultrasound can answer this question rapidly and accurately. If the baby's heart is beating, the baby is alive. The fetus, and its heartbeat, can be seen by seven weeks after the mother's last menstrual period.

Why is this important? Well, if you start bleeding in the first few months of pregnancy, you can quickly find out what is going on. If the baby has died, you know that you are going to miscarry. Without an ultrasound, you might have gone through weeks of spotting and bleeding, wondering the whole time if your baby was already gone or if there was still hope that the pregnancy might continue.

Jill seemed to be having a miscarriage at about 10 weeks of pregnancy. "I was bleeding and cramping a lot and had passed some tissue. My doctor suggested doing an ultrasound just to be sure before I had a **D&C** (a procedure to remove any tissue remaining in the uterus). To our surprise they found I had been pregnant with twins and only one had miscarried—the other one was doing fine. The second baby kept growing and was born at term and healthy."

HOW MANY WEEKS PREGNANT ARE YOU?

The average pregnancy lasts 40 weeks from the date of the last menstrual period. This assumes that **ovulation** (the release of the egg from the ovary) and conception occurred two weeks after menstruation began; for women with regular periods of 28 days this assumption is usually true. For women who have very irregular periods, menstrual cycles that are longer or shorter than average, or who don't remember when their last period was, ultrasound can provide a good estimate of when their baby will be born. Research has shown that early ultrasound for women who are not sure of when the baby was conceived can reduce the rates of induction for post-term pregnancies.

The age of the baby can be estimated by ultrasound by measuring its size. In the first 12 weeks, the measurements are usually accurate within a week. From 13 to 18 weeks of pregnancy, measurements usually predict the date of delivery to within two weeks. Measurement of the baby is not useful *at all* in predicting delivery date if it's done after 30 weeks.

Colleen went for an ultrasound when she became pregnant with her second baby. Her older daughter, Sophie, was 18 months old and still breastfeeding when Colleen began to suspect she had conceived again. "Because Sophie was still nursing a lot, I hadn't had a period at all since she was born; I really didn't think I could be pregnant," Colleen says. "But I noticed my nipples were getting sore, and I'd been feeling queasy. I did one of those drugstore tests and it came back positive. I didn't have any idea when I had gotten pregnant, so I went for an ultrasound.

It told us I was 13 weeks and the baby was due around the first week of August."

IS THE BABY GROWING NORMALLY?

Ultrasound is a fairly accurate way of estimating fetal size. Measurements of the head, the body, and the upper leg give good estimates of the weight of the fetus at any time during the pregnancy. The individual baby's measurements can be plotted on a chart that shows the average weights at each week of pregnancy. Estimating the fetal weight by ultrasound is least accurate for the biggest and the smallest babies. The newer 3-D ultrasounds give more accurate estimates of the baby's weight.

Size does not show the baby's growth. A fetus who is small for gestational age through the whole pregnancy may be growing normally, even though it is smaller than average. The growth of the fetus can only be observed by doing ultrasounds two to three weeks apart (see Chapter 16).

WHERE IS THE PLACENTA?

The placenta looks like a large slab of liver attached along one surface to the inside of the uterus and linked by the umbilical cord to the baby. Its position gradually shifts during pregnancy and usually it ends up at the top or on one side of the uterus.

It can be a problem, though, if the placenta is across the bottom of the uterus, where the cervix is. (This is called **placenta previa**.) The cervix is the entrance to the vagina that the baby has to pass through to be born, and when labour contractions start to open the cervix, the placenta will be torn and will start to bleed heavily; a Caesarean section will be necessary to safely deliver the baby.

An ultrasound is the best and easiest way to determine the location of the placenta. If you have bleeding in the third trimester of pregnancy (a sign that the placenta may be at the bottom of the uterus), an ultrasound can confirm or rule out placenta previa.

This diagnosis can only be made in the third trimester of pregnancy—many placentas are "low-lying" in early pregnancy ultrasounds but move to a normal position by the end of the pregnancy.

If part of the placenta has separated from the wall of the uterus this is called abruption of the placenta, accidental hemorrhage, or premature separation of the placenta. This will cause pain and usually vaginal bleeding. An ultrasound will show where the placenta is and the technician may be able to see blood behind the placenta or membranes. Small separations may not show up on ultrasound.

Ultrasound also makes **amniocentesis** and **chorionic villus biopsy** (tests that we discuss later) safer by showing where the placenta is, so that the biopsy needle can avoid it.

OTHER QUESTIONS

There are many other specific situations in which ultrasound can be helpful during pregnancy. These include suspected twins (because of a larger than average uterus), suspected abnormalities in the baby (because of family history or maternal serum screening), or suspected abnormal positions of the fetus such as **breech** (baby is head up instead of head down in the uterus) or **transverse lie** (baby is lying sideways in the uterus). Most of these will be discussed in more detail in later chapters.

Ultrasound for Everyone?

The greatest controversy surrounding ultrasound is whether it should be used on all pregnant women. This will benefit pregnant women only if it shows situations which can be treated, and if this treatment will improve outcomes for mothers and babies.

Benefits from routine ultrasound for everyone have not been demonstrated in research studies to date.

Should we continue doing it anyway, even if there are no demonstrated benefits? There are two problems with this approach: first, while ultrasounds are apparently safe in the short term, long-term studies to rule out long-term harmful effects are lacking; second, every ultrasound adds to the overall cost of health care. This is reasonable and justifiable if there are benefits to mother and baby, but if no benefits can be demonstrated, then the cost of routine ultrasounds is an unnecessary expense.

ULTRASOUND FOR EVERYONE IN THE FIRST TRIMESTER

Ultrasound in early pregnancy is very accurate at establishing the number of weeks of pregnancy. These early pregnancy ultrasounds do seem to

WHAT AN ULTRASOUND CAN TELL YOU

- Is the fetus alive? (From four weeks after conception)
- How old is the fetus? (Only accurate in early pregnancy)
- Is there more than one baby?
- What is the position of the baby? (Is it head down, breech, etc.?)
- Are there certain abnormalities of the brain or heart? (Can be detected after 18 to 22 weeks)
- How big is the baby?
- Where is the placenta?
- Is the baby growing? (Requires two ultrasounds at least two or three weeks apart)

reduce the numbers of women who were induced at the end of the pregnancy for being "overdue" or post-term.

Since about 80 per cent of women's expected due dates can be predicted just as accurately by their menstrual history as by ultrasound, it is more efficient to use ultrasound only selectively for women with uncertain menstrual dates.

ULTRASOUND FOR EVERYONE IN THE THIRD TRIMESTER

Studies found that women who had ultrasound in the third trimester without a specific reason showed no improvement in perinatal mortality, low Apgar score at birth, or admission to the special care nursery over the group who had not had routine ultrasound. However, late routine ultrasound is associated with a higher rate of Caesarean section.

How Do Women Feel about Ultrasounds?

Women's feelings about ultrasounds have not been widely studied. In the studies that have been done, most women had positive feelings about having an early pregnancy ultrasound. It confirmed the reality of the baby, reduced their anxiety, and increased their confidence. Some women hope to learn the sex of the child. Many like the idea of having a picture to show people. Fathers sometimes say the pregnancy feels more real to them after they see an ultrasound of the baby, and that they are reassured about the health of the baby.

Parents are often not aware of the limitations of ultrasound, and assume that a "normal" ultrasound means the baby is guaranteed to be healthy (which is not the case). Not all abnormalities can be seen in a routine ultrasound.

One area that often creates anxiety is that some ultrasound technicians either are not allowed or do not wish to discuss the ultrasound results with the pregnant woman or her partner. Many women find this very frustrating and upsetting. When the person doing the ultrasound says, "I can't tell you anything, you'll have to ask your doctor," it's quite natural for the couple to react with fear and assume that something is wrong—even though the ultrasound may actually be quite normal.

Is Ultrasound Safe?

The benefit of any treatment must be weighed against the risks. There has been surprisingly little research to evaluate possible harm from ultrasound exposure to fetuses, especially considering how commonly it is used in early pregnancy. What research has been done so far is reassuring about short-term safety, although the studies have been too small to pick up any rare complications, and long-term risks have not been studied.

Discussing Ultrasound with Your Doctor

What if your doctor has simply assumed that you will have an ultrasound, as many do? How can you discuss this topic with him or her if you would prefer not to have one?

- Ask if your doctor is looking for any specific information from the test. If, for example, he says he wants to confirm your due date, you can point out that you have accurate records of your last period (if you do) or other information (such as temperature charts) to determine when your baby was conceived.
- Ask your doctor what could happen if you don't have an ultrasound. What would the potential problems be? Are there other ways that these could be diagnosed?
- You can simply tell your doctor, during an early pregnancy visit, that you would prefer not to have an ultrasound unless there is a specific reason.

The Evidence About...
Ultrasound

Ultrasound has been very helpful to doctors and pregnant women in many specific situations.

On the other hand, the value of ultrasound for all pregnancies has not been demonstrated.

Short-term safety of ultrasound, although little researched, seems to be established. Long-term safety has not been studied.

-8-
The Discomforts of Early Pregnancy

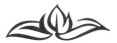

After all you'd heard about pregnant women glowing, you're finding you mostly look green. Why do they call it "morning sickness" when it seems to last all day? And you hate waking up in the middle of the night with terrible cramps in your legs.

Pregnancy is a state of health, not disease. Yet pregnancy often brings with it symptoms that at any other time might be considered signs of illness. Elizabeth, a physician, remembers that when she was three months pregnant, "I was sure I had a brain tumour. I knew I was pregnant as well, but I didn't believe just being pregnant could cause such bad headaches, or make me vomit so much. I kept thinking: my poor baby, after I die of my brain tumour, it will have no mother. Not very rational, I now realize, but that was how awful I felt."

Few studies have looked at treatments for the so-called minor symptoms of pregnancy. Yet some symptoms are fairly common, and may make women feel too unwell to go to work, or to take care of their homes and families.

Because pregnancy symptoms go away either during or after pregnancy, almost any treatment is going to appear to "work" some of the time. To really see if a treatment is effective, we need controlled studies where the treatment is measured against either another treatment or doing nothing at all.

Morning Sickness

Watch any soap opera, and if one of the characters rushes into the bathroom to throw up, or complains of a queasy feeling at breakfast, you know the pregnancy test is going to be positive. Morning sickness is so common and such a well-known symptom that pregnant women who don't feel nauseated are surprised.

"Morning sickness" isn't the best name for it. While some women are especially queasy when they first wake up in the morning, others feel sick all day long. At least half of pregnant women have some nausea, with or without actual vomiting, in early pregnancy. (Feeling queasy is much more common that actually vomiting.)

Elizabeth says, "This is how it went every morning for about two months. I'd get out of bed, rush to the bathroom and throw up. Then I'd have a shower, and get out just in time to throw up again. I'd get dressed, stagger downstairs and try to eat a little toast even though I was feeling terrible. Usually I'd throw the toast up again as soon as I got to the office. But by lunch time it was usually a bit better, and I could eat a little more. Then I could usually eat a normal supper."

The cause or causes of nausea and vomiting during pregnancy are not yet known. This has hindered the development of effective treatments.

For women who have mild nausea and queasiness, eating small, frequent meals may be the best way to reduce the unpleasant feelings. (This can be easier said than done for women who have to go to work and may not have easy access to quick snacks.)

For a small percentage of women, vomiting is so severe that they become dehydrated and lose weight. This is called **hyperemesis** (which means excessive vomiting). These women may need to be hospitalized temporarily to be given intravenous fluids.

Other treatments that have been studied are discussed below.

ACUPRESSURE

Two small studies with controls looked at acupressure on a specific point (P6) on the mother's wrist. While the studies were small, they both found that the acupressure significantly reduced the nausea. Since this treatment doesn't involve any drugs and harmful effects are unlikely, it's something pregnant women could consider trying. Wrist straps sold for carsickness and seasickness are widely available in drugstores and will put pressure on the appropriate area of the mother's wrist.

DIETARY SUPPLEMENTS

Ginger has been shown to reduce nausea, and one small study found that extra vitamin B6 was also helpful. Mothers can easily add these to their diet, and there are no known side effects.

MEDICATIONS FOR NAUSEA

A number of medications have been tested to stop severe vomiting in early pregnancy.

Bendectin: Bendectin was once the most widely prescribed drug in pregnancy, and studies showed it was highly effective in treating nausea and vomiting. The manufacturers took it off the North American market in 1983 because of lawsuits by parents whose babies were born with abnormalities after the mothers had taken the drug. Since a certain percentage of birth defects always occurs in the general population, and because Bendectin was so frequently prescribed, it was inevitable that some babies whose mothers had taken the drug would be born with birth defects. That doesn't mean that the Bendectin *caused* the problem, and, in fact, 19 large studies showed that mothers who took the drug had no higher risk of babies with birth defects than mothers who didn't take it. However, the company making the drug did not want to fight all the lawsuits and decided to stop selling Bendectin. It is unfortunate that this effective and safe medication became unavailable to pregnant women.

Diclectin: Diclectin is a drug combining **doxylamine** (an antihistamine) and **pyridoxine** (vitamin B6). It is the only drug licensed by the

Health Protection Branch (Canada) to be sold
specifically to treat the nausea and vomiting of
pregnancy and is prescribed for more than 20
per cent of pregnant women in Canada. Its ingredients are two of the three drugs that were in
Bendectin. While Diclectin is not available in the
United States, the two components are readily
available so some caregivers will prescribe them
separately for mothers.

Antihistamines: These are commonly used to
treat nausea and vomiting. They are effective,
and although their safety for the baby has not
been as widely studied as was done for
Bendectin, there is no evidence that they cause
any harm.

Constipation

Women who tend to be constipated when not
pregnant usually become worse with pregnancy.

Eating lots of fruit, vegetables, beans, whole
grains and bran, drinking more water, and getting more exercise will help constipation in
one-third of pregnant women.

If constipation persists after trying these
remedies, laxatives can be used. The safest laxatives to use during pregnancy are the ones that
are either bulking agents or stool softeners. Ask
your caregiver to recommend a brand name.
These are not absorbed into the body and will
not affect the baby. They can be used safely
throughout pregnancy. Other laxatives act by irritating the bowel and are absorbed into the body
and cross the placenta. They should be used only
on a short-term basis, if at all, because their
safety in pregnancy has not been established.
They also tend to cause more side effects, such as
painful cramping and diarrhea.

Iron supplements can also cause constipation. Since iron supplements have not been
shown to be helpful during pregnancy (see
Chapter 51), if you are taking iron and suffering
from constipation, stopping the supplement
may help.

Fatigue

Many women feel extremely tired, particularly
during the early months of pregnancy, even if
they are not anemic or malnourished. Minimal
research has been done on this symptom.
Apparently, creating a baby uses a lot of energy
and the only treatment is rest and time.

The Evidence About…
Discomforts during Early Pregnancy

Some of these discomforts can be very unpleasant for the woman who is experiencing them, yet potential treatments have not been very widely researched. Pregnancy symptoms are common, but at present, women need to rely on trial and error to find something that eases their discomfort, and it is quite possible that many of the remedies used are no better than placebo.

Yeast Infection

Yeast infections of the vagina are common in non-pregnant women, and are two to ten times more common during pregnancy. **Yeast vaginitis** can cause a heavy, white curdy discharge, itching, and a sore, tender vagina, but it will not infect the uterus, harm the baby, or cause any pregnancy complications.

If yeast is causing soreness or itching, it is safe to treat it with vaginal suppositories or cream containing either **imidazole** or **nystatin**. Imidazole has been found to be more effective than nystatin. There is a tendency for yeast to come back again, even after treatment, and the treatment can be repeated during the pregnancy.

Yeast can be present in the vagina without causing symptoms (about 25 per cent of women do have yeast in their vagina at the end of their pregnancy). If it isn't causing bothersome symptoms, it doesn't need to be treated.

Yeast present in the vagina during labour will not harm the baby. Babies can develop a yeast rash in their diaper area or patches of yeast in their mouths, called **thrush**. These are minor problems that are easily treated. There is no evidence that treating yeast in the mother's vagina during pregnancy reduces the chance of the baby developing either of these problems.

-9-
Sex during Early Pregnancy

"If I could stop feeling sick to my stomach all day long, I might feel like having sex," says Becky.

"Well, I'm not barfing or anything, but I'm exhausted. I get home from work, eat supper, and then all I want to do is go to sleep. Jeff says he can't understand why I'm so tired. I don't even look pregnant at this point, but it is sure taking up all my energy," says Vicki.

Avida shakes her head. "I actually wish Veejay was more interested. He's afraid he'll hurt the baby or that I'll have a miscarriage if we have sex. I'm embarrassed to even ask my doctor about it."

Women do vary quite a lot in how they feel about sex when they are pregnant. Many, however, find their level of sexual desire is quite low during the first trimester. Some of this is definitely related to feeling nauseated and tired. Breast changes during the first few months—an increase in blood supply and the growth of ducts inside the breasts preparing to make milk for the new baby—make many women's breasts so sensitive that even gentle touch can be painful. And while the woman may not look obviously pregnant, any pressure on her stomach or abdomen may still be very uncomfortable, so sexual positions with her partner on top may be a problem. If the baby's position is putting a lot of pressure on the mother's bladder, sexual intercourse can make that discomfort worse.

Of course, every pregnancy is different. Some women find their breasts are more sensitive in a positive way, and the increased blood flow to the pelvis can make orgasms feel more intense. For these women, sex may be even more enjoyable than usual during pregnancy.

Will sex increase the risk of miscarriage? No. The baby is well-protected in the uterus and not affected during sexual intercourse. While an orgasm will cause uterine contractions, these are mild (compared to labour) and soon stop.

Some tips for sex in early pregnancy:

- Good positions include "spooning" with the man behind the woman, woman on top, and other similar positions that don't put pressure on the woman's abdomen or breasts.
- If the woman's breasts are too sensitive for stimulation, this is a great time to discover and explore other erogenous zones.

- Oral sex is safe but your partner should avoid blowing air into your vagina.
- A small amount of bleeding (**spotting**) after intercourse during pregnancy is not unusual and is usually not a problem. Avoid having sex if you are experiencing vaginal bleeding.
- Remember that there are many ways to express love without sex if one or both of you is not comfortable—cuddling, kissing, massaging.
- Your body will change as the pregnancy progresses; what feels comfortable today may not next week. Experiment and try different approaches, and be patient with each other.

-10-
Rubella (German Measles)

Rubella is a viral infection that causes a mild illness—a fever and a rash—in children and adults. About a quarter of the cases show no symptoms at all. Because it is very contagious, most people catch rubella in childhood, and after that are immune to it. Rubella infection gives immunity for life.

While it is a minor disease for most people, in early pregnancy rubella can be very serious. The rubella virus is **teratogenic**, meaning that it causes the fetus to develop abnormally.

The earlier in the pregnancy that the infection develops, the more serious the consequences to the fetus. *Eighty per cent of women who catch rubella in the first three months of pregnancy will either miscarry or have a baby with birth defects* (called **congenital rubella syndrome**). After four months of pregnancy, rubella does not seem to cause any problems.

Congenital rubella syndrome is serious; the babies have significant problems, such as blindness and deafness. They also carry the virus in their bodies and can pass it on to other babies and to adults. There is no treatment; rubella is a virus and is not killed by antibiotics.

Rubella can, however, be prevented through vaccination. If all women were immunized against rubella before they became pregnant, congenital rubella syndrome could be eliminated. In Canada, this vaccination is recommended for all children at 13 to 14 months with a second dose at five years of age. This is an extremely safe vaccine; in rare cases it causes a slight fever, rash, and temporary joint pain.

Women who are thinking about getting pregnant in the future can have their blood checked to see if they are immune to rubella; if they are not, they can have rubella vaccine before they become pregnant (it takes about three months to be sure the antibodies have developed). At the first prenatal visit (as early as possible in pregnancy), blood testing for rubella antibodies is usually done. If rubella antibodies are present, there is no concern about exposure to rubella during pregnancy, because you can't get it again.

Rubella vaccine is not recommended for pregnant women, but when it has been given accidentally, none of the infants developed congenital rubella syndrome. If a pregnant woman is not immune to rubella, rubella vaccine can be given right after the baby is born, to prevent the disease in any future pregnancies. This vaccine is safe for breastfeeding mothers and their babies.

Ellen remembers, "I was sure I must have had German measles; I certainly seemed to have had everything else that was going around when I was a kid. But when they tested my blood at my first prenatal appointment, it came back negative. That had me worried—I'm a teacher, and I was terrified that I might catch it from one of the kids in my class."

Fortunately, Ellen didn't get the infection, and she arranged to be vaccinated as soon as her baby was born. "I'm glad I don't have to worry about catching German measles during this pregnancy."

While the names are similar, red measles (**rubeola**) is not the same as German measles. The red measles virus makes children and adults much sicker than rubella, and there is a vaccine against it as well, but red measles does not cause birth defects.

Toxoplasmosis

Toxoplasmosis is an infection caused by a parasite called **Toxoplasma gondii**. It can't be passed from one person to another; instead it is caught by eating the parasite, which is found in raw or undercooked meat or in cat feces. If, for example, you change your cat's litter box, wash your hands less than thoroughly, and then pick up some food with your fingers and eat it, it is possible (disgusting as it sounds) to have some small particles of cat feces transferred to your food.

You can't catch toxoplasmosis just by petting or picking up a cat.

In adults, toxoplasmosis is a mild illness, like having the flu. If you have it once, you become immune to it for life (like rubella). If you catch it during pregnancy, though, toxoplasmosis can be passed on to the baby and cause serious birth defects.

When mothers get toxoplasmosis in the first three months of pregnancy, about 10 to 15 per cent of their babies are affected. The babies who are infected will usually have small heads, developmental delays, seizures, and sometimes liver problems as well.

If the mother develops toxoplasmosis later in

> *The Evidence About…*
> **Toxoplasmosis**
>
> Pregnant women,
>
> * should not eat raw or undercooked meat, including steak tartare, rare steaks and burgers, raw fish (as in some sushi), uncooked hot dogs, etc.;
> * should wash their hands thoroughly after handling raw meat; and
> * should wear gloves if handling cat litter or working in a garden where cats may have been, and should wash their hands thoroughly afterwards.

pregnancy—after six months—the baby is much more likely to be affected (60 per cent risk). However, the effects at this stage are less severe. The baby may seem normal at birth but later in childhood may develop an eye condition called **chorioretinitis**, which can cause blindness.

In Europe, antibiotics are now being used to treat toxoplasmosis, and there is some evidence that this is effective.

-12-
Rh-negative Mother

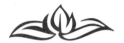

At your first prenatal appointment, a sample of your blood was taken for your blood type. Today, when you sit down beside your doctor's desk, she says, "I see that you're Rh-negative. We should talk about giving you the **Rh gammaglobulin**. Do you know the blood type of the baby's father?"

"No," you say, puzzled. "I can ask him. But why does it matter?"

Your doctor explains: "If he is Rh-negative like you, we don't need to worry, because your baby has to be Rh-negative as well. If he is Rh-positive, then your baby might be Rh-positive, and there may be a problem in that situation."

What does it mean to be Rh-negative, and how will this affect your baby?

You might have heard about babies who died in the past because their mothers were Rh-negative when the baby was Rh-positive. Today a drug called **anti-D gammaglobulin** can prevent almost all Rh problems.

If you have ever donated blood, you will have a card listing your blood type. In one category, you can be A, B, AB, or O. In another category you can be Rh-positive (this means you have a substance called **factor D** in your blood) or Rh-

negative (you don't have factor D). Your card will describe your blood type as, for example, A negative or O positive.

About 15 per cent of white North Americans are Rh-negative; among African-Americans, only 7 to 8 per cent are Rh-negative.

If the mother is Rh-positive, and the baby is Rh-negative, there is no problem. If the mother and the baby are both Rh-negative, or both Rh-positive, that does not cause a problem, either.

The *only* time there may be a problem is if the mother is Rh-negative and the baby is Rh-positive.

When Jennifer found out that she was Rh-negative, she asked her husband what his blood type was. He turned out to be Rh-negative as well. "Great," Jennifer's doctor told her. "You two are obviously a good match! We don't need to worry about the gammaglobulin in this situation."

But Trudy's case was different. Her husband tested Rh-positive, and the doctor explained that there might be a problem. "Your baby could inherit the Rh-positive blood type from Eric," the doctor pointed out, "and then there is a risk of you developing antibodies against the Rh-positive blood cells."

The problem with the Rh-negative mother and her Rh-positive baby develops when blood from the baby gets into the mother's blood. The mother's and fetus' blood circulations are in completely separate blood vessels, but these vessels are very close to one another in the placenta. Little ruptures can occur in the placenta, and blood cells from the baby can enter the mother's circulation.

If the baby's Rh-positive blood cells get into the mother's Rh-negative circulation, the mother's immune system will recognize them as foreign to her and make antibodies against them: these are called **anti-D antibodies**. Like the antibodies we make to kill germs, anti-D antibodies attack cells—in this case, Rh-positive red blood cells.

The time when this mingling of the blood cells is most likely to happen is at the time right after delivery, when the placenta is separating from the wall of the uterus. The baby is already born, so even if these antibodies do form, the baby can't be harmed by them.

There is almost no risk to the first baby, even if he or she is Rh-positive and the mother is Rh-negative. However, these antibodies stay in the mother's circulation, so if she gets pregnant again with another Rh-positive baby, they can easily cross the placenta and attack that baby's red blood cells, causing a disease called **hemolytic disease of the newborn**.

This problem was more serious in the past, when women tended to have larger families: with each baby, the risks increased. The smaller families common today, and the availability of effective preventive treatment, mean that Rh incompatibility problems are far less likely.

Preventing Anti-D Antibodies from Forming

Anti-D gammaglobulin is a concentrated, purified blood product that is given to the Rh-negative mother. It coats the Rh-positive cells entering her circulation and keeps them from causing the production of antibodies.

When the Rh-negative mother gives birth, a sample of the baby's blood is taken from the umbilical cord and tested. If the baby is Rh-negative, there is no problem and nothing needs to be done.

If the baby is Rh-positive, an injection of anti-D gammaglobulin is given to the mother. This should be given within 72 hours of delivery. Before the development of anti-D gammaglobulin, about 17 per cent of Rh-negative women who delivered an Rh-positive baby would show anti-D antibodies in their blood at the beginning of their next pregnancy.

With the use of anti-D gammaglobulin, the risk of antibodies in the next pregnancy is reduced from 17 per cent to 0.2 per cent.

There are other times when the mother's and baby's blood can mix. Anti-D gammaglobulin given at these other times reduces still further the chance of antibody production. Risky situations include the following scenarios.

AFTER A MISCARRIAGE OR INDUCED ABORTION

If it is given after an abortion or miscarriage to all Rh-negative mothers, anti-D gammaglobulin reduces the risk of sensitization from around 3 per cent to 0.2 per cent. Obviously, this is

HEMOLYTIC DISEASE OF THE NEWBORN

In the days before anti-D gammaglobulin, not all Rh-negative women had problems. In fact, the majority did not. Only about 17 per cent of Rh-negative women develop antibodies, and only some of their babies become ill. However, this is still a substantial number, and the disease is very serious.

While the antibodies in her blood will cause no symptoms in the mother, they can cross the placenta during her next pregnancy, get into her baby's blood system, and break down (**hemolyze**) its red cells.

In the most severe cases, the baby dies in the uterus. In less severe illness, the fetus becomes very anemic. This can be discovered by **amniocentesis**, and is treated with blood transfusions. If the baby is too premature to be born, it can be given transfu-

sions inside the uterus. As soon as the baby is mature enough, labour is induced so the baby can be treated outside the uterus.

Babies born with severe hemolytic disease often need immediate resuscitation and blood transfusions. Less severely affected babies are well at birth, but quickly develop **jaundice** (yellowness of the skin) as **bilirubin** accumulates in their blood. Bilirubin is produced when the red blood cells are broken down. To prevent brain damage from high levels of bilirubin, jaundice *above a certain level* is treated with special fluorescent lights that reduce the level of bilirubin in the blood. (Mild jaundice is common and normal in newborns, and does not usually require treatment.) If this **phototherapy** is not sufficient, blood transfusion is required.

treating all the women who had Rh-negative fetuses as well, but since the blood type of the fetus is unobtainable, the safest course is to treat everyone.

"I couldn't understand why my doctor wanted me to have this shot after my miscarriage," Eleanor says. "It seemed like one more thing to cope with when I was feeling so miserable about losing the baby." But when she thought it over, she decided to take the gammaglobulin. "It got me thinking about my next baby and doing what I could to protect him or her," Eleanor recalls. "In a funny way, it gave me some hope."

AFTER BLEEDING DURING THE PREGNANCY

Anti-D gammaglobulin is recommended after any procedure that might cause bleeding from

the placenta during the pregnancy. These include amniocentesis, **chorionic villus biopsy** (see Chapter 16, page 92), significant abdominal injury to the mother, abruption of the placenta, or the manual turning around of a breech baby.

Because the blood type of the fetus is not known during the pregnancy, this also treats some mothers with Rh-negative fetuses. The gammaglobulin is not dangerous or harmful to the baby whether it is Rh-negative or Rh-positive.

Treating All Rh-negative Mothers Routinely during Pregnancy

A small number of Rh-negative women carrying an Rh-positive baby will develop Rh antibodies during their first pregnancy, even before they

The Evidence About...
Rh-negative Mothers

With the use of anti-D gammaglobulin, the risk of antibody production in Rh-negative women can be reduced to 0.06 per cent.

All women should have their blood tested in early pregnancy to see if they are Rh-negative and if they have any anti-D antibodies.

For Rh-negative women without antibodies, treatment with anti-D gammaglobulin after a miscarriage or after delivery of an Rh-positive baby can prevent antibody formation and dramatically reduce the risk of hemolytic disease of the newborn in another pregnancy.

In situations where the fetal blood and maternal blood may mix, such as amniocentesis or a **placental abruption** (when the placenta separates from the wall of the uterus during the pregnancy), anti-D gammaglobulin given as soon as possible can significantly reduce the risk to this baby and subsequent babies.

Routine treatment of all Rh-negative pregnancies at 28 weeks does give a small further benefit.

Women who already have antibodies (fortunately rare since the introduction of the gammaglobulin) need to have their pregnancies carefully followed in a specialized centre where the baby's need for **intrauterine transfusion**, premature delivery, or transfusion after birth can be assessed.

deliver. Some researchers have tried giving all the Rh-negative women anti-D gammaglobulin at 28 weeks of pregnancy. Then the blood type of the baby was checked at birth, and those mothers who had an Rh-positive baby were given a second injection of anti-D gammaglobulin within 72 hours of birth.

Adding this 28-week injection further reduced the risk of sensitization from 0.2 per cent to 0.06 per cent.

Is Anti-D Gammaglobulin Safe?

Anti-D gammaglobulin is a blood product and must be screened for hepatitis and HIV, as other blood products are. The method of extraction of the gammaglobulin kills the HIV virus. Women who have religious objections to blood products must make their own decisions about its use. Otherwise, there are no known complications from this treatment.

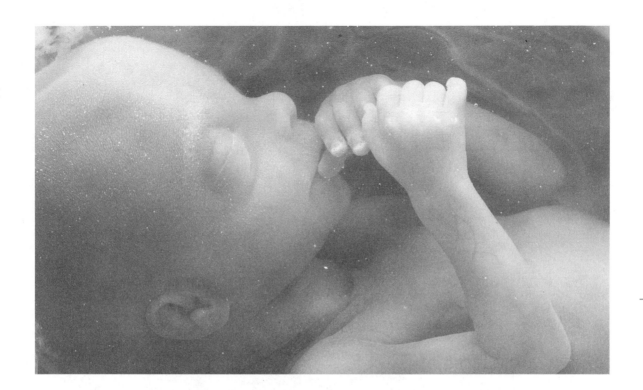

Three Months
❧ *Nine to Twelve Weeks* ❧

Pregnancy is usually divided into three trimesters lasting roughly three months each, and by 12 weeks you'll have reached the end of the first trimester. You're beginning to get used to the idea of being pregnant and expecting a baby.

Some of the early discomforts of pregnancy may be decreasing by now, although morning sickness often continues for the full 12 weeks and may sometimes last throughout pregnancy. You'll have begun regular prenatal checkups, and you may be wondering about whether your baby has any genetic problems or whether you should have some tests done to see if all is well.

13

What Happens at a Prenatal Checkup?

Sherry heads off for her first midwife's appointment, not quite sure what to expect.

When she had called to book the first appointment, the receptionist said she'd set aside an hour, but explained that this first visit was usually longer than later ones.

Sherry's midwife, Allison, confirmed this when she arrived. "Usually this first visit takes longer because I need to get your medical history and discuss some tests and things with you. But if you ever want more time at a future visit, just tell the receptionist when you book your appointment."

Allison made notes as Sherry told her about her past illnesses. She showed Sherry the form she'd be using to record information as the pregnancy progressed, and explained some of the things they would be keeping track of.

"I'm going to give you a form now to go and have some blood tests done," she said. "The lab will test for infections of various kinds, including some sexually transmitted diseases, anemia, and antibodies to rubella. They'll also check your blood type. Then you'll give them a urine sample, and they'll test that for bacterial infections, for sugar, and for protein. I'll ask you to do another urine sample each time you come for an appointment, so we can check again for protein."

Allison then asked Sherry to step on the scales in her office, and wrote down her weight. "We'll record your weight at each visit, too," she said. Using a **blood pressure cuff**, she measured and wrote down Sherry's blood pressure. This was also something she'd repeat at each visit.

"It's too early at this point to hear the baby's heartbeat," Allison said. "But at the later visits I should be able to hear it, and I'll count how fast it is beating. Once you are about five months along, I'll start measuring your uterus each month to track how the baby is growing. To do that, I put one end of the measuring tape here, just at the top of your pubic bone, and measure to where I feel the top of the uterus to be. It's not highly accurate in terms of determining the size of the baby, but it helps to give us a rough idea of how the baby is growing." (While this measuring of the uterus is commonly done, there is no evidence that it improves outcomes. If you find it uncomfortable, you can certainly decline.)

A big part of each visit, Allison emphasized, would be talking about how the pregnancy was going. They would want to discuss the various prenatal tests that Sherry could choose to have done, as well as Sherry's plans for the birth. They discussed nutrition and supplements during pregnancy and Allison explained how they calculated Sherry's due date.

"And what do you know about breastfeeding?" Allison asked.

"Well, my sister breastfed her baby," Sherry said. "So I think I know something about it."

"Your sister might be a great support to you, but I'd also encourage you to consider attending La Leche League meetings while you're pregnant. That's a great way to learn more about breastfeeding and feel really prepared when your baby is born." Allison gave Sherry a piece of paper with meeting times and dates and phone numbers for the La Leche League leaders.

Then she handed her a second piece of paper. "I know it seems early to be thinking of the birth, but I'd encourage you to sign up for prenatal classes soon as they tend to fill up. The ones we've listed here are the teachers our midwifery practice recommends."

Sherry took the papers and the forms for the blood tests and started to stand up. "Oh, I forgot to ask—when do I come back?"

"For the first seven months, you would come once a month, unless there are concerns that need to be followed more closely. After you are about 30 weeks, we'll have you make appointments every two weeks, and then for the last month you'll come in every week," Allison explained.

She told Sherry that she'd call her if there were any concerns when the results of the blood and urine tests came back, but otherwise they'd get together again in four weeks.

Each caregiver, of course, will handle prenatal visits a little differently. In some midwifery or obstetrics practices, you may have your visits scheduled with a different caregiver each time. This is to give you a chance to meet all of them, since your birth will be attended by whomever is on call at the time. In others, you will see the same doctor at every visit but may get a different doctor when you give birth.

In some clinics, you will be weighed and have your blood pressure checked by a nurse or assistant before you see the doctor. The doctor will have the results of these checks and will be able to discuss them with you if there are any concerns.

You might find it helpful to make a list of the questions you want to ask before you go to the appointment; it's easy to forget what you were concerned about if you don't write it down. If you are worried about having enough time, ask to have a longer appointment booked when you set it up. Sometimes it works best to ask to be the last appointment of the day.

14

Weight Gain in Pregnancy

At each prenatal visit, you'll probably be asked to step on the scales and have your weight recorded on your chart. In a society that tends to be obsessed with weight anyway, many women find this one of the more stressful parts of a prenatal visit. Why does your caregiver want to know how much you weigh and how that weight changes from visit to visit? And how does it affect your pregnancy and your baby?

How Big Will that Belly Grow?

In the past, women were usually urged to limit their weight gain. More recently, higher weight gains—between 25 and 35 pounds (11.5 and 16 kg) have been encouraged for women of normal weight. This is probably a positive move away from the earlier emphasis on restricting weight, but may not allow enough for the variations in experience of normal women. As Margaret found: "I am only 5-foot-3 (160 cm) and usually weigh about 100 pounds (45 kg). I felt like I was stuffing myself all the time trying to gain enough weight, and I'd only managed 22 pounds (10 kg) by the end of my pregnancy. My doctor kept nagging me to eat more, but it was impossible." Margaret's baby girl weighed a healthy 7 pounds, 6 ounces (3,345 g) when she was born.

Overweight women are still frequently told to restrict their weight gain during pregnancy. Debbie, who weighed 200 pounds (91 kg) pre-pregnancy, was told to gain no more than 15 pounds (7 kg) during her first pregnancy; when she hit 14 pounds (6.3 kg) at six months, she knew she was in trouble. "I wouldn't eat anything at all the day before my doctor's appointment," she says. "But then I'd have to do the same thing the next month, and it was pretty stressful." In the end, Debbie gained 26 pounds (11.8 kg), dreaded every doctor's appointment, and had an 8-pound, 8 ounce (3,855 g) healthy baby boy.

There is no justification for allowing healthy pregnant women to go hungry, or for imposing dietary restrictions upon them. In other words, it is important to pay attention to your appetite, and not to be ruled by the numbers on the bathroom scale at home or in your doctor's office.

Weight Gain Guidelines for Pregnancy

In 1990, the American Institute of Medicine published weight gain guidelines for pregnant women, which are still widely used today. They are based on your pre-pregnancy **body mass index or BMI** (see sidebar). Their recommended weight gains are:

- For underweight women (BMI less than 19.8), between 28 and 40 pounds (12.5 and 18 kg)
- For normal weight women (BMI between 19.8 and 26), between 25 and 35 pounds (11.5 and 16 kg)
- For overweight women (BMI between 26 and 29), between 15 and 25 pounds (7 and 11.5 kg)
- For obese women (BMI over 29), 13 pounds (6 kg)

This was a change from previous guidelines that had emphasized restricting weight gains, and was an attempt to reduce the number of low–birth weight babies by improving their mother's diets. The number of low–birth weight babies decreases as the mother's weight gain increases.

However, low birth weight is not only determined by the mother's weight gain. In fact, low weight gain by a pregnant woman can be a marker or sign of other problems. Women who gain very little weight during pregnancy are more often young, thin, less educated, poor, under stress, and smokers. These are all factors known to increase the risk of having a low–birth weight baby.

WHAT'S YOUR BMI?

This is a simple calculation of the ratio between your height and weight to give you an estimate of whether you are underweight, in a healthy weight range, or overweight. Because muscle adds weight, it may give you inaccurate results if you are very muscular.

Your BMI is your weight in kilograms divided by your height in metres squared. There are also many BMI calculators on the Internet in which you enter your height and weight, and automatically tell you the number and whether this means you are underweight, overweight, etc.

At the opposite end of the scale, women who gain a lot of weight during pregnancy are more likely to have a larger-than-average baby and this may result in difficulties during the birth. Studies suggest, though, that the number of very large babies (more than 10 pounds/4.5 kg) is only increased in mothers who gain 35 pounds (16 kg) or more during pregnancy.

Women who gain more than the guidelines during pregnancy are more likely to be tall and overweight or obese before they become pregnant. In fact, more than 75 per cent of obese and overweight women gained more than the recommended amounts in some studies.

With growing concerns about obesity and its related health problems, researchers have also looked at the problem of weight loss after pregnancy. They've found that when women gain more weight while pregnant, they tend to have a harder time losing it after the baby is born. Breastfeeding does help to increase the amount of weight lost, as does exercise in the first year after the baby's birth.

Researchers have found that only about 30 to 40 per cent of women will gain the amount of weight suggested in the guidelines—most will gain more or less.

Overweight and Pregnant

Ellen, pregnant with her third baby, was shocked when the midwife told her that she might not be able to have a home birth this time. Ellen had retained some of the weight she gained with each pregnancy and put on a little more weight in between, and the midwife was concerned that Ellen was now overweight enough to be considered high risk.

What are the pregnancy-related risks of being overweight or obese? Research suggests that obese women are more likely to miscarry, to experience pre-eclampsia, or to have blood clots. Caesarean births are much more common in obese women. There is also a higher risk of having a very large baby—which can lead to difficulties in giving birth—and of having **anemia** (low iron in the blood) after the baby is born. Overweight and obese women are also more likely to gain more during pregnancy and the **postpartum** period.

Obesity can be described as "a risk factor for risk factors." In other words, if you are obese, you are at higher risk of having, for example, high blood pressure, which is linked to pre-eclampsia and other pregnancy problems.

The number of women who are overweight or obese is significantly increasing. In 1980, about 7 per cent of women in the United States weighed more than 200 pounds (91 kg) at their first prenatal visit; 20 years later, more than 24 per cent of women weighed more than that when they became pregnant. Over the same time period, the percentage of women weighing more than 300 pounds (136 kg) at the first prenatal visit increased from 2 to 11 per cent. That rate of increase does not seem to be ending yet, as another U.S. study found the percentage of overweight women between 2000 and 2003 went up by another 11 per cent.

Certain groups of women are at higher risk when it comes to weight. In the United States, for example, more than 80 per cent of African-American women are either overweight or obese, according to several studies. Women living in low-income households, or who have lower education levels, are more likely to be overweight or obese as well.

Losing weight before becoming pregnant would reduce the risks, but the evidence is clear that weight loss is rarely easy or simple. A systematic review of weight-loss programs found that most produced minimal weight loss for the majority of those involved, and in those programs that did achieve a greater amount, only 3.2 per cent still kept the weight off two years later.

Some intensive programs for obese or overweight pregnant women have been able to reduce the amount of weight gained during the first year after the pregnancy. These programs usually involve several components including one-to-one counselling, group sessions, home visits, and other supports.

For the obese woman who is already pregnant, the question is "what now?" How can you minimize the risks?

It is clear that attempting to lose weight or severely restrict weight gain during pregnancy is not helpful. A study of more than 7,000 women who had "good outcomes" (healthy, full-term babies and vaginal deliveries) found that there were wide variations in weight-gain patterns among women. About 70 per cent of the overweight women and 57 per cent of the obese women in this study gained more than 25 pounds (11.5 kg) during their pregnancies; only 7 per cent of the overweight women and 16 per cent of the obese women who had good outcomes gained less than 15 pounds (7 kg). In other words, the majority of the larger-sized women who had good outcomes gained a significant amount of weight.

Restricting food can decrease the size of the baby, which may sound like a good thing until you look at the ways these restrictions increase the child's risk for later health problems. During World War II, the Netherlands experienced a prolonged famine where food was in short supply for everyone, including the pregnant women. Compared to babies who were born before the famine, the babies whose mothers had inadequate amounts of food during their pregnancies had higher rates of diabetes, heart disease, blood clotting problems, problems with stress, breathing difficulties, and obesity as adults.

Some studies have been done with overweight women who were placed on low-calorie diets during pregnancy, but these have not shown any clear effects on the size of the baby or the health of the mother.

There is no justification for making pregnant women go hungry or imposing dietary restrictions upon them.

The Value of Exercise

Good research on exercise during pregnancy is hard to do because women who exercise are often different in other ways from women who don't exercise (they may eat differently, for example). Most of the studies that have been done compare women who participate in regular exercise with the general population of pregnant women. The conclusions from these studies are:

- Exercise in pregnancy is a good thing! It is good to continue exercising if you were doing it before you got pregnant, and it's good to start in pregnancy even if you haven't exercised before.
- Exercise can help pregnant women sleep better and feel less depressed.
- Women who exercise have faster labours, fewer inductions, fewer forceps deliveries, and fewer Caesarean births. Since these are all areas where overweight and obese women are at higher risk, regular exercise can help to minimize those risks.
- Exercise does not cause miscarriage.
- Exercise is associated with uterine contractions, but is not associated with an increased risk of premature birth.

These benefits make adding exercise a helpful strategy for all pregnant women, including obese or overweight women.

Of course, you may need to modify your activities during pregnancy (this is probably not a good time to take up horseback riding, for example!). If running makes you feel like you have to urinate with every step because the baby

The Evidence About...
Weight Gain

Weight gain and food intake should not be restricted during pregnancy.

Overweight and obese women are at a higher risk of problems during pregnancy and when giving birth.

With appropriate safety precautions, exercise during pregnancy is beneficial to the mother and safe for the baby.

keeps bouncing against your bladder, try walking or swimming instead.

Because your body changes during pregnancy, additional safety precautions are recommended.

- Talk to your caregiver about any individual risk factors you should be aware of.
- Warm up thoroughly before you exercise. This is important because your ligaments are more lax, your joints are looser than normal, and your abdominal and back muscles are stretched. All these factors increase your risk of injury if you are not warmed up.

- Avoid exercising to the point of breathlessness or until your heart rate is over 100 to 120 beats per minute. Intense exercise will divert your blood and oxygen to your muscles and away from the baby.
- In the third trimester, you should avoid floor exercises where you are lying on your back, as this position reduces the blood flow to your uterus and your baby.

Ellen decided to incorporate more exercise into her life. She took a long walk each evening when her husband was at home and could watch her older children, and went swimming in the local pool two or three times a week. Her blood pressure stayed within the normal range and she did not show any signs of other problems.

After some discussions with other midwives, Ellen was able to find one who felt comfortable attending her birth at home. Her baby daughter was born after a fairly short, straightforward labour, weighing just under 8 pounds (3,625 g). Ellen is hoping to have more children, and this has motivated her to increase her exercise program and make sure her diet is healthy.

"I want to be in good shape next time before I conceive," she explains.

-15-
Miscarriage and Tubal (Ectopic) Pregnancy

"I'm bleeding!" Carole called her doctor in a panic. "There's blood in my underpants. It looks like the start of my period."

At her first pregnancy appointment, at six weeks, everything had seemed fine. Now, just two weeks later, she was bleeding.

In the office, her doctor looked at her cervix with a speculum. The blood was definitely coming from inside the uterus.

"I had hoped it might just be some irritation on your cervix bleeding, but it isn't," said her doctor. "You might be starting to miscarry."

Carole started to cry. "What can I do to stop it? I can't lose my baby."

Her doctor took her hand sympathetically. "If your baby is going to be fine, it is. If you are going to have a miscarriage, you are. There is nothing you or I can do to change that."

Carole said, "I'll go home and go to bed for a couple of days. I'll just take the time off work. I'll do anything to keep from losing my baby."

Again her doctor tried to comfort her. "Carole, I know you would do anything; I know you really want this baby. But going to bed isn't going to keep you from having a miscarriage. If you start having heavier bleeding and cramps you might want to stay in bed for your own comfort, but it isn't going to keep you from miscarrying."

Carole called her doctor again the next day. "I'm still bleeding, sort of like a light period. I don't have any bad pain though. That's a good sign, isn't it?"

Her doctor suggested having an ultrasound to see if the baby was still alive or not.

Carole was upset. "How will that help? I didn't want to have any ultrasounds during my pregnancy."

Her doctor explained that having an ultrasound would tell them whether the baby was alive or not, but it wouldn't change the fact that there was no treatment that would help. Carole decided to wait a few more days.

That night, Carole barely slept. The bleeding was heavier and she had painful cramps. Towards morning, her husband drove her to the hospital. "I guess I'm having a miscarriage—surely I couldn't have cramps and bleeding this bad and the baby still be OK," she said to her doctor when he arrived.

Her doctor examined her again. "Yes, you are having a miscarriage. There is a lot of blood and clots here now, and I think your uterus feels a little smaller than it did. I don't know what will happen from here. You may finish miscarrying and the bleeding will stop on its own. Or you may keep on bleeding and cramping for days, until you have a **D&C**, a dilation and curettage, to scrape out all the tissue that is left in your uterus."

Carole's doctor again suggested having an ultrasound: "It will tell for sure that you don't have a live baby. And it will also show how much tissue is left in the uterus. If there isn't much, you are probably fine just to go home and let your body handle this by itself, without having a D&C."

Carole decided to have the ultrasound: "I cried all the way through it. The technician was so business-like, and didn't say anything to me at all. My friends had told me about ultrasounds where they had seen the baby and seen its heart beat. When I asked the technician, he said he couldn't tell me anything, I would have to ask my doctor."

The ultrasound showed no live baby, and very little tissue left in the uterus. Carole went home. She stopped bleeding about four days later, and got her normal period six weeks after that.

A miscarriage (also called a **spontaneous abortion**) is the death of a fetus before 20 weeks of pregnancy. Miscarriage is common—probably about 35 per cent of all pregnancies end in miscarriage. About 25 per cent of pregnancies miscarry before the woman even knows she is pregnant. She may think her period is just a little late, or a little heavier than usual, but in fact she did have a fertilized egg and is having an early miscarriage. Another 10 per cent of pregnancies miscarry after the woman has missed her period and realizes she is pregnant.

At least 85 per cent of miscarriages happen before 12 weeks of pregnancy.

Causes of Miscarriage

There is probably more misinformation concerning the cause of miscarriage than about any other area of pregnancy. Many women worry that they caused their miscarriage by having sex, moving heavy furniture, or exercising too much—none of which are related to miscarriage. Often women blame whatever they did the day before the bleeding started, when in fact, the baby has usually died several days before the bleeding of miscarriage begins.

There is *no* increased association of miscarriage with bad nutrition, vigorous exercise, sedentary lifestyle, video display terminals, or pregnancies that happen as a result of failures of oral contraceptives or spermicidal creams and jellies. Pregnancies that are planned and wanted miscarry just as often as pregnancies that are unwanted.

About 50 per cent of miscarried fetuses have genetic problems. The miscarriage could be regarded as nature's solution to a totally abnormal embryo. The other 50 per cent miscarry for various reasons, many of them unknown. It may not have been a perfect egg or a perfect sperm, or perhaps the developing embryo did not implant itself in a good spot in the wall of the uterus.

There are some situations where miscarriages are more common:

- When mothers smoke, or drink more than two alcoholic drinks per day, or use recreational drugs, miscarriage is slightly more common.
- If the mother becomes pregnant with an IUD in place, she is more likely to miscarry.
- Women with diabetes have a higher rate of miscarriage. If the mother's blood sugar is perfectly controlled during the weeks before conception and in the early weeks of the pregnancy, this risk is reduced.
- Older mothers (over 35) are slightly more likely to miscarry, because older mothers are more likely to have babies with abnormal chromosomes.
- Infections such as **German measles** or **syphilis** in early pregnancy can cause miscarriage.

Terms Used to Discuss Miscarriage

THREATENING TO MISCARRY

Any woman who has bleeding in early pregnancy is likely to be described as "threatening to miscarry," although that isn't very accurate. About half the women who have vaginal bleeding in early pregnancy will miscarry, but for the other half the bleeding may have nothing at all to do with miscarriage.

Rita says, "In three out of my four pregnancies, I had two or three days of bleeding about two weeks after my period was due. The first time I worried about it, but after that, I thought it was normal for me. My sister had the same experience when she was pregnant, and I know

DID I CAUSE MY MISCARRIAGE?

Miscarriage is NOT caused by:

- too much exercise
- too little exercise
- eating junk food
- dancing
- using computers or video display terminals
- not wanting to be pregnant
- having sex
- whatever you did the day before you started bleeding

You CANNOT prevent a miscarriage by:

- resting in bed
- eating really well
- taking **estrogen** or **progesterone** pills
- taking vitamins, minerals, or herbal supplements

this sounds weird, but for both of us, it only happened when we were carrying boys."

Leslie remembers her first 10 weeks of pregnancy with anger. "I had some bleeding at six weeks and at seven weeks and at nine weeks. Each time it stopped by itself, and each time I had an ultrasound. The doctor said I was 'OK for now, we'll see how things go in the next couple of weeks.'

"Finally, when I bled again at 11 weeks, my doctor examined me and found that I had a **polyp** (a small, benign growth) on my cervix, which was bleeding. It had nothing to do with the pregnancy at all. He removed it and I never bled again. It makes me mad that I worried for

10 weeks about my baby and had three ultrasounds for nothing."

Leslie says that if she had this kind of bleeding again during pregnancy, she would insist on having it more thoroughly investigated.

INEVITABLE MISCARRIAGE OR INEVITABLE ABORTION

The woman who is having heavy bleeding with clots, has leaked amniotic fluid, and has a soft open cervix is having an inevitable miscarriage. The fetus is already dead, and is in the process of being passed from the uterus.

An inevitable miscarriage may also be diagnosed by an ultrasound, which shows that the baby has died or was never formed. Even though the woman may not be bleeding very heavily at that moment, she is eventually going to miscarry.

The diagnosis of inevitable miscarriage can also be made by repeating the blood test for pregnancy. If the levels of pregnancy hormone are lower than average, and are getting lower rather than higher in the first 12 weeks of pregnancy, the pregnancy is going to miscarry.

Many women who are going to miscarry will comment that they don't "feel pregnant" anymore even if they are only bleeding lightly (or sometimes not at all). This is because they are no longer producing pregnancy hormones, and they will eventually miscarry.

Mary says, "I knew something was wrong when I got up in the morning and started dressing my kids to take them to the playground. I was doing up Paul's coat when I realized that I didn't feel queasy at all. I felt normal. When I met my friend at the park, I told her I thought

I was going to miscarry, because I didn't feel pregnant any more. And I was right. The bleeding started the next day."

INCOMPLETE MISCARRIAGE OR INCOMPLETE ABORTION

This means that the miscarriage is inevitable but there is still tissue in the uterus, which may cause the woman to keep on bleeding and cramping.

MISSED ABORTION

This means that the fetus has died, sometimes weeks earlier, but has not been expelled from the uterus. Usually the woman doesn't feel pregnant any more, her uterus isn't growing, and her breasts are back to normal, but she hasn't had the bleeding and cramping to expel the dead fetus. A missed abortion will expel itself eventually, or if it is diagnosed by ultrasound, the woman may choose to have a D&C.

BLIGHTED OVUM

A blighted ovum is a miscarriage in which there has been a fertilized egg, but it has died so early that no actual fetus has formed. An ultrasound will show a small empty sac in the uterus with no fetus in it. Often in this situation, the woman has never felt very pregnant, but did miss a period and have a positive pregnancy test. This miscarriage usually doesn't cause a lot of bleeding, and usually doesn't need a D&C.

RECURRENT MISCARRIAGE

A recurrent miscarriage is one which occurs in a woman who has already had a miscarriage. Many researchers have studied women who have more than one miscarriage, to see if they have some common problem. To date, there seems to be nothing that women who have more than one miscarriage have in common except bad luck. In some individual cases, there may be physical problems that make it more difficult for the mother to carry a baby full term.

A small subgroup of women who have three or more consecutive miscarriages, without ever having a full-term pregnancy, have been studied for the possibility of immunity problems between the woman and her partner. This work looks promising, but is as yet inconclusive.

Ultrasound and Miscarriage

Ultrasound has been extremely helpful to mothers who are concerned that they are having a miscarriage. Ultrasound can detect a fetal sac by 35 days after the last period, and a fetal heartbeat by 45 days after the last menstrual period. If the woman is unsure of her dates, sometimes two ultrasounds about a week apart are needed to distinguish a blighted ovum from a very early pregnancy.

The ultrasound can also help in decision-making about the need for a D&C by showing how much tissue is left in the uterus.

Prevention of Miscarriage

There is almost as much misinformation about the prevention of miscarriage as there is about its causes. The research can be summarized quickly: *nothing* so far has been demonstrated to prevent miscarriage.

Two main approaches to preventing miscarriage have been tried: bed rest and hormones.

BED REST

For years, women who had any bleeding in early pregnancy were told to rest in bed. Studies have shown that women who rest in bed miscarry just as often as women who continue their usual activities. Unfortunately, bed rest continues to be advised on the basis that "it can't do any harm." This is not exactly true; bed rest disrupts women's lives, their households, and their jobs, for no benefit. Women who don't confine themselves to bed (and how many women can?) and then miscarry, often feel guilty unnecessarily, believing that if they had rested more, they could have saved their babies.

HORMONE THERAPY

Diethylstilboestrol (DES) is a hormone that was given to women in countries all over the world for over 30 years (from the 1940s to the 1970s) in the belief that it prevented miscarriage. By the 1950s, the research trials had clearly shown that it was not effective: it did not prevent miscarriage.

The tragic result of that unsuccessful attempt to prevent miscarriage is that children born to women who took DES during their pregnancy are at a higher risk of serious health problems (among them, infertility and vaginal cancer).

What makes this truly tragic is that DES continued to be widely used for 15 years after the research had demonstrated that it didn't work to prevent miscarriage. It was only stopped when the early reports of the harm it had done to the children were made public.

Hormone treatment with progesterone-like drugs is currently being used to try to prevent miscarriage. There are good reasons to think that progesterone is needed to maintain the growth of the fetus in the first 12 to 20 weeks. To date, there are no studies that have demonstrated the usefulness of progesterone-like drugs in preventing miscarriage, although this research is ongoing.

Tubal (Ectopic) Pregnancy

When Lesley became pregnant for the fourth time, she expected everything to go as smoothly as it had with her first three. A week after her first prenatal visit, though, she got a pain in her side, bad enough to make her call her doctor and say she needed to be seen that day. "I knew I had never felt anything like it with my other pregnancies." As soon as the doctor examined her, he sent her for an ultrasound that showed what he had suspected: Lesley had a tubal (ectopic) pregnancy.

The father's sperm and the mother's **ovum** (or egg) normally meet and combine to start the growth of the embryo inside the mother's

Fallopian tube (this tube runs between the **ovary**, where the eggs are produced, and the **uterus**). Over the next few days, this embryo continues on down the Fallopian tube and into the uterus. There it makes a home in the uterine lining and starts developing into the fetus and placenta.

In a tubal pregnancy, the embryo doesn't make it all the way to the uterus. Instead it grows right inside the Fallopian tube. This is dangerous because although the uterus can grow very dramatically throughout pregnancy, the Fallopian tube can't. That means that soon the rapidly growing embryo will rupture the tube, causing internal bleeding and pain.

Lesley had surgery that night to remove the tubal pregnancy, and while the operation and her recovery went well, the experience was difficult emotionally. She says, "First, I found out I was pregnant, and we started planning for the new baby. We were feeling excited and positive. Then the next thing I know, I'm having major surgery—and there's no baby. I was worried, too, that this would affect my chances of getting pregnant again."

Tubal pregnancies occur in about 1 pregnancy out of 100. They are more common in these situations:

- If a woman has had a previous pelvic infection which has scarred her tubes, tubal pregnancy is more likely.
- If a woman has had one tubal pregnancy, her risk of having another one is from 7 to 15 per cent.
- Women who become pregnant with an IUD in place, or after a tubal ligation, are more likely to have a tubal pregnancy.

- Women who become pregnant using fertility treatments are at higher risk for tubal pregnancy.

TREATMENT OF TUBAL PREGNANCY

Possibly 40 per cent of tubal pregnancies will end spontaneously without the woman ever knowing she is pregnant. The fetus dies very early on and is gradually reabsorbed without the woman having any pain or bleeding. Her period may be a little bit late or a little bit heavier than usual, but that is all.

When tubal pregnancy causes pain and bleeding enough to be diagnosed, it is usually treated with surgery, either through the **laparoscope**, which only requires a small incision in the abdomen, or through surgery with a full abdominal incision.

Another treatment has recently been developed to try to avoid surgery for tubal pregnancy. With this treatment, a drug called **methotrexate** is injected **intramuscularly** into the mother. More than one injection may be needed. It works about 90 per cent of the time, and is most successful when the diagnosis is made early in pregnancy and the embryo is still small. If this drug treatment is not successful, then surgery will be required.

When there is surgery after a tubal pregnancy, the tube is usually removed, and that may make it more difficult for a women to get pregnant again, because only one ovary can send eggs into the uterus. It's important to talk to the doctor and let him or her know if you are hoping to have more children in the future.

Grieving after a Miscarriage

Often family or friends consider a miscarriage to be a fairly minor loss, certainly not as significant as a stillbirth or the death of a newborn. Yet for the mother, and sometimes the father, a miscarriage can be very traumatic. Once a pregnancy is confirmed, parents may begin to make plans for the new addition to their family, and a miscarriage may be the loss of a very real baby.

Leanne says, "One day we were all excited about the baby, picking out names and planning how we'd decorate the nursery. Then the next day the bleeding started and by Friday, there was no baby. Nothing. I could hardly bring myself to leave the house—I was afraid that if I saw someone with a baby I'd just break down and cry."

Besides the physical care provided, women who have experienced a threatened or an actual miscarriage will also need emotional support.

Amanda remembers being appalled by the attitude of the emergency ward doctor who treated her miscarriage. "She told me to be grateful, that the baby probably wouldn't have been normal. How could she say that? I wanted that baby so much. She just made me feel awful, like I couldn't have a normal baby. I needed her to at least say she was sorry, not to tell me to be grateful."

Charlene felt she coped quite well after experiencing an early miscarriage, but when her due date arrived, she felt sad all day. "I couldn't get it out of my mind that this was the day my baby was supposed to be born," she says.

Women may benefit at some time from information about miscarriage, most particularly from the knowledge that it is common, and that nothing they did caused it or could have prevented it.

The Evidence About...
Miscarriage

Miscarriage is a common pregnancy complication that cannot be prevented. Women who miscarry need emotional support as well as physical care.

The tragedy of DES should remind all of us about the importance of research. The research showed DES did not prevent miscarriage, yet many doctors continued using it. As well, this hormone was assumed to be safe because babies appeared normal at birth; it was only years later when researchers discovered the tragic, long-term effects.

But they also need an acknowledgment of their grief, that this has been a loss which they can mourn.

Fathers, too, can be deeply affected by a miscarriage. Early on, the pregnancy may not seem entirely real to some fathers, but dads also join in the planning and the excitement and feel the loss when a pregnancy ends unexpectedly.

"It was seeing the ultrasound that did it for me," says Rod. "I was so impressed when I could see his little heart beating. I knew he was real, I knew he was alive. And then we lost him. I think I felt as bad as Janine, even though I didn't have to go through the physical stuff."

Julie had two miscarriages and then gave birth to a healthy, full-term baby. "I was just devastated when I had the second miscarriage. The first time I made out that it was no big deal, miscarriages are pretty common. But when it happened again I began to feel like I would never have a baby. When I told my doctor how miserable I was feeling—I'd go to work and end up crying in the washroom—she referred me to a support group and that helped a lot."

Support groups such as the one Julie joined are available in many communities; other women have found comfort through making connections in newsletters, books, and online support groups with other women who have had miscarriages. Ask your physician or midwife about what is available in your area, if you would like some extra support.

-16-
Tests to Assess the Baby during Pregnancy

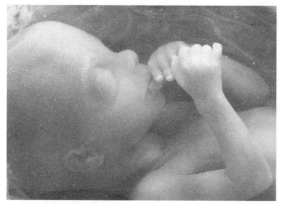

It's natural to wonder how the baby is doing while you're waiting for it to be born. (Why don't pregnant women have windows in their bellies?) Most mothers worry, at some point, whether the baby is healthy and developing normally. If someone asks you if you want a girl or a boy, you're likely to say, "I just want a healthy baby." You're probably faithfully attending your prenatal visits primarily to be reassured that your baby is doing well.

But sometimes the tests and checks of the baby's well-being are anything but reassuring. Sharon, for example, was expecting her first

TESTS DISCUSSED IN THIS CHAPTER

1. Testing for **genetic** (chromosome) abnormalities:
    a) **chorionic villus biopsy** (a sampling of the placenta done at 10 to 12 weeks)
    b) **amniocentesis** (a sampling of the amniotic fluid done at 15.5 or 16 weeks)
    c) **nuchal translucency screening** (a detailed ultrasound in which part of the baby's neck is measured)
    d) **maternal serum screening** (a blood test done on the mother at 16 weeks)
2. Testing the baby's well-being:
    a) ultrasound to assess size and growth
    b) biochemical tests of blood and urine
    c) fetal kick counting
    d) non-stress testing and contraction stress testing
    e) **fetal biophysical profile** and **Doppler ultrasound**

baby. She was in good health and expected her pregnancy to go well. She began monthly appointments with her doctor soon after she found out she was pregnant, and was put through a whole set of testing and assessment procedures that her doctor assured her were "routine." First, the doctor suggested an ultrasound to "confirm her dates," even though Sharon keeps careful track of her menstrual cycles and knew when her last period was. Then she had the maternal serum screening, which placed her in the "high-risk" group, followed by an amniocentesis to see if her baby had Down's syndrome (it didn't). By the time Sharon actually went into labour, she'd had three more ultrasounds to make sure her baby was growing normally, and had been through a stress test to see if her baby would be able to cope with labour.

Sharon's experience may not be typical, but it's certainly not uncommon. And now Sharon definitely feels anxious about pregnancy and birth. She's spent a lot of time worrying about this baby and sees it as a vulnerable little person in a risky situation.

Sharon's extra stress (and the costs of her tests to the medical system) will be worth it if the procedures she had help her to have a healthier baby. Will they? That's the question the researchers have tried to answer as they looked at various methods of assessing the baby before birth.

How can parents and professionals determine if the baby is, in fact, growing as it should be and doing well? In the past, mothers watched their abdomens grow larger each month and felt the baby move. That didn't provide a lot of information, but it did show that the baby was alive and getting bigger. Since the late 1960s, several methods of assessing the health of the fetus have been developed. These tests can be used for women with health problems that make their babies more at risk of certain problems, or they can be offered to all pregnant women.

Testing for Genetic Abnormalities

Some of the tests are to diagnose genetic (chromosomal) abnormalities in the fetus. There are no treatments for these problems, but you can be offered the option of therapeutic abortion if the fetus is found to be abnormal.

Abortion is a topic that can generate strong emotions, and the decision about whether or not to have an abortion is a very personal one. Some parents choose to have these tests done because they know that if the fetus is abnormal, they will have an abortion. Parents who would not choose an abortion may still want to know if their child has genetic abnormalities, to help them prepare. In any case, parents who choose to have any of these screening tests done should spend some time beforehand discussing what they will do with the information if their baby does have a genetic abnormality. How do they feel about abortion? How do they feel about caring for a disabled child?

CHORIONIC VILLUS BIOPSY AND AMNIOCENTESIS

Chorionic villus biopsy is a method of obtaining fetal cells early in pregnancy (usually 10 to 12 weeks) to test for any chromosome abnormality (such as those causing Down's syndrome, **sickle cell anemia, hemophilia**, etc.). To perform this test, a needle is inserted either through the mother's abdomen into the uterus, or through the vagina and cervix into the uterus, to take a sample from the **chorion** (a membrane that will develop into the placenta). Ultrasound is used to help the doctor performing the biopsy guide the needle to the right place. Since these cells are actually part of the baby, they can be examined to see if there are any chromosome abnormalities.

Chorionic villus biopsy is usually done before 12 weeks of pregnancy and this is an advantage for women who may decide to have an abortion if there is a chromosome abnormality, because an abortion is a simpler procedure at this point. However, many fetuses with chromosomal abnormalities will spontaneously miscarry early in the pregnancy. If the mother had opted to wait and have amniocentesis instead, she might have miscarried the baby before the time for the testing arrived.

Amniocentesis is the withdrawal of a small amount of amniotic fluid from the uterus by a needle (again, with ultrasound images to help the doctor get the needle in exactly the right place). This fluid contains cells from the fetus, and these are analyzed for chromosomal defects as in the previous tests. Amniocentesis is usually done between 15 and 16 weeks of pregnancy and the analysis takes two or three weeks (much longer than for chorionic villus biopsy) This can be significant if an abnormality is found and the mother decides to have an abortion; the pregnancy will now be between 17 and 19 weeks. This makes the abortion itself more complicated, and it can be more emotionally distressing for the

mother than if it was done during the first trimester.

Mothers over the age of 35 are most likely to have this testing because they are, statistically, at higher-than-average risk of having a child with a chromosome abnormality. You may also be offered the test if you have already had a child with a chromosome abnormality, or have a close relative with an abnormality.

Amniocentesis will also be offered to women who get a "positive" result on the maternal serum screening for Down's syndrome, but it will not be offered to those who screen negative—see below.

In any of these situations, you can simply refuse the test if you prefer not to have it done. Some women know they don't want to have an abortion even if the baby has Down's syndrome or other problems. They feel that having a positive test result will make the pregnancy more stressful and are more comfortable just waiting to see what happens.

What are the risks to these procedures? Chorionic villus biopsies and amniocentesis both have a low complication rate. Chorionic villus biopsy needs a repeat test (because the first one didn't give clear results) in a little more than 2 per cent of cases. Amniocentesis needs to be repeated between 1 and 2 per cent of the time. The actual rate of failures varies with the experience of the centre doing the testing. The rate of miscarriage after amniocentesis is about 1 in 300, and the risk of a very low–birth weight baby or a baby with breathing problems is about 1 in 200. Chorionic villus biopsy has a higher rate of pregnancy loss than amniocentesis, but the exact risk is very difficult to state because many of the studies include in the pregnancy loss numbers the therapeutic abortion figures as well as miscarriages. Different research trials have reported different figures, and, for both procedures, the complication rates seem to be lowest for centres with the most experience.

NUCHAL TRANSLUCENCY SCREENING

This test is a detailed ultrasound that must be done at a certain stage of gestation: between 11 weeks and 13 weeks, 6 days. While it is commonly used in Europe, it is less widely available in North America. During the ultrasound, the technician measures two things: the baby's length (to estimate the baby's age) and the thickness of an area on the back of the baby's neck, which shows up dark on the ultrasound. This is actually fluid under the skin. If this is thicker than usual, there is a greater likelihood that the baby will have Down's syndrome or another birth defect (including problems with the baby's heart). A positive result on this test does not mean for certain that the baby will have any particular defect; it simply means that the baby is at a higher risk. A risk of greater than 1 in 300 is considered "high risk," so if your baby has a 1 in 150 chance of a birth defect, then this pregnancy would be high risk (even though 149 of 150 babies given these odds will be just fine). An amniocentesis would need to be done to confirm whether or not your baby actually has Down's syndrome or another genetic abnormality. You might also want another detailed ultrasound later in the pregnancy to see if the baby has heart problems.

MATERNAL SERUM SCREENING

"Now, when you come back next month you will be 16 weeks along, and we can do the maternal serum screening," says your doctor.

"What's that?"

"Just a blood test. It will tell us if the baby is okay."

You are handed a pamphlet to read and you walk out wondering what this test is all about. Most of the pregnant women you know have had it done, and the doctor certainly seems to think it's just routine. It might be reassuring to know that the baby is healthy...

Despite what you may be told, though, the maternal serum screening does not "tell you if the baby is okay." It is a screening test, which means it tells you the risk of your baby having certain abnormalities. It does *not* tell you whether or not your baby, in fact, does have these abnormalities.

The MSS is a popular test, primarily because it is simple to do; it is almost routinely offered to all pregnant women. It isn't, however, simple to explain, and when the information is simplified it is usually not accurate and leaves out important details. Before deciding to have this test done, you should understand the information the test can give.

To perform the MSS test, a sample of the mother's blood is taken when she is between 15 and 17 weeks pregnant. It is important for the accuracy of the results that the dates be precise. This sample is then analyzed in a lab. There is no risk to either mother or baby when the test is done.

The test is done to determine the risk of two separate abnormalities in your baby. One is

Down's syndrome, a chromosome abnormality that causes mental retardation and can cause physical problems in the baby as well. The other is an abnormality in the development of the baby's brain or spinal cord called an **open neural tube defect**. This can be either **anencephaly**, in which the baby's brain does not develop (and the baby will not live), or an abnormality of the spinal cord called **spina bifida**, in which the spinal cord does not fuse. Spina bifida can cause different degrees of disability, from complete paralysis below the waist to varying degrees of leg weakness.

The test does not tell you whether or not your baby has one of these problems. It tells you the relative *risk* of your baby having either Down's syndrome or a neural tube defect. The results for the two tests are determined from the same blood sample but are quite separate. If your results fall into a risk category above a certain level for either abnormality, this is called a high-risk or positive screen.

In the general population, the overall risk for any woman of having a baby with a neural tube defect is 1 or 2 per 1,000 pregnancies. For women who have already had a baby with a neural tube defect, or who have a close family relative with this condition, the risk increases to 10 per 1,000. Calculating the risk of Down's syndrome is more complicated because it increases with the mother's age: at age 20, the risk of having a baby with Down's syndrome is 1 in 1,500; at age 40, the risk is 1 in 130. Also, a woman who has already had a baby with Down's syndrome has a higher risk of having another baby with the condition.

The MSS test results come back to your doctor as a number (1 out of 1,000, or 1 out of 110),

which is your risk of having a baby with that abnormality. In Ontario, for example, the positive or high-risk screen for Down's syndrome has been arbitrarily defined as a risk of 1 in 385 or greater. So a risk of 1 in 400 would be negative, a risk of 1 in 300 would be positive. A positive or high-risk screen for neural tube defects has been arbitrarily defined as a risk of 1 per 100.

Obviously, a positive screen does not mean your baby has the problem for which he or she is being tested—as the numbers show, in most cases the baby does not. Cases in which the screen is positive but the baby does not have the condition are called false positives. On the other hand, a negative screen or test result does not mean the baby won't have these problems; the MSS will screen positive for only 70 per cent of Down's syndrome cases and 80 per cent of open neural tube defects. The cases missed by the screen are called false negatives.

Deciding what the results of the test mean for you as an individual can be very difficult. What can you do to further clarify the situation if your test is positive, as it is for about 8 per cent of the women who are tested?

You can, if you like, have further testing to follow up on these results. First, you should confirm that you actually were 16 weeks pregnant when the test was done, as it is only accurate at that time.

If your screen is positive for Down's syndrome, you can have an amniocentesis, which can give you a definite answer about whether your baby has this condition, but carries a risk of miscarriage of about 1 in 300.

If your test has been positive for neural tube defect, you can have a detailed ultrasound, which will diagnose anencephaly and possibly spina bifida. You can also have the serum **AFP** (alpha-fetal protein, a substance produced in the baby's liver) repeated or have an amniocentesis to test the AFP levels in the amniotic fluid. If these tests are positive, the risk of a neural tube defect is higher.

Parents should also recognize that no test guarantees a perfect baby. Tracy says, "I had the MSS test done, and was so reassured when the results came back low-risk. I thought they meant the baby was healthy. It shocked me when he was born and had a rare condition that causes developmental delays and other physical handicaps. His syndrome doesn't show up on the test."

Remember as well that 30 per cent of babies with Down's syndrome are born to mothers whose MSS tests came back negative.

Katherine had the maternal serum screening done for the first time when she was pregnant with her fourth child. She decided to have the screening—which she had not bothered with during her first three pregnancies—because she was now 36, and her doctor advised her that she had a higher risk of having a baby with Down's syndrome. When the test came back positive, Katherine and her husband didn't know what to do.

"Did it mean we had a baby with Down's syndrome? I asked the doctor. No, just that I was in a higher risk group. Well, I knew I was in a higher risk group because of my age, so that wasn't very helpful. We couldn't figure out what this meant. I was confused, Jack was confused, and we didn't know what we should do next."

After discussing it with her husband and her doctor, Katherine decided to repeat the test. Again the results were positive. The doctor explained Katherine's options but none of them appealed to her very much. Even if she had an amniocentesis and found out that the baby had Down's syndrome, she wasn't sure that having an abortion would be a possible choice for her. "It already felt like a real baby to me," she says.

Katherine decided not to have an amniocentesis, but she continued worrying about her baby. To her relief, Devon was born quite normal and healthy.

"We hadn't really thought it out enough," she says now. "We had the test because the doctor recommended it, but Jack and I never discussed what we'd do if the test came back positive."

What will it mean if your test is negative? It doesn't mean that your baby is guaranteed to be normal. This test only covers two possible conditions, and your baby might have some other problem. It is also possible that your baby will have either Down's syndrome or an open neural tube defect even though your test was negative. The negative test simply means that you are considered to be in a lower risk group.

What does it mean if your baby does have one of the disabilities mentioned? Both Down's syndrome and open neural tube defects have a range of severities. Some people with Down's syndrome, for example, have serious disabilities, while others, with some assistance, lead productive and happy lives. The tests can't tell you how severe—or how mild—the problem will be.

Even if you initially requested the screening because you planned to have an abortion if the results were positive, you can change your mind. You may also decide that an abortion is the right choice for you and your family even though it hadn't seemed like an option before you had any tests done. Counselling to discuss your options is

INFORMED CONSENT

Informed consent is considered to be an important part of ethical medical care, but it can be harder to achieve than it sounds. If a medical test (or a medical treatment) is offered or recommended, you should be given information about the test that allows you to decide if you want to have it done or not.

That sounds straightforward. But when you are pregnant, you generally have to rely on your doctor or midwife as the source of information, and it's easy for them to present even accurate information in a slanted or biased manner. They may emphasize the potential risks or emphasize the potential benefits, for example.

In some cases—and maternal serum screening is one of them—the information is fairly complicated and can take a long time to explain.

To be truly informed about prenatal tests and other aspects of your medical care, you may want to seek out additional sources of information such as books like this one, your childbirth educator, Internet resources, or a genetic counsellor.

available; you might also want to contact one of the support groups for parents of children with Down's syndrome or neural tube problems to get a realistic picture of the range of disability.

Just because a test is easy to do doesn't mean it should be done. Before you choose to have maternal serum screening, be sure you understand what it is testing for and the uncertainty of the results. Discuss with your partner now whether you will have further testing if you have a positive screen result. It's also important to discuss your feelings about abortion even if you don't make a hard and fast decision, because if abortion is being considered, further testing must be proceeded with immediately.

How Is the Baby Doing in the Uterus?

Beyond these tests for genetic problems, which can be diagnosed but can't be treated, physicians and researchers have looked for ways to assess the baby's health as it grows inside the uterus.

There are two goals: to find ways of identifying babies who are not growing well before birth, and to find effective ways of improving the situation for these babies.

MEASURING THE SIZE AND GROWTH OF THE FETUS

One of the things that doctors and researchers try to determine is the size of the baby. Their concerns are that a very big baby might be prone to problems if it doesn't fit through the mother's pelvis at birth; a very small baby may be weak and malnourished and not able to cope with the stress of labour and birth. This isn't always true: some women give birth without difficulty to large babies, and some healthy babies are just genetically smaller than average.

At each prenatal visit, you will probably have your abdomen measured from your pubic bone to the top of the uterus. This is called the **fundal height**. Is this an accurate measurement? If you have two different doctors measure your abdomen, they're likely to come up with different numbers; however, despite these limitations, the method does predict fairly accurately which babies will be large and which will be very small.

Ultrasound is much more reliable in measuring the size of the baby. Researchers have done hundreds of ultrasounds at various stages of pregnancy, measured the fetuses, and worked out the expected average size of the baby for every week of pregnancy. These charts of weights have become the "gold standard" for assessing situations where the fetus is thought to be too small.

If your baby seems to be smaller than expected when your doctor or midwife measures your abdomen, your caregiver will probably recommend having an ultrasound done to check the size more accurately.

However, there is a big difference between fetal size and fetal growth. Assessment of the size of the fetus can be done with one ultrasound. The technician just looks at the baby, measures it, and compares it to the average. To determine how the baby is actually growing requires at least two ultrasounds performed long enough apart for the baby to have grown.

When the fetus is below the 10th percentile of the average weights determined by ultrasound, it is described as "light for dates," "small for dates," or "small for gestational age." If you are told that your baby is "small for dates," you will probably feel very concerned. Is your baby in trouble? Not necessarily. Not all small babies are small for the same reasons.

For example, your baby may simply be meant to be small. Perhaps you weighed less than 6 pounds (2,720 g) at birth, even though you were full-term, and your brother was 2 ounces (57 g) smaller than you when he arrived. In this case, it's not surprising that the baby you are carrying is also a bit smaller than average, and he

will likely remain small throughout your pregnancy.

Some babies are smaller than average because they have picked up an infection such as rubella or toxoplasmosis early in the pregnancy. This is a concern, but there is no treatment that will make these babies bigger or healthier.

Another group of babies start out growing at an average rate but then their rate of growth begins to lag behind. A baby in this group is not necessarily small for dates. For example, if the fetus was at the 90th percentile and has now dropped to the 40th percentile, it would still be considered within the normal, average range of size. However, the dramatic drop in growth means the fetus is probably at some risk—there is likely a problem that has caused this sudden change.

It is impossible to tell if your baby is in this group unless you have at least two ultrasounds. If your baby's growth has slowed down, he is described as having "**intrauterine growth restriction**." Most researchers believe this is caused by a problem with the blood supply to the placenta, which is preventing the baby from getting enough nutrition.

This situation can be dangerous for your baby, who is at a higher risk of serious problems before, during, and after birth. The baby's risk of health problems during childhood and adult life is also higher.

What can be done to help these babies? Here are some common recommendations and what research tells us about how helpful or not helpful they are:

- **Quit smoking:** Many babies with intrauterine growth restriction have mothers who smoke. If you quit smoking, your baby's rate of growth will improve.

- **Add more calories to your diet:** If you are thin and undernourished, you have a higher risk of having a low–birth weight baby. According to the research, though, eating more will only cause a slight improvement in your baby's growth. This probably means that women need to be eating well before they conceive to help their babies grow.

- **Rest in bed:** Women with small babies have been advised to rest in bed, but when compared with groups of similar women going about their usual activities, there is no evidence that the bed rest helps the baby to grow.

- **Try abdominal decompression:** One interesting approach used abdominal decompression as a way of increasing the blood flow to the placenta. A large plastic dome is placed over the woman's abdomen and the air is pumped out, leaving a partial vacuum over her abdomen. If this technique is used repeatedly during pregnancy with a small-for-dates baby, the studies found a significant increase in birth weight (on average, more than 1 pound [450 g] heavier than the babies in the control group). This method has not been widely adopted, perhaps because when it was first introduced it was with unfounded claims of benefit for all babies, not just small ones. Larger studies would provide a better evaluation of this approach, which seems to have potential.

If your baby has intrauterine growth restriction, you could certainly ask your doctor if this option is available where you live.

- **Drugs:** Another potentially helpful treatment is the use of certain drugs: **calcium channel blockers** and **betamimetics**. Some small studies have been done which show promising results but, again, larger studies need to be done before these medications can be recommended.

- **Induction of labour:** It is common for doctors to suggest induction of labour for these small-for-date or growth-restricted babies as soon as the pregnancy is far enough along so that prematurity is not a major risk. The theory behind this is that the baby will grow better on the outside than it is on the inside. The timing of induction has not been studied enough to make any recommendations and additional research is needed. At present, each situation must be evaluated individually.

FETAL MOVEMENT COUNTING

The baby who is not doing well in the uterus may move much less for a day or so before it dies. Knowing this, some researchers suggested that pregnant women could count how often the baby kicked for a set time period each day. If the baby wasn't moving as much as it had in the past, the mother would call her doctor, and tests would be done to find out what was going on with the baby.

This was such a simple and easily done test that it became very popular. However, when the research studies were completed, they found that counting the baby's movements did not improve the outcomes. Even worse, when the mother reported that her baby was moving less frequently, she was likely to undergo further testing, be admitted to hospital, and have labour induced. Each of these procedures has complications and costs, and there were no overall benefits to the babies.

NON-STRESS TESTING

In the 1960s, **electronic fetal monitors** were introduced into the care of pregnant woman. The EFM measures the baby's heartbeat right through the mother's abdomen, and records it on a continuous printout.

While the EFM is most often used in labour, a "non-stress" test for pregnant women was soon developed. For a non-stress test, the EFM belts are strapped across the woman's belly, and the machine records the baby's heartbeats for 20 minutes.

What are the doctors who analyze the print-out looking for? A normal or "reactive" test shows the baby's heartbeat occasionally speeding up and slowing down, rather than staying the same all the time. If the baby kicks, or the mother drinks something cold, you would expect to see a change in the heart rate.

The researchers hoped that a reactive test would show that the baby was healthy and likely to do well through the rest of pregnancy and during labour. If the baby's non-stress test was not reactive, then the doctor would intervene, most often by inducing labour. However, the controlled studies found that the number of babies who died was actually higher in the study groups where the doctors had access to the non-stress test results than in the control groups where doctors did not have this information.

Diana says, "I think the name 'non-stress' test is inaccurate. It was pretty stressful for me!

Having to go down to the hospital, wait until I was called, and lie there while they ran the monitor, and then wait while they studied the results was not my idea of a good way to spend an afternoon. I sort of worried the whole time the monitor was running. Some days they would leave it running a long time and I would think something was wrong and then my nurse would tell me she got held up with another patient. Then she would say, 'It looks fine today, but your doctor wants you to come back and have another one next week.' So I never really stopped worrying. It's discouraging to realize that, after all I went through, my doctor really didn't get any useful information."

CONTRACTION STRESS TESTING

The contraction stress test is also called an **oxytocin challenge test**. It is done exactly the same way as a non-stress test, except that the mother is given the drug **oxytocin** (through an IV) to cause contractions.

Just as in the non-stress test, the doctor is looking to see if the baby's heartbeat changes when there is a contraction. This test is performed at or near the end of pregnancy, and is intended to determine which babies will cope well with labour and which will be at risk of problems or death during labour.

However, when studies were done comparing the outcomes for babies who had the test done with those who did not have the test, there were no benefits for the babies. Any information the test gave did not help the doctors in delivering the babies safely.

FETAL BIOPHYSICAL PROFILE

The biophysical profile of the fetus is a specialized ultrasound that looks at five things: fetal movement, muscle tone, breathing movements, heart rate, and the volume of amniotic fluid. It brings more information into the picture than just the recording of the baby's heartbeat.

The test is more useful in one way: it does a better job than the previous tests of predicting which babies will get into trouble during labour.

Unfortunately, using the profile did not result in better outcomes for the babies in the small studies done so far. This is a good area to research further, as at least the test does identify babies at risk.

DOPPLER ULTRASOUND

This method of checking on the baby can be helpful in some specific cases. The Doppler ultrasound (a small, handheld ultrasound scanner) can be used to measure how much blood is flowing through the **umbilical artery** (the major blood vessel in the umbilical cord, carrying nutrients and oxygen from the placenta to the baby). Doing this test routinely on all pregnancies did not lead to better outcomes for the babies.

However, when the test was done on mothers who had high blood pressure and babies who had intrauterine growth restriction, it was very good at picking out which babies were seriously at risk of problems during labour and birth. (These babies are at a higher risk anyway, because of the hypertension or growth restriction—the Doppler ultrasound narrows it down still further.)

Delivering the babies at risk right away has been shown to reduce the number of babies who die or suffer other complications.

Prenatal Fetal Assessment: What Have We Learned?

If you are feeling a little discouraged as you read this section, you're not alone. The research summarized here is pretty disappointing.

Everyone involved in caring for pregnant women—and, of course, the expectant parents themselves—would like to be able to identify potential problems and solve them so that more babies are born healthy. A number of methods of testing for the well-being of the fetus have been introduced and some have been very widely used. Many have been used as the basis for making decisions about care for the pregnant woman and her baby. Yet a careful assessment of the research and clinical trials shows that most of these tests have not improved the outcome for babies.

In many cases, we got more information. We learned a lot about fetal growth and development and about the placenta. But, so far, little of this information has been demonstrated to improve the outcomes for mothers and babies.

We've also learned that:

- more information does not necessarily mean better outcomes for mothers and babies;
- recognizing situations where the fetus is at risk does not always mean there is anything we can do to reduce that risk; and
- large-scale clinical trials to assess the effectiveness of these tests and interventions

> ### The Evidence About...
> ### Assessing the Baby during Pregnancy
>
> The more sophisticated ultrasound techniques do identify fetuses at risk, so there is hope that treatments to improve the outcomes for these babies will be found.
>
> Selectively using Doppler ultrasound on certain women has been demonstrated to improve outcomes for these babies.

should be done first, before they become widely used on pregnant women.

Discussing Tests during Pregnancy with Your Doctor

Some tests—for example, the MSS—are offered routinely by many doctors. Others will be recommended if you fit certain categories. For example, your doctor may recommend an amniocentesis if you are over 35, or a biophysical profile if you have gone more than a week past your due date.

You can weigh your doctor's recommendation against the research results cited in this book and decide if you want to have the test or not.

You may want to have an amniocentesis even though you have ruled out the option of abortion, for example, because you would like time to prepare for a disabled child. Or you may have decided that you would rather not know, and can therefore tell your doctor that you don't want any of these screening tests.

What if your doctor wants to have a biophysical profile done? You can ask how the information obtained will be used, and let him know you are concerned that research hasn't shown any benefits to this procedure—other than predicting which babies will have problems.

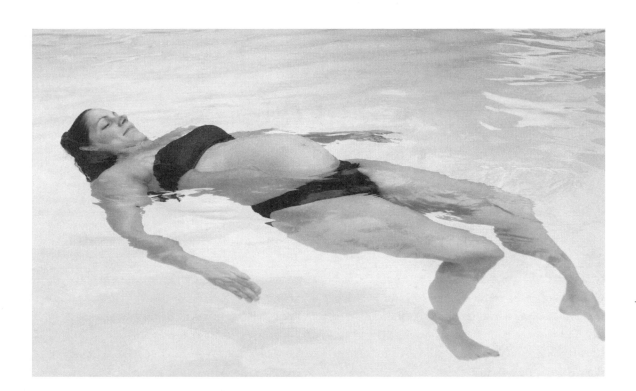

Four Months
❧ *Thirteen to Seventeen Weeks* ❧

With any luck, that early pregnancy fatigue and nausea will be easing by now. In fact, most women find this middle trimester the most enjoyable part of pregnancy. The initial discomforts are past, the baby isn't so big that you feel awkward, and you can start to prepare in earnest. Now is the time to investigate prenatal classes, and begin to think about how you will care for your baby when he or she arrives.

-17-
Prenatal Classes: Do They Help?

Forty years ago, there were very few prenatal classes. Pregnant women gathered information from their sisters and friends, from their mothers, and from their medical caregivers. Often they were simply told not to worry—after all, the doctor would take care of everything.

The earliest prenatal classes were like present-day school health classes: teaching women about their bodies and the changes that occur in pregnancy. For the labour and birth, women were told that the doctor and nurses would tell them what to do.

In the 1960s, prenatal class teachers focused on avoiding the pain-killing drugs that were widely used at the time during labour. These classes emphasized breathing patterns to help women "stay in control" and not make noises during the contractions. These lessons were important because if the labouring woman showed signs of pain or distress, the hospital staff were likely to urge her to take medication.

Through the 1970s and 1980s, prenatal classes gave more information to pregnant women and their partners. Women learned about nutrition, alcohol and smoking in pregnancy, the growth of the fetus, and the different stages of labour. The classes also taught that many hospital policies in place at the time were not necessary: you don't need to be shaved, you don't need an enema, you don't need an intravenous. Avoidance of pain medication during labour was accepted as a good thing, and pain-relieving techniques such as massage and "patterned breathing" were encouraged. Some classes concentrated on **vaginal birth after Caesarean section** (VBAC). Prenatal classes became a force for change from rigid hospital birthing policies to the adoption of family-centred maternity care.

At present, most prenatal classes have some things in common. They provide accurate information about pregnancy, fetal development, and stages of labour. They teach techniques like position change, massage, and breathing patterns to help cope with labour pain. Most discuss common interventions in labour, including those for pain relief. Care of the new baby, and changing relationships between the couple, any older children, and the new baby, are discussed.

Beyond those basics, though, there are a variety of special prenatal classes that may be available in your community. Each will have a different focus and approach.

Steffi attended a prenatal class for single teen mothers. "We only had one class about the birth, and that was mostly to tell us what to expect at the hospital. I liked the hospital tour; it helps to see the rooms before you actually go. We had a lot of stuff about nutrition, getting welfare, finding a place to live, and birth control."

Jeanine's prenatal classes were taught by an independent childbirth educator who taught in a room at the local Y. "I have to confess that Jack didn't like them much because after each class I'd go back and argue with our doctor. A lot of the things the teacher talked about were different than what our doctor usually did. Jack thought the teacher was pretty much against the whole medical system. But it opened my eyes. I found out there were other ways of doing things."

She adds, "We did do some breathing and relaxation stuff, too, and we practised quite a bit. When I was in labour, what I had learned in the classes helped me a lot. I had a lot of back pain in labour, but I knew from the classes it was pretty common, and we'd learned some things that helped, like having Jack press hard on my back."

Manuela's classes were taught by the nurses at the hospital. "We learned about what happens during labour and birth. The nurses were able to show us how the fetal monitor works and they brought in the vacuum extractor and the forceps, so we had a chance to get familiar with everything. I liked knowing what was available for pain, and what would happen to me in labour."

Sherry's classes were taught by her midwife. "We'd actually discussed most of the issues during my prenatal visits, so I didn't learn all that

much. The best parts were watching the videos of birth, and getting to know other pregnant couples who were going through the same things we were. We talked a lot about our fears, our feelings about becoming parents, our relationships."

No class can cover everything in detail. Lee Ann says, "My prenatal classes had mentioned that one in five moms don't deliver naturally, but instead of educating us on Caesareans, the class focused on the four moms who would deliver vaginally. But there we were, I was Mom number five, who needed a Caesarean."

Some classes teach a wide variety of labour skills that include relaxation techniques, breathing patterns, distraction, comfort measures, movements, etc. Others will cover these briefly but focus more on the medications (such as narcotics and epidurals) available for pain relief.

Some place a lot of emphasis on teaching labour-support skills to the woman's labour partner, while others barely discuss the partner's role.

Classes vary in their overall attitude towards labour and birth. In some classes, labour is approached as something that women are taught to manage through breathing and relaxation techniques. As the coach, the father is to remind the mother what to do. In other classes, the approach to labour is that it is something that women instinctively know how to do. The other people present are not seen as coaches, but as a source of support. Some classes treat birth as a normal event with profound spiritual and emotional aspects. These classes are likely to encourage questioning of medical routines and interventions. Other classes encourage cooperation with medical personnel and acceptance of a more technological approach.

CHOOSING A PRENATAL CLASS

What should you be looking for when you choose your prenatal classes?

In a small community, you may not have much choice; there may only be one set of classes available. Then it becomes particularly important to supplement the classes with outside reading, and through discussions with your caregiver and your friends.

If you do have a choice of classes, here are some points you might consider:

- Ask your caregiver. Your doctor or midwife will know what classes are available and may feel one is preferable.
- Do you have some special circumstances that might point you towards a particular class? Single mothers, for example, sometimes feel more comfortable in a class specifically for single parents. Some communities will also offer separate classes for couples who are expecting twins or other multiples, for those planning a vaginal birth after a previous Caesarean section (**VBAC**), for those planning a home birth, or for survivors of sexual abuse.

  If you are considering one of these special classes, discuss the course outline with the teacher to be sure it meets your needs. Not all single mothers, for example, need information on applying for welfare and public housing, and some may prefer a class where the emphasis is on preparing to give birth.
- What books does the class teacher recommend for further reading? Checking out the book list will help you identify the teacher's philosophy and approach so that you can decide if it fits with yours.
- What do new parents say about the classes they attended? When people tell you the classes they attended were "great" and "wonderful," don't just accept that at face value. What is great for one person might be boring and frustrating for another. Ask them what they found helpful, what they learned that was useful during labour, anything they wished was included in the class but wasn't. This will give you information that will help you decide if the class is right for you.

  Even with a prenatal class that matches your needs and philosophy, don't forget the other resources available to you: books, magazines, videos (your public library probably has a number of videos on childbirth that you can borrow), and more.

If you have access to the Internet, there are newsgroups, bulletin boards, and chatrooms on all aspects of pregnancy, childbirth, and parenting where people share experiences and offer answers to questions.

The Effects of Prenatal Classes

Because of these wide variations, it is very difficult to research any benefits or disadvantages of prenatal classes.

As well, the group of women who choose to take prenatal classes may be inherently different than the group who don't, so different outcomes in the two groups may be from factors other than the classes.

However, there have been studies done, and the one clear difference that has emerged from the

PRENATAL EDUCATION: WHAT ARE YOUR OPTIONS?

Depending on where you live, you may have many choices in prenatal education or only a few. Some possibilities:

- preparation for home birth (may be taught by your midwife)
- International Childbirth Education Association classes (independent classes taught by certified instructors)
- preparation for Caesarean section classes
- early pregnancy classes (focus on nutrition, exercise and healthy pregnancy)
- VBAC classes
- hospital-based classes taught by nurses
- single parent or teen mother classes
- classes for parents expecting twins or multiples
- refresher classes for people expecting a second or later baby
- classes dealing with a particular approach to birth: Bradley Method (husband-coached childbirth), Lamaze, Hypno-birthing, Birthing from Within, etc.
- weekend all-day workshop classes (for people who find it difficult to attend evening classes on a regular basis)
- breastfeeding preparation (often offered as an extra class)

Concern has been expressed that prenatal classes create expectations of a "natural birth," which is impossible for some women, and that these women consequently either suffer unnecessary pain in labour, or suffer feelings of guilt and failure if they decide to ask for pain medication. This possibility—that classes may do harm—has not been evaluated by research in any systematic way.

When prenatal classes make women aware of options and choices and pass along accurate information, they can be a vital agent for change. It was because many women learned about their choices in prenatal classes that hospitals began to change their policies around allowing labour support people, changing positions for birth, walking during labour, etc.

As Jeanine says, "Talking to the other women in my prenatal classes was very enlightening. At my hospital, the rule was that every woman in labour got an IV. Well, if that's medically necessary, how come at Linda's hospital it was *not* part of the routine? Why did babies at my hospital go to the nursery for eight hours after birth for observation, while the babies at Daria's hospital stayed with their mothers? If I hadn't been to the classes I wouldn't even have known about those possibilities."

When parents like Jeanine talk to their doctors and write letters to the hospital asking for changes, they can have a real and significant influence on the practice of obstetrics in their community.

Prenatal classes can also have the opposite effect. Ask Manuela if anyone questioned the nurses who taught her class, and she says, "Yes, a couple of people asked about stuff they'd read or heard about. But the nurses explained that some

research is that women who have attended prenatal classes use significantly less pain-relieving medication during labour than those who have not attended any classes. This is a very important positive outcome, because all the pain-relieving medications currently available can cause side effects to the mother and risks to the baby.

The Evidence About...
Prenatal Classes

Attending prenatal classes is likely to reduce your need for pain medications during labour. The classes will also provide you with information and opportunities to meet other expectant parents.

---

of these books are really radical and the people who write them aren't nurses or doctors and don't really know what they're writing about. On the other hand, there are hundreds of babies born at this hospital every year, so they obviously know what they're doing." This kind of class discourages questioning of medical routines and will probably reduce the level of change at that hospital.

-18-
Preparing to Breastfeed

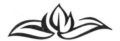

You've probably dreamed of holding your new-born in your arms and nurturing him or her at your breast. But you may also have heard about women who found getting started with breastfeeding somewhat challenging. How can you prepare for breastfeeding? Are there things you can do to make the experience more successful? Yes, there are!

Getting Ready to Breastfeed

The most important steps you can take during pregnancy are:

- Seek out a support system. Find out in advance who the breastfeeding experts in your community are, or where you can go if you need some advice or practical help.
- Prepare for being very busy in the first few weeks after your baby is born! Babies need to eat frequently, and learning to breastfeed takes a lot of time. You might want to arrange for a cleaning service for the first six weeks, stock your freezer with prepared meals, and take other steps to buy yourself extra time to focus on learning to breastfeed.

- Watch other mothers breastfeeding. A great way to do this is to attend La Leche League meetings, where you will see mothers with babies of all ages at the breast. Pregnant women are always welcome at LLL meetings, and in some places your partner may be able to attend as well. You may also find it helpful to watch DVDs such as *Dr. Jack Newman's Visual Guide to Breastfeeding*, which gives you close-up shots of babies at the breast and explains how to know when the baby is feeding well.
- Look for reliable sources of information. When mothers are given information booklets on breastfeeding distributed by formula companies, they are much more likely to not breastfeed or to wean early. Make sure the information you rely on is written by someone who is not trying to sell you formula!

Special Situations

If you have had previous breast surgery—for example, breast reduction surgery or breast implants—you might find it helpful to consult with a lactation consultant or other expert while you are pregnant. The book *Defining Your Own Success: Breastfeeding after Breast Surgery* by Diana West (her website www.bfar.org is also very helpful) may help you understand more about how your surgery may affect your breastfeeding experience. Almost all women who have had breast surgery can breastfeed, although some may need to supplement their babies as well.

You may be told by your doctor that your breasts have not developed normally either during puberty or during the pregnancy. Breastfeeding experts have noticed that sometimes when women have widely spaced, tubular shaped breasts and few or no changes during pregnancy, they have a lower than usual milk supply. While this may be a risk factor, many women whose breasts look this way do produce plenty of milk. You may want to make sure you have extra help when your baby is born to give you the best chance.

If you had problems breastfeeding a previous baby, are you likely to have the same problems with this baby? During each pregnancy, the ducts in the breast grow, and new ducts are formed. A mother who did not have enough milk to breast-feed exclusively with her first baby may find she has plenty of milk for her second or third child.

This also applies to women who have had previous breast surgery. So even if you had some difficulties last time, you can be optimistic about breastfeeding this time around.

What Doesn't Help

At one time, women were often told they needed to "toughen up" their nipples during pregnancy by rubbing them with towels or repeatedly pulling at them. In fact, nipples never "toughen up" and this kind of treatment during pregnancy doesn't prevent sore nipples. Sore nipples are most frequently caused by difficulties with latching on the baby.

Sometimes pregnant women are told they have inverted nipples, meaning nipples that are sunken into the breast rather than standing up from the surface of the breast. Some inverted nipples will protrude when pressure is applied to the skin around the nipples while others will sink further into the breast when this pressure is applied. Women with inverted nipples may be advised to wear nipple shells during pregnancy or manipulate their nipples to try to get them to protrude, but research does not support these techniques. Instead, you might find it helpful to contact a lactation consultant who can help teach you how to effectively latch your baby on. Babies "breast" feed rather than "nipple" feed so they are usually able to breastfeed just fine even if you have inverted nipples.

-19-
More Than One Baby: Multiple Pregnancy

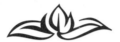

When Diane's first son Craig was 10 months old, she and her husband decided to try for another baby. She conceived almost immediately, and early in the pregnancy her doctor noticed how big she was getting and recommended an ultrasound. The ultrasound, Diane says, "began an adventure which still seems quite incredible" when it showed that she was carrying four (yes, four!) babies.

Although she had not been sick at all during her first pregnancy, Diane experienced severe nausea and vomiting the second time. Her mother came to stay with the family and help care for Diane's toddler over the next few stressful months.

Diane was admitted to hospital at 24 weeks gestation because she was having occasional contractions. "I was told I'd have a Caesarean for the delivery because there were just too many things that could get tangled up, but the doctors waited until I went into labour." Her quadruplets, two boys (Harrison and Kenny) and two girls (Alison and Jessica), were born at 27 weeks gestation. They weighed 2 pounds, 5½ ounces (1,063 g); 2 pounds, 6 ounces (1,077 g); 2 pounds, 8 ounces (1,134 g); and 3 pounds, ½ ounce (1,205 g).

"All four of them needed respirators," Diane says, "and before they were born the nurses would say to me that I couldn't go in labour today because there were only three respirators available. Fortunately, I went into labour on a four-respirator day."

The quadruplets stayed in the hospital for two and a half months, and, as Diane says, "They experienced practically every problem you can think of that a premature baby could have." But all four arrived home healthy and have continued to do very well.

Diane says people meeting their family often say, "I'm glad it's you and not me." When she hears those words she thinks to herself, "I'm glad it's me, too." She tells other parents expecting multiples, "Yes, it's hard, it's not what you had planned, but it's also very joyous and very special."

Diane's story is a dramatic and uncommon one. Quadruplets are very rare, although they (and other multiple births, from twins and triplets to septuplets) are becoming more

FERTILITY TREATMENTS AND MULTIPLE BIRTHS

When women are having trouble conceiving, they may be given medications to encourage ovulation—but this medication often causes more than one egg to be released during each menstrual cycle. This increases the chances of having at least one egg fertilized, but if several eggs are fertilized, the women will become pregnant with twins, triplets, or more babies.

Another approach to treating infertility involves removing eggs from the mother's ovaries during surgery, fertilizing the eggs with sperm outside her body, and then implanting these fertilized eggs in her uterus. Because many of these implanted eggs will not survive, usually several are implanted at the same time. If two or more do survive, though, the mother will find herself with a multiple pregnancy.

The increased use of these treatments is the main reason we are seeing multiple births more frequently.

common with the increasing use of fertility drugs. (Diane, however, did not use any fertility drugs.)

The most common multiple pregnancy, of course, produces twins.

Twins are born about 1 out of every 90 births in North America. Identical twins arise from a single fertilized egg that divides in the first few days after conception. The number of identical twins is about 1 out of every 250 births; this is remarkably constant worldwide and seems unrelated to age, heredity, number of other children, or race. Identical twins are truly chance occurrences.

Fraternal twins arise from the separate fertilization of two eggs, both of which are released in the same menstrual cycle. The frequency of fraternal twins varies considerably. In rural Nigeria, twinning occurs once in 20 births. In Japan, twinning only occurs once in 155 births. Heredity is important; a mother who is a twin is much more likely to have twins. Fraternal twinning is more common the older the mother is and the more children she has had. Fraternal twinning is more common in big, tall women. Fertility treatments are more likely to cause fraternal twins. And yes, fraternal twins can have two different fathers.

The number of twin pregnancies is far higher than the number of twin births. The introduction of very early ultrasound has shown that many twin pregnancies end early on with the spontaneous death and re-absorption of one twin. Probably, some cases of threatened miscarriage actually were the miscarriage of a twin while the other twin survived and went on to a full-term delivery. There have been rare cases of twins delivering at different times, occasionally weeks apart, but almost always both were very premature.

A multiple birth is both exciting and stressful. A woman carrying more than one baby is likely to experience the common pregnancy symptoms (heartburn, nausea, tiredness, etc.) more severely than one carrying a single child. She may also feel anxious about the emotional and financial aspects of taking care of more than one infant.

Multiple pregnancies are at a higher risk for a number of pregnancy problems. If you are expecting twins, triplets, or more you are much more likely to go into labour prematurely. You are more likely to develop pre-eclampsia. Your babies are more likely to be small for gestational age, as well as being premature. The combination of prematurity and being small for gestational age makes the risk of perinatal death and cerebral palsy higher than in single births.

If you discover that you are expecting more than one baby, you may find linking up with a support group extremely helpful. Knowing other parents who have survived (and enjoyed) the experience of caring for more than one newborn will be reassuring, and these parents will probably have plenty of tips on getting through the pregnancy as well.

Can We Prevent Premature Labour in Multiple Pregnancies?

For many years, bed rest has been recommended for women with a multiple pregnancy. The goal is to help the babies to grow bigger and to reduce premature labour. Bed rest, either in or out of hospital, was introduced into clinical practice before its risks or benefits were ever evaluated by research.

Very little research has been conducted on bed rest, and most of it deals with twins rather than pregnancies with more than two babies. The research that has been done has not produced clear or consistent results.

Some studies have shown that hospitalization reduces the rate of high blood pressure in the mothers, but causes no improvement in any other outcome.

A study involving women who had shown some early dilation of the cervix (which would suggest they were more likely to go into

The Evidence About...
Twins and Higher Multiples

Additional advice and support is helpful for parents who find they are having more than one baby.

No evidence supports the widely given advice to women pregnant with twins to rest more, or to be admitted to hospital to rest.

Research does not support the routine use of Caesarean section for all twin births.

Research on the best care for higher multiple birth is minimal, due in part to the difficulty in studying a relatively rare occurrence. However, the use of fertility drugs means that these multiple births are becoming more common.

labour prematurely) did not show any differences in rate of premature birth between the "bed rest in hospital" group and the control group.

The research also suggests that the number of babies born prematurely as well as the number with a very low birth weight is actually higher when mothers are routinely hospitalized.

Bed rest seems like an impossible goal for some. Maureen had two-year-old twins when she became pregnant again—with twins. "I was advised to rest as much as possible," she says, "but how much rest can you get with a couple of two-year-olds to look after? It didn't seem to make a lot of difference. I went into labour at 37 weeks—just like the first time—and the babies were both a good size and healthy."

Various medications to prevent premature labour in multiple pregnancies have also been tested, and none have been shown to be effective.

How should your twins or other multiples be born: vaginally or by Caesarean? Again, this has not been well researched, although there is more information about twins than other multiple births.

One study compared Caesarean section to vaginal birth when the second twin was breech. The researchers found that the mothers who had Caesarean sections were more likely to have complications, and there were no benefits in terms of the outcomes for the babies. Triplets and higher multiples are almost always delivered by Caesarean section, but this is not on the basis of any research evidence.

Because multiple births—especially those involving more than two babies—are less common than single pregnancies, it is harder to conduct research on them, and there are no definitive answers to many questions. This means that parents expecting multiples, and the caregivers who are working with them, have less concrete information on which to base decisions.

-20-
Urinary Tract Infections

Wendy got a call from her doctor's nurse a few days after her first pregnancy appointment. "You've got some infection in your urine. The doctor wants you to take an antibiotic to clear it up."

Wendy was puzzled and unhappy. "But I feel fine. I really don't want to take any drugs while I'm pregnant."

"Well, your urine culture definitely shows infection. You'd better come in and talk to the doctor."

Wendy went back to the office later that week, and explained to her doctor that she felt fine and would prefer to avoid taking medication.

Her doctor responded, "I understand that you don't feel any burning or pain when you are going to the bathroom, but your urine culture definitely shows lots of bacteria. If you take antibiotics to clear them up now, they won't make you really sick with a bladder or kidney infection later in the pregnancy."

"Can this infection hurt my baby?" Wendy asked. "I really don't want to take any drugs in this pregnancy unless I absolutely have to."

"No, the baby's not at risk," said the doctor. "The bacteria in your urine can't affect your baby's development the way German measles or thalidomide can. They can just make *you* sick, sometimes really sick. And there is a very small chance that this kind of infection will start premature labour." Since Wendy was still reluctant to take antibiotics, her doctor suggested they repeat the test on her urine to be sure it was accurate.

Forty-eight hours later, Wendy got another call from her doctor: "The second culture shows exactly the same results. I think you should take the antibiotics."

What does the research say about Wendy's risks in this situation?

Three to 8 per cent of pregnant women have significant numbers of bacteria in their urine, without being ill or having any symptoms. This is called **asymptomatic bacteriuria** (urine bacteria). Studies show that women with urine bacteria, despite having no symptoms at this point, have a higher chance of becoming ill with a urinary tract infection during the pregnancy, as well as a slightly higher chance of a premature delivery and low–birth weight baby.

The same studies also found that the treatment of bacteria in the urine with antibiotics, even when there are no symptoms, reduces the risk of the mother becoming ill with bladder or kidney infection during the pregnancy by about 50 per cent. Treatment with antibiotics also reduces the risk of premature delivery.

A number of effective antibiotics are available that are safe for use in pregnancy. The length of time needed for treatment is uncertain—in studies, continuous therapy until delivery, seven to ten days of therapy, and three days of therapy have all been equally effective.

But Wendy decided not to take antibiotics for her urine bacteria. "I drank tons of water every day and kept my bladder really flushed out. I didn't get any signs of infection ever. If I had gotten sick, then I would have taken the antibiotics. I don't think my doctor was too pleased about my decision, but it was right for me."

Bladder Infections

The woman with a bladder infection and the woman with urine bacteria have the same urine culture results. But they don't feel the same. The woman with urine bacteria feels fine—she wouldn't know she had it. The woman with **acute cystitis** (a bladder infection) definitely feels uncomfortable!

The symptoms of a bladder infection are frequent or urgent urination, burning pain when you do urinate, and bloody or cloudy urine. You may have all or just some of these symptoms. Frequent urination by itself is a normal part of being pregnant and not a sign of infection.

Urinary tract infections are common in pregnant women. One to 3 per cent of women will have either a bladder infection or a kidney infection (**pyelonephritis**) during pregnancy. Drinking lots of water seems to help prevent them.

Treating bladder infections with the appropriate antibiotic relieves the symptoms of burning and frequent urination, and probably also reduces the chances of it developing into a more serious kidney infection. Studies suggest that three-day treatment in pregnancy may be as effective as taking antibiotics for a longer period of time, but the data is too skimpy to make firm recommendations.

Kidney Infections

Kidney infections are, like bladder infections, more common in pregnant than non-pregnant women. This is because the collecting system of the kidney and the tubes leading from the kidneys to the bladder become wider during pregnancy. This dilation lets urine sit longer and allows the bacteria to multiply.

Women with kidney infections are often acutely ill. If you get a kidney infection, you may feel pain when you urinate for a couple of days before more severe symptoms develop, but not all women experience this. When the kidney infection has flared up, you will have pain in your back or side, a fever, and cloudy or bloody urine. Admission to hospital for intravenous antibiotics for 48 hours has been the usual treatment, with a switch over to antibiotics taken by mouth after that.

The Evidence About...
Bladder and Kidney Infections

One to 3 per cent of women will become ill with a bladder or kidney infection sometime during their pregnancy. These can be effectively treated with antibiotics.

The treatment of bacteria in the urine with antibiotics, even when there are no symptoms, reduces the risk of the mother subsequently becoming ill with bladder or kidney infection during the pregnancy by about 50 per cent.

Recent studies have suggested that if the woman is not vomiting and can keep medication and fluids down, treatment with oral antibiotics is just as effective as intravenous antibiotics. Because intravenous is not required, hospitaliza-tion may not be required either—as long as the woman is able to get the rest and care her illness requires.

About 30 per cent of women who are treated for a kidney infection during pregnancy will get another kidney infection during the same pregnancy. To try to prevent these recurrences, studies have compared taking antibiotics every day until the end of the pregnancy with regular urine cultures followed by antibiotic treatment if any bacteria are found. Both of these strategies reduce the risk of repeated kidney infections equally to about 8 per cent.

The bacteria which infect the bladder and kidneys do not cause infection or illness in the fetus or newborn, except in the case of **beta strep** (see Chapter 31).

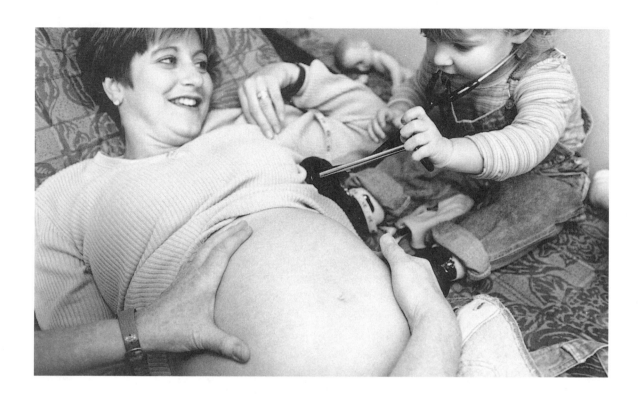

Five Months
❧ *Eighteen to Twenty-one Weeks* ❧

What's that funny feeling in your stomach? Gas? Nope, there it is again and it feels more like a flutter than gas. Yes, that's your baby. Sometime this month or soon after, you'll begin to feel your baby moving. Of course, your baby has been moving around for quite some time but at this stage he or she is big enough that you'll be aware of the movements. At first, it may feel more like gas bubbles in your tummy, or a fluttering sensation. But before long you'll recognize definite kicks or the entire baby rolling over, or maybe a series of hiccups.

You're also probably very conscious that you're halfway there—and there's plenty to be aware of and plan for.

-21-
Your Developing Baby

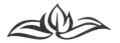

Although your belly doesn't come with a window, advances in ultrasound technology have helped us learn more about how babies develop in utero. It's quite remarkable, really, as in nine months your baby grows from a single cell to a 7- to 8-pound (3,175- to 3,625-g) infant. Here are some of the milestones your baby passes along the way:

At five weeks, your baby is about one-tenth of an inch (2.5 mm) long and his heart, the size of a period on this page, is already beating.

By eight weeks, your baby has grown rapidly and is an inch (2.5 cm) long! The placenta and amniotic sac have formed, and he has a mouth with lips (and teeth buds inside) and distinct but webbed fingers and toes.

By 10 weeks, your baby's fingers already have the unique pattern of ridges and grooves that will be his fingerprints throughout his life, and he can turn his head from side to side.

By 12 weeks, your baby is 3 inches (7.6 cm) long and all his organs are formed. He swallows the amniotic fluid and urinates, kicks his feet and waves his hands (even though you can't feel those movements yet). If something touches the palm of his hand, he will curl his fingers around it.

By 18 weeks (that's now!), you may be feeling your baby kick, even though he's only about 6 inches (15.2 cm) long. Your caregiver can usually hear the heartbeat during checkups. The baby now shows sleep cycles and may even dream.

By 22 weeks, your baby can suck his thumb and have hiccups. He's about 7.5 inches (19 cm) long, and babies born this early (occasionally even a little earlier) have survived.

At 27 weeks, your baby's eyebrows and eyelids are visible and your baby can blink. He's "breathing" amniotic fluid now, inhaling in and out. He'll respond to your familiar voice when you talk and be startled by loud noises. Twins will look at each other's faces and deliberately touch each other, even hold hands.

By week 31, he's more than 15 inches (38 cm) long and will respond to light shining on your belly (if you go outside in the sunlight wearing a bikini, for example). His kicks and movements may be strong enough to make you catch your breath. His tastebuds have been working for some time, and he is becoming familiar with the tastes of the foods you eat as he drinks the amniotic fluid.

From week 32, all your baby's vital organs are formed. His lungs will continue to mature until he is at term. He will also practically double his weight!

-22-
Preparing for Baby: What You Need

Maybe this is your first baby, and you are trying to imagine yourself as a mother. Or maybe you already have one or more children, and the challenge is to imagine how this new addition will affect your family and how you will get things done with a new baby to care for. Either way, there is some preparation to do—and more decisions to make than just about your pregnancy and birth.

Part of it is practical. What equipment and other items will you need for your new baby? It's impossible to come up with a precise list, because the item one person describes as absolutely essential will be another person's "complete waste of money." Remember, too, that often other parents will lend or give you equipment their babies are finished with, and that buying second-hand is also a good option for many items. But here are some of the basics that many people purchase, and some things to think about in deciding what to buy:

- **Diapers.** Babies pee and poop a lot. Most parents use disposable diapers, and there are many types to choose from. While you'll want to stock up on some, don't buy too many in newborn size because your baby may grow more quickly than you expect. Cloth diapers are less expensive and put less strain on the environment. Again there are many styles from which to choose, from plain flat diapers that can be folded in different ways as the baby grows, to fitted, multi-layered diapers that come in various size ranges. You might want a mixture of flat and fitted diapers to start with, to give you more flexibility. (A few parents also choose the diaper-free option, in which parents learn their babies' cues and carry them to the toilet when they need to "go.")

- **Car seat.** If you have a car, you need a car seat for your baby. Check with your local automobile association to see if workshops are offered to teach parents about how to install and use car seats—police checks find that many car seats are not properly installed or the baby isn't properly buckled in. Even if you don't have a car, you may want to get an approved car seat for the times you ride in a taxi with your baby. If finances are an issue, there are some agencies that will provide car seats for families in need. (Avoid buying a second-hand car seat; if it has been in an accident or is older than five years, it may not be safe.)

- **Baby clothes.** One of the great pleasures of pregnancy can be spending time picking out clothes for the new baby. Everything looks so tiny! While it can be tempting to purchase tons of cute sleepers and T-shirts, remember that new babies grow quickly—and a big baby may not even fit the newborn-size outfits at birth. On the other hand, a reasonable supply of basic clothing—at least seven or eight each of sleepers and undershirts, plus a couple of dress-up items—will mean you can do laundry less often. You can also stock up on some bigger sizes that your baby will soon grow into (and can wear now if you get desperate after a day when every diaper seems to leak). Babies can go through a lot of clothes in a short time. If this will be a cold-weather baby, you may also want a snowsuit and some sweaters.

- **A place for baby to sleep.** A crib should meet current safety standards. If you are planning to use a second-hand one, ask your caregiver or public health nurse to help you determine if it meets the standards (which include having the bars close enough together that baby's head can't get stuck, and a mattress that fits snugly so baby can't get stuck between the mattress and the sides). Don't add bumper pads, pillows, or fluffy duvets. **SIDS** experts recommend that you keep the crib in your room for at least the first year. Other sleep options preferred by some parents include having the baby in a sidecar-type arrangement with a special bed that attaches to the parents' bed, and bringing the baby into bed with them. (See sidebar on "Safe Sleep" on page 280.)

- **A sling or soft baby carrier.** A sling, wrap-type carrier or front-pack carrier allows parents to walk around with baby yet have both hands free to tackle housework, help other children, or push a shopping cart. Studies have shown that carrying your baby in one of these carriers will significantly reduce the amount of crying and distress for the baby. It's also easier on your back and shoulders than trying to carry the baby in your arms. It's worth researching the different types; some are easier to use than others, and some are more adjustable so your partner can use them too. (At least one sling manufacturer uses fabric with hockey team logos on it—very popular with dads!)

Other Items You Might Be Considering

- **A pacifier.** Babies suck differently on a pacifier than at the breast, and research has shown that the early introduction of a pacifier may lead to earlier weaning. (Letting the baby suck on your finger doesn't seem to have the same effect, as the baby sucks more like she would at the breast. According to several studies, pacifiers also seem to increase the risk of ear infections, and may encourage the baby to bite while breastfeeding when teething begins. If you do decide to use a pacifier, it's best to wait until breastfeeding is well established—about six weeks.

- **A mechanical swing or bouncy seat.** Some parents swear by these to calm a fussy baby, but others find their babies hate them. See if you can borrow one from a friend for a while after your baby is born before buying one.
- **A stroller.** Until they can sit up alone, babies need a stroller where they can lie flat as you push them. In the early months, most will be happier if they are in a carrier or in your arms. Think about what you will be doing with the stroller before making a purchase. If you will mostly be using public transport and want to bring a stroller with you, look for one that is easy to fold up (remember you'll be holding the baby in one hand). If you'll mostly be walking from your home and bringing back shopping items, a larger stroller with more room for bags might be good. This is another purchase that can probably wait until baby is a bit older.
- **A breast pump.** If you have a premature or ill baby who isn't able to suck, a good breast pump can allow you to provide your baby with the milk she needs. For these situations, a hospital-grade electric pump that allows you to pump both breasts at the same time is the best choice (these can be rented). You might also want a pump if you are going to be returning to work within a few months of your baby's birth. Otherwise, a breast pump is not really necessary. Sometimes mothers begin using a breast pump early on, even

though their babies are nursing well, and end up creating an oversupply of milk that can be a challenge for the baby to cope with and cause problems with plugged ducts and **mastitis** (breast infections) for them.

- **A nursing pillow.** These large-sized pillows are designed to fit across the mother's lap, raising the baby up to make breastfeeding easier. Some are crescent-shaped, others have Velcro straps that go around the mother's waist. Some mothers find these very helpful, but others find they make nursing harder and not easier. For women who are short-waisted, the pillows tend to raise the baby too high. Small babies often roll down the slope of the pillow, making it hard to get the baby positioned properly. And using a pillow makes it difficult for the mother to go out with the baby—who wants to drag along a huge pillow as well? Usually mothers find they can use a pillow or two from their beds or sofas if they need something to help them support the baby's weight while breastfeeding.

While advertising tries to convince parents that babies require a lot of stuff, in fact what your baby needs most of all is you: the milk from your breasts, the warmth of your body, your loving touch, and the sounds and movement he'll experience with you as you go about your daily tasks.

-23-
Caesarean Birth

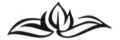

You might be wondering why you'd want to be thinking about Caesareans this early in your pregnancy. In fact, you might have been planning not to think about them at all! But the percentage of women whose babies are born through this type of surgery has been increasing steadily over the past 20 years. In Canada, the rate is now more than 20 per cent and in the United States, it's over 26 per cent. That's why it's a good idea to familiarize yourself now with the reasons for Caesareans, the controversial issues, and what happens if you do need this procedure.

Mary Elizabeth knows that the Caesarean section she had saved her life and that of her baby. "Towards the end of my pregnancy, I started having some bleeding from my vagina. I had an ultrasound done and the doctor discovered that my placenta was at the bottom of my uterus, right over my cervix. If I had gone in labour and my cervix had started to dilate, I could have bled to death. We scheduled a Caesarean for two weeks before my due date. I'm glad I had my baby now, rather than in the 'olden days,' when we might both have died."

Situations like the one Mary Elizabeth faced

are pretty clear-cut: there was really no other choice for her and her baby except Caesarean section. There are other cases where the need for a Caesarean is absolute and definite: a baby in a transverse position that won't shift even after an attempt at **external version**, for example.

Most of the time, though, the reasons for Caesarean sections are less clear. In most parts of North America, about 20 to 25 per cent of all babies are born by C-section. The rates in other parts of the world vary from about 5 to almost 50 per cent.

Looking at the international statistics from various countries about outcomes for both baby and mother, we find that when the Caesarean rate is lower than about 7 per cent, there are more problems. But when the rate is higher than 7 per cent, there is no corresponding improvement in outcomes. *A country where about 7 per cent of babies are delivered by C-section will see just as many healthy babies and mothers as a country where 25 per cent are delivered surgically.*

Why is this important? A Caesarean section, like any surgery, carries risks, and only when these risks are outweighed by the benefits should

AVOIDING UNNECESSARY CAESAREANS

Some things you can do to help prevent a Caesarean section:

* arrange for a doula or other trained labour support person
* walk around as much as possible during labour
* avoid routine continuous electronic fetal monitoring
* avoid induction unless medically indicated
* use alternate methods of pain relief rather than an epidural; delay having an epidural as long as possible
* if you've had a previous Caesarean section, plan to have your next baby vaginally
* if your baby is breech or transverse, ask to have an **external version** after 37 weeks (see page 176)

a Caesarean be done. If this surgery is not leading to healthier mothers and babies, it is unnecessary and potentially dangerous (as well as costly).

Caesarean section is more dangerous for the mother than a vaginal birth. The complication rate from Caesareans for the mother is two to five times higher than with a vaginal birth. Infections in the incision, **hemorrhage** (severe bleeding), bladder and kidney infections, and clots forming in the legs which can go to the lungs are all more frequent with Caesareans.

The rate of mothers dying from Caesareans (40 per 100,000 live births) is also higher than from vaginal births (10 to 14 per 100,000 live births). Some, but not all, of the increase in the Caesarean death rate, though, is related to the complication for which it was performed in the first place.

Even when all goes well, the mother faces a longer period of recovery after a Caesarean birth than after a vaginal delivery, and may find it harder to begin caring for her baby and breast-feeding.

Caesarean section does not guarantee a good outcome for babies, as some people think. Rates of Caesarean section and infant mortality rates are not shown by research to be particularly related; hospitals with a Caesarean rate of 10 per cent have the same infant mortality rate as those with a Caesarean rate of 25 per cent.

There are risks to the baby, too. Caesarean babies are four times more likely than vaginal birth babies to breathe fast for a few hours after they are born. This is called **transient tachypnoea of the newborn**. This condition goes away with no treatment, but it does mean the baby needs more careful observation for the first few hours to make sure that she is improving. This fast breathing may be mistakenly interpreted as an early sign of infection so the baby will be more likely to be treated with antibiotics. As well, Caesarean babies are slightly more likely to develop a more serious breathing problem called **respiratory distress syndrome**, which does need treatment.

If the Caesarean benefits the mother or baby, then these risks can be accepted as necessary. But if the Caesarean does not benefit mother or baby, then these complications are unnecessary as well. North American Caesarean rates are considerably higher than 7 per cent, and that strongly suggests that some of these Caesareans do not benefit mother or baby.

The tough question is: *Which Caesareans are unnecessary?* There are some definite answers to that, and there are still some grey areas. The next section looks at some factors that contribute to high Caesarean rates.

Why So Many Caesareans?

PREVIOUS CAESAREAN

At one time, the motto was "once a Caesarean, always a Caesarean" and any mother who had one Caesarean birth was told that any subsequent babies would require surgical delivery as well. Solid research has clearly demonstrated that in most cases these mothers are quite capable of giving birth vaginally. Routine repeat Caesareans, done just because the mother had a previous section, will lead to a large number of unnecessary operations. (See Chapter 24 "Vaginal Birth After Caesarean Section.")

FAILURE TO PROGRESS

The diagnosis of **dystocia**, (or "failure to progress in labour") often leads to Caesarean section. Dystocia is a general word meaning abnormal labour—doctors almost always use it to refer to labour that is progressing very slowly. The Society for Obstetricians and Gynaecologists of Canada (SOGC) has published guidelines to try to prevent labours from receiving this label too quickly, with the goal of avoiding unnecessary Caesareans. Their advice:

- A woman should not be said to be "in *active* labour" unless her cervix is 3 to 4 centimetres dilated and at least 80 per cent effaced. Contractions, of course, may have begun many hours or even days before this point is reached. Until the cervix has effaced and dilated to this point, the mother is considered to be in early or latent labour. Latent labour can be very long but still normal.
- Once active labour is underway, then labour needs to be observed for at least four hours to see if progress is being made. A diagnosis of dystocia can be *considered* when less than 0.5 centimetres of dilation per hour occurs over a four-hour time period.
- If labour is progressing slowly but mother and baby are both doing well, no treatment may be needed. The mother can be encouraged to walk and she should have a support person with her at all times. Before considering a Caesarean section, rupturing the membranes or using oxytocin to speed up the contractions should be tried. If the mother is exhausted and in a lot of pain, an epidural might help.

Using the SOGC's guidelines for diagnosing and treating dystocia has been shown to reduce the number of Caesarean sections done for this reason, with equally good outcomes for the babies.

After 10 hours of strong contractions, Picku and her husband drove to the hospital. To Picku's surprise, the nurse told her she wasn't in active labour. "All those contractions," Picku says, "and I wasn't even 2 centimetres dilated. I thought something was definitely wrong, but the nurse said it was normal for this stage to go slowly.

They sent us home, and we went back about 12 hours later. By then I was about 5 centimetres dilated and things started moving after that."

It was only afterwards that Picku's doctor explained the guidelines to her, and then she was pleased that the nurse had sent her home. "I was disappointed at the time, because we were so excited about being in labour. It's discouraging to be sent home again, but in reality I was more relaxed at home. And I'm glad I didn't end up with a Caesarean just because my labour started out so slowly."

NON-REASSURING FETAL HEART PATTERNS (FETAL DISTRESS)

Fetal distress is diagnosed when the baby shows signs of not getting enough oxygen or otherwise having trouble coping with labour, and is another common reason for Caesarean delivery.

Using an electronic fetal monitor to continuously monitor the heart rates of babies during labour definitely has been found to increase the rate of Caesarean section without improving the outcome for the babies. That means that some of the babies who were continuously monitored were delivered by Caesarean unnecessarily. Unfortunately, we don't know which ones. At present, research is trying to clarify which fetal heart rate patterns do truly indicate fetal distress. To date, all the patterns identified as "non-reassuring" still include many babies who are doing well.

The best recommendation to reduce unnecessary Caesarean sections for fetal distress seems to be: don't use continuous monitoring during labour for normal pregnancies.

LABOUR INTERVENTIONS

While research studies usually try to measure the effects of each intervention separately, in real life often the interventions are interconnected, with one leading to another. It can be difficult to tell whether a single intervention or a whole series actually led to the situation that required a Caesarean.

Consider Terry's experience, for example. Three days after her due date, she started having contractions in the middle of the night. "They were very irregular and short, lasting about 30 seconds each. I thought I probably had a long way to go, but I called my doctor anyway to let her know that I thought labour had started. The contractions continued pretty much the same way all day and through the next night and I was tired from not sleeping very much. I went for my regular doctor's appointment, and, after more than 24 hours of contractions, I was only 1 centimetre dilated. My doctor called it failure to progress."

The kind of long latent phase of labour that Terry experienced is common. It isn't unusual for women to go through days of short, irregular contractions without the cervix dilating very much. Sometimes the labour will stop altogether and then start again at a later date. In most cases, labour will gradually or suddenly get stronger without any intervention.

Terry's doctor, however, recommended that she go to the hospital to have her labour augmented. She was put in bed, given **pitocin** (a hormone which can speed up labour) by IV, attached to a fetal monitor, and shortly after that given an epidural. Four hours after this process was begun, Terry's doctor ruptured her membranes. At this point the baby's heart rate began to show some episodes of slowing during contractions. The pitocin level was turned up higher.

"I remember my doctor saying she wanted to get this baby born before suppertime," Terry says.

The baby's heartbeat on the fetal monitor then became more erratic, and Terry's doctor told her that the baby was in distress and a Caesarean would be necessary at once. "All I could think was that I was willing to do whatever was needed to have a healthy baby." Terry developed a fever and infection after the Caesarean and wasn't able to care for her new son (who was fine) for two days.

It's hard to second-guess a mother's birth experience, but Terry's story does show how different interventions are often related. Because she agreed to the augmentation of her labour (even though the research shows that the slow latent phase she was experiencing is quite normal), her labour became more painful. (Eighty per cent of women who have their labour induced or strengthened by oxytocin feel that it increases the amount of pain they experience and find it unpleasant.) She then decided on an epidural to help with the pain.

Was it her slow early labour that led to Terry's Caesarean section, or was it the combination of the induction, fetal monitoring, restriction to bed, and epidural anaesthetic? Would the results have been different if her doctor had encouraged her to rest and wait at home until her contractions became stronger and more regular, or suggested walking to make the contractions more effective?

Since many interventions carry with them an increased risk of Caesarean section, one of the best things a woman in labour can do to mini-mize her risk is to avoid interventions as much as possible.

PLANNED CAESAREAN SECTION

If a Caesarean is recommended before labour even begins (for example, because your baby is in a breech position, or because you had a previous Caesarean section, or because your baby is "too big") you can ask for a second opinion, just as you can for any major operation.

THE PHYSICIAN'S FEAR OF LAWSUITS

Half of the lawsuits filed against doctors practising obstetrics claim that a Caesarean section should have been done to avoid whatever damage the baby suffered during delivery. These claims are made despite the complete lack of evidence that Caesarean delivery reduces childhood neurological problems, cerebral palsy, or seizures.

Even when the doctor is found not to be at fault, dealing with a lawsuit is expensive, time-consuming and stressful.

It is impossible to quantify how much the fear of being sued affects doctors' decision-making about doing Caesareans. However, as one example, although the research shows that careful forceps deliveries are just as safe as Caesarean section, the rate of forceps deliveries has decreased and the rate of Caesarean section has increased. Doctors feel that if something does go wrong, they are less likely to be sued if it happens after a Caesarean section rather than a forceps delivery.

CAESAREAN INCISIONS

The **incision in the skin** is most often **transverse** (from side to side), just at the top of your pubic hair. This is sometimes called a **bikini cut**, because it won't show if you wear a bikini. The skin incision may also be vertical, going from just below the belly button to the top of the pubic hair.

The **incision on the uterus** is almost always transverse across the bottom of the uterus. This incision is stronger when it heals and safer during the next pregnancy. In rare cases, because of the position of the baby or the placenta, a vertical incision must be used. In a few cases, the doctor starts off by doing a transverse incision, but has to add a vertical one to get the baby out. Then the mother has a scar like an upside-down T on her uterus.

The direction of the skin incision has nothing to do with the direction of the incision in the uterus. They may be the same, or different. A transverse incision on the uterus is definitely preferable because it will be stronger during subsequent pregnancies and births.

Since the fear of being sued is impossible to measure or research, hard data on this is not available. However, it is definitely an issue for doctors today.

When a Caesarean Is Required

ANAESTHETIC

Let's say you and your doctor have decided that a Caesarean is required to safely deliver your baby.

This decision may have been made before labour, because of the baby's position, placenta previa, or other complications, or it may be made during labour because the baby is in distress or the cord has slipped below the baby's head and is seen in the vagina (**prolapsed**), for example, or it may be made at the end of labour when attempts to deliver the baby with forceps have failed or there are other problems. Just as for any other surgery, you will need to have anaesthetic to stop you from feeling the pain.

Modern anaesthetic techniques, with special modifications for pregnancy, make anaesthesia for Caesarean section for both mother and baby extremely safe. To try to put it in perspective, the risk of the mother dying from having a baby (Caesarean or not) is between 10 and 14 per 100,000 live births. Anaesthesia complications will cause only one of these deaths—a very low number.

For Caesareans, the most common type of anaesthetic is regional—usually either an epidural or a spinal. Both of these involve injecting anaesthetic into the mother's back; the difference is in the placement of the injection. Mothers usually like the idea of being awake to see the baby as soon as it is born. Sometimes mothers are interested in being awake but are worried about seeing the surgery. You might be reassured to know that a drape will be hung up over your chest so that you won't see any of the gory parts. With regional anaesthesia, you will often feel touch and pressure during the surgery. If you feel pain, the anaesthetist can give you more painkillers or a general anaesthetic.

Regional anaesthetics avoid the risk of the mother vomiting while she is unconscious. The biggest concern with these regional anaesthetics is that the mother's blood pressure will drop, so she is given extra fluids through an IV before the surgery.

A general anaesthetic, which makes the mother unconscious during the operation, may be a better choice in a few situations. Mothers with bleeding problems are likely to have more serious complications if they have an epidural, so a general anaesthetic would be recommended. A general can also be given more quickly than an epidural, so it's the best choice when speed is critical. The biggest risk of general anaesthetic is **aspiration pneumonia**, which develops when the unconscious mother vomits stomach fluids and then inhales them into her lungs. Giving antacids immediately before putting the mother to sleep cuts down on the risk of severe aspiration pneumonia.

Many women who have an epidural or spinal anaesthetic during a Caesarean want to have their partners or support people with them. The experience of surgery is pretty stressful, and having that emotional support can make a big difference. Your partner can hold the baby once he is born and bring him to you so you can touch the baby and have a good look. Most hospitals now permit at least one support person during Caesareans, but a few still restrict them to planned and pre-scheduled Caesareans only.

Some mothers also want their partners there even if they have a general anaesthetic. The partner will be able to tell the mother afterwards what happened, and will be able to hold the baby. However, most hospitals discourage or forbid the partner's presence when the mother is having a general anaesthetic.

STEP BY STEP THROUGH A CAESAREAN

Once the decision is made to deliver the baby by Caesarean section, you will have an intravenous started, a **catheter** put in your bladder to drain the urine, and the top part of your pubic hair shaved.

You will be moved to an operating room (usually right in the labour and delivery department, but occasionally in another part of the hospital). This room is brightly lit, stocked with surgical instruments and sterile gowns, and has a table with a heater over it for the baby. During your surgery, all the medical personnel will wear gowns, hats, and facemasks.

If you are having a spinal or epidural, the anaesthetist will put it in now. Then your abdomen will be washed with soap and you will be covered with clean sheets, leaving a gap in the middle for your belly. The sheets are pinned up on poles by your chest so that if you are awake you won't see the actual surgery. If you are having a general, the sheets will be put in place first, then the anaesthetist will put you to sleep (this is done at the last minute so the baby gets as little anaesthesia as possible).

The first cut goes through the skin and fat down to the muscle. Then the abdominal muscles are pulled apart and cut to get down to the **peritoneum**, a membrane that lines the entire inside of the abdomen. This is cut, too, and right underneath is the uterus, filling the whole abdomen. Another incision is made in the uterus—some amniotic fluid will gush out at this point—and the baby is pulled out through the incision, the cord is clamped and cut, and the baby immediately handed to the **pediatrician**. Then the placenta is pulled out through the

RECOVERING FROM A CAESAREAN SECTION

- You have had major surgery, so expect your recovery to be slower than if you'd had a vaginal birth.
- About one in five women will have a fever and infection; antibiotics given at the time of the surgery reduce this.
- You may have gas pains and bowel problems. Eat lightly for the first two days, and walk around as much as possible.
- You will have a catheter in your bladder for several hours at least. It may be difficult and uncomfortable to urinate at first when the catheter comes out.
- You will probably have an IV for a day or two, to provide fluids and pain medication.
- You will feel pain at the incision site—some women say it feels like their insides are falling out! It can help to press your hands or a small pillow against the incision when you get up or walk around.
- It can be a challenge to find a comfortable position for breastfeeding. Put a pillow under the baby to protect the incision, or ask your nurse or a lactation consultant to show you how to nurse on your side or using a **football hold**.
- Your emotional reactions may be quite intense. Some women are extremely disappointed about having a Caesarean, even when they know it was necessary. Ask your caregivers about support groups in your community; it often helps to talk to other new mothers about your feelings.

incision. This whole part—from giving the anaesthetic to delivering the baby—takes about 10 minutes.

The baby is out, but now the doctor has to stitch you back together. First, the incision in the uterus has to be carefully sewed up in layers. Then the peritoneum is closed up. The muscle layer is tacked back together, and the skin is closed either with stitches, staples, or tiny bandages called **steristrips**. This part of the birth takes 30 to 45 minutes.

If you have had a general, the anaesthetic will be stopped at this point and you will start to wake up. If you have had a regional anaesthetic, you have probably been admiring your new baby during the process. You will now move to a recovery room, where a nurse will make frequent checks of your breathing and blood pressure. Usually the catheter is left in for several hours, until you are able to get up to use the bathroom, and the IV is left in for a day or two to make it easier to administer medications and keep you hydrated.

Alex remembers: "They rushed Shirley into the operating room for the Caesarean and told me I'd have to wait outside because they were giving her a general. It seemed like just a couple of minutes when the nurse came out with my baby girl. I picked her up for a second and admired her, and then the nurse took her away to be weighed and everything. I stood there waiting for Shirley to come out, and I didn't know why it was taking so long. Nobody told me that it was normal. I was convinced that something terrible had happened to her and began trying to figure out how I'd cope as a single father. It was more than 45 minutes before they wheeled Shirley out, and I was so relieved to find out she was okay."

After the surgery is over, the mother faces a recovery period just as she would after any operation. One common complication from Caesareans is infection, and about one in five mothers will have a fever and other signs of infection during the first few days after they have given birth; some of these mothers will be seriously ill. The risk of infection is higher for women who have been in labour for some time before the surgery, for those whose membranes ruptured before the surgery, and for obese women.

Because post-Caesarean infections are so common, they have been studied carefully. The research has now clearly established that giving antibiotics to the mother at the time of the Caesarean will significantly reduce the rate of infection. This is most often done through the IV after the baby is born and the cord has been clamped, so the drug isn't passed on to the baby.

Jennifer's advice to mothers who have Caesareans: "Make sure you have help when you get home. With the shorter hospital stays that seem to be the rule now, it's essential. When I got home I still couldn't stand up straight and walk. I'd lean my elbows on the change table to change the baby's diapers. I was so tired, I definitely needed more sleep than the baby. Remember that you've been through surgery, and get the help and rest you need."

Elective Caesareans

"We tried to get pregnant on our own for several years," recalls Lisa. "It didn't work. Finally we went for infertility treatments, and it took eight

---

The Evidence About…
Caesarean Sections

In some situations Caesarean sections can save the lives of mothers and babies.

However, when the rates of Caesareans are higher than about 7 per cent, there is no improvement in outcomes for mothers or babies. The North American rate of 20 to 25 per cent clearly puts mothers at risk without improving outcomes for babies.

Using the SOGC's guidelines for **VBACs** and **dystocia** will reduce the rate of Caesarean section. Avoiding the use of continuous monitoring will also reduce the number of Caesareans.

Giving antibiotics to the mother who is having a Caesarean during the procedure will significantly reduce her risks of developing an infection.

---

more months before I finally conceived. After all I'd been through, I didn't want to take any chances with this birth so I asked the doctor to schedule me for a Caesarean."

Her doctor agreed. Lisa's surgery went smoothly and she was thrilled to deliver a healthy baby boy.

But her reasons for wanting a surgical birth were based on misinformation. A Caesarean delivery when no medical indications are present is not safer than a vaginal birth. Research from Brazil, where Caesareans have been readily available to women who request them for some time, found that in these low-risk cases, both mother and baby experienced more problems and complications after a surgical birth than after a vaginal birth.

-24-
Vaginal Birth after Caesarean Section (VBAC)

Rose's baby girl Shannon, now four, was delivered by Caesarean section because she was in a breech position. When she became pregnant again, Rose assumed she'd plan for a second Caesarean. But one of the mothers at Shannon's daycare told her she'd had a VBAC with her second pregnancy.

"What's a VBAC?" Rose asked.

"It stands for vaginal birth after Caesarean section. For me, it was a million times better than having another C-section. You should talk to your doctor about it."

With her doctor's appointment several weeks away, Rose decided to do some research on her own, and discovered there was a VBAC support group in her community. The group leaders had some interesting information, and she began to wonder if she would like to give birth vaginally.

For many years, obstetricians in North America have been very ready to perform a Caesarean section on all women who have had a previous Caesarean section. Generally, the mother was scheduled for her next Caesarean section between 38 and 40 weeks of pregnancy, without waiting for labour to start. This is called

a booked, elective, or repeat Caesarean section. If labour did start before the scheduled date, the mother was instructed to come to the hospital immediately, and a Caesarean section would be performed at once without waiting to see if labour would progress.

Doctors planned these repeat Caesareans because they believed that to have a second surgical delivery was safer than the mother going into labour and trying to give birth vaginally. They were concerned that the scar on her uterus might rupture. They also assumed that most women who have had a Caesarean section would wind up needing one again with their next labour.

Both of these assumptions have been shown to be false.

It wasn't, initially, physicians who doubted these assumptions. While many women with Caesareans accepted the advice they were given and arranged for repeat sections, some women decided to try giving birth vaginally. At first, there were no studies and few statistics to support their choices. It was often difficult to find a doctor willing to attend a VBAC birth, and many hospitals set up procedures that made it difficult. Women persisted, though—sometimes by deciding to do a VBAC at home—and gradually the statistics accumulated.

Randomized controlled studies have not been performed to compare the outcome of elective Caesarean section with a **trial of labour** (the mother going into labour, and only having a Caesarean for the usual reasons). These studies have not been done because women will not agree to be randomly assigned to Caesarean section or labour. The information we have comes from studying two large groups of similar women. One group had trials of labour after Caesarean section, and the other group had elective repeat Caesarean section.

Initially, these studies concluded that:

- trial of labour after Caesarean section (with a lower uterine segment transverse incision) is safer for the mother, and as safe for the baby as repeat elective Caesarean section; and
- with trial of labour, almost 80 per cent of women deliver vaginally.

These results led to an increase in the number of VBACs. In more recent years, additional studies on similar groups of women have suggested that there are more slightly more complications for women having VBACs and for their babies, although the total numbers in both groups is very low. These studies led to recommendations by doctor's associations in North America that discouraged many women from attempting VBACs.

The biggest concern that has been raised about having a VBAC is that there may be a risk of uterine rupture. This does not mean the uterus explodes (despite the way it sounds); it means the scar from the previous Caesarean splits open. This is very serious. It causes immediate pain, shock, internal bleeding, and fetal distress, and the baby must be delivered promptly by an emergency Caesarean section.

The risk of this complication is very low provided the previous Caesarean left a **lower uterine segment transverse incision**. What's a "lower uterine segment transverse incision"? For the past 40 years, the vast majority of Caesarean sections have been done with this kind of cut. It means that the obstetrician has cut sideways across the bottom of the uterus (the lower uterine segment), which isn't very muscular and does not contract during labour.

The older "classical" incision is cut vertically in the uterus and goes through the more muscular upper part of the uterus, which does contract during labour. This kind of incision is now very rarely used.

Occasionally, an **inverted-T** incision may be used, in which first a transverse lower uterine incision is made, and then, if there is difficulty in getting the baby out (as can happen with a breech position), the doctor creates extra room by adding a vertical incision up through the lower uterine segment and into the muscular upper segment.

The appearance of the skin incision—up and down or across the abdomen—has nothing to do with the uterine incision.

With a lower uterine segment transverse incision the chance of rupture of the uterus is very small: the risk is from 0.09 to 0.22 per cent.

There is very little data on women who have laboured after having a classical incision in their upper uterine segment. The best estimates of the risk of rupture range from 2.2 to 14 per cent. Data on women labouring with an inverted-T incision are also limited: the current best estimate suggests a risk of rupture of about 1.3 per cent.

Rupture with a vertical incision is not only more likely than with a transverse lower segment incision, it is much more dangerous for the baby. The baby is more likely to be expelled from the uterus into the abdominal cavity, and there is more likely to be significant separation of the placenta. This rupture is just as likely to occur before the onset of labour as it is during labour, making it difficult to prevent by elective Caesarean section unless it is performed well before term.

OTHER SAFETY CONSIDERATIONS

There are other complications, besides the rather dramatic one of uterine rupture, to be considered in comparing VBACs and repeat Caesareans.

Very few women die having babies, but more women die having Caesarean sections than having vaginal births. Because some of these deaths are from the conditions that prompted the Caesarean (such as severe pre-eclampsia) and not the surgery itself, it is difficult to estimate the actual risk from Caesarean section itself. When researchers sift out other factors, they conclude that the risk of a mother dying from an elective Caesarean section is two to four times the risk of dying from a vaginal birth.

Mothers having Caesarean sections are more likely to develop wound infections, pneumonia, bleeding requiring blood transfusion, urinary

tract infections, and uterine infections. These are all lumped together and called **morbidity**. The morbidity rate is higher among women who have elective repeat sections than among those who have a trial of labour—and the trial of labour group includes both those who do deliver vaginally and those who end up having a second Caesarean section.

It's clear from these statistics that a planned VBAC is safer than a repeat Caesarean section for the mother.

What about the safety of the baby? The death rates and complication rates for the babies are the same for both groups in the studies that report this data.

The main risk of Caesarean delivery for the baby is that it will develop either a fast breathing rate, or a more serious breathing problem called **respiratory distress syndrome**, in the first few hours after birth. Both are more common after Caesarean section than after vaginal birth. Since 80 per cent of the babies whose mothers choose to have a trial of labour will be born vaginally, this reduces their risk of both conditions.

Also, there is always a risk of doing the elective Caesarean prematurely as a result of mistaken dates or inaccurate ultrasound estimates.

In 1999, the American College of Obstetricians and Gynecologists adopted more restrictive guidelines for VBACs. After the new guidelines were implemented, the rate in California fell from 24 per cent VBAC to 13.5 per cent. Researchers studied the records of nearly 400,000 women who had one previous Caesarean birth during the three years prior to the change and the three years following the change. They found that the newborn and maternal mortality rates did not improve despite the changes but were about the same as when more babies were born by VBAC.

Thinking about VBAC

What should Rose consider as she plans the birth of her second baby?

First, she needs to know what kind of incision she has in her uterus. The risk of uterine rupture is about 0.1 to 0.2 per cent with a lower uterine segment transverse incision, about 1.3 per cent with an inverted-T incision, and from 2.2 to 14 per cent with a classical incision vertically in the upper uterine segment.

She doesn't need to think too much about the reason for her first Caesarean. The reason for the previous Caesarean section makes only a marginal difference in the success rate of VBAC.

Researchers originally thought that some reasons for Caesarean section—like labour that stops progressing, or a baby too big to fit through the pelvis—were more likely to recur and require a second Caesarean than complications like a breech presentation. But this theory has not proved true. Even with a previous diagnosis of abnormal labour causing the first C-section, 75 per cent of women were able to deliver vaginally during a trial of labour. Many women have vaginally delivered bigger babies than the one for which they had a Caesarean.

Rose had only one previous Caesarean delivery, but some women have had two or three before planning a VBAC. The studies to date, although small, do not suggest any significant differences in success rate or complication rate for women who have a trial of labour after more than one Caesarean section.

A previous vaginal delivery as well as the previous Caesarean does increase the chances of a successful trial of labour.

Diane, for example, had two normal vaginal births. When she went into labour with her third baby, he was in a transverse position—lying sideways—and was delivered by Caesarean section. With her fourth pregnancy, she confidently planned a VBAC. "I knew I could have a baby vaginally," Diane says. "I'd done it twice. So having a VBAC didn't seem like a big deal to me."

For Rose and other women contemplating a VBAC, there are often emotional issues as well.

Hanna was in labour for more than 30 hours before she had a Caesarean because her baby was in distress. She vividly remembers how painful and exhausting her long labour was, and how scared she felt at the end when they rushed her into the operating room. It's an experience she won't risk repeating; she plans to have an elective repeat C-section with her next baby.

Iris also had a long and difficult labour before her surgery, and she was very disappointed when it ended up in a Caesarean. When she became pregnant again, she decided to plan for a VBAC. But it wasn't easy making that choice.

"I had so many conflicting feelings," Iris says. "I really didn't want another Caesarean, but I was terrified of another long, hard labour. And what if I went through it again and then had another Caesarean after all? Even with support from the VBAC group I belonged to, I felt pretty anxious about the whole thing."

Knowing that labour is safe after a Caesarean doesn't always balance out the mother's fears of having to go through a painful experience that might end up, once again, with surgery. If the Caesarean was done part way through their first

A DIFFICULT DECISION: ANN'S VBAC

For some women, the VBAC decision is readily supported. For others, it is more challenging.

Ann's first baby was in a breech position. When her labour seemed to be progressing very slowly, her doctor became concerned and strongly recommended a Caesarean. During the surgery, he had trouble getting the baby out. He had initially done a transverse incision across the bottom of Ann's uterus; now he added a vertical one so that the whole incision looked like an upside-down T on her uterus.

Before Ann left the hospital, the obstetrician met with her and explained how the surgery had gone. "If you have another baby, it will have to be delivered by Caesarean because of that incision," he told her.

Ann recalls, "I didn't get pregnant again for four years because I couldn't bear the idea of another section. I still feel that I didn't need that first Caesarean, I just let myself get talked into it."

When she did conceive again, Ann was determined to have a VBAC. But it turned out to be much harder than she had expected: "I went to see eight different doctors. As soon as they heard about my incision, they stopped talking to me. They all said I had to have a Caesarean and that was it. One doctor told me I had a 50 per cent risk of my uterus rupturing and me and the baby dying. Most of the others just said it was unacceptable."

Ann felt strongly that she was not being irrational or unreasonable. She had carefully researched her situation. Since incisions like hers are rare, she did not have a lot to go on, but the rate of uterine rupture seems to be between 1 and 2 per cent. This is certainly higher than the risks of a repeat Caesarean, but Ann felt the risk was acceptable to her.

The ninth doctor Ann spoke to agreed to provide her care during this pregnancy. They discussed the risks and the doctor reminded Ann that the choice she was making was not the safest route.

But it was Ann's choice. As she points out, "We know that the safest choice for a woman with a lower transverse incision is to have a VBAC, yet many women choose to have a repeat Caesarean. It's not the safest choice, but those women rarely have any problems finding a doctor who is prepared to do another C-section for them."

Ann was by then 32 weeks. The rest of her pregnancy went smoothly—her baby was head down and average in size. When labour started, Ann and her husband went to the hospital right away. Ann had a five-hour labour (most of it spent in the shower) and a straightforward delivery of a lovely little girl.

It's not surprising that Ann gave birth to a healthy baby vaginally, despite having an inverted-T incision. The statistics tell us that between 98 and 99 per cent of the women in her situation will do exactly that.

What's significant about Ann's story is that she made her own decision, despite running up against some opposition. She understood the research, assessed the risks, and made a responsible choice. Anne says, "Even if I had had a complication, I wouldn't have thought my decision to have a vaginal birth was wrong. I know it was the right choice for me."

labour, women wonder just how much worse it can get. Will they be able to cope with the end of labour and pushing out a baby? First-time mothers wonder about these questions, too, but the Caesarean mother often feels like her body didn't work properly the first time, and might fail her again.

As Iris found, support groups for VBAC mothers can help work through those fears. Other women have found information and support by reading books such as *Silent Knife* by Nancy Wainer Cohen or by contacting others on the Internet.

The VBAC Labour

When mothers decide to have a VBAC, should their labours be handled differently than "normal" labours?

Inducing labour may be riskier for VBAC labours. Using oxytocin to induce labour seems to have the least effect on risk, but it should still be used cautiously. (Using oxytocin to speed up or augment labour once it has already started does not seem to increase the risk.) Inductions with prostaglandin (see Chapter 41) are associated with an increased risk of uterine rupture and should be avoided.

Women in VBAC labours can have epidurals if they want, without increased risk. Although the mother doesn't feel pain, her caregivers will be able to figure out if the scar on her uterus does rupture because the baby will show signs of distress.

It does not improve outcomes for women having VBACs to have their babies in "high-risk" or teaching hospitals rather than their own com-

The Evidence About...
VBAC

A woman who has had a previous Caesarean section with a lower uterine segment transverse incision should be encouraged to have a trial of labour with her next pregnancy. National consensus statements in both Canada and the United States recommend trial of labour.

The likelihood of a successful vaginal birth is not significantly changed by the reason for the first Caesarean section or the number of previous Caesarean sections.

The woman who is considering a trial of labour after a Caesarean section in which a classical incision was performed has a higher risk of uterine rupture, and increased risk over elective Caesarean section.

munity hospitals. (Some communities designate certain hospitals to take high-risk pregnancies and births, and these have additional facilities for caring for premature babies, for example. Teaching hospitals include medical students, interns, and residents on staff and often take more high-risk cases.) Some women may choose to have VBACs at home.

Monica says, "When I was pregnant with Eric (after having a Caesarean with her first baby, Adam), the doctor told me I had to come to the hospital as soon as I had a contraction to be hooked up to an IV and a fetal monitor. I was told I couldn't have any painkillers so that I'd notice right away if my uterus ruptured. I don't know anything that makes it harder to relax during contractions than trying to feel if your uterus is rupturing! My labour took quite a while, but I did manage to give birth vaginally."

When Monica conceived again, she read more about the research results on how VBAC labours should be treated. "This time I decided to labour at home most of the time, where I was more comfortable and relaxed. I was only at the hospital for two hours—with no IV or monitor—when the baby was born."

-25-
Sexually Transmitted Diseases

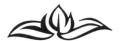

There are several infections that are often passed from one person to another during sexual activity. It can be embarrassing to discuss these diseases with your doctor, yet diagnosis is important because some have significant effects on your unborn baby and can be treated.

Screening for Sexually Transmitted Diseases (STDs)

STDs such as syphilis, herpes, AIDS, and hepatitis B are common in our society, and so are common in pregnant women. It is true that any woman who is sexually active (and this obviously

includes all pregnant women) can get an STD, but some women are more at risk than others. The more sexual partners a woman ever has, the higher her risk of coming in contact with one or more STDs.

Some other risk factors for having an STD have do with lifestyle. Young, single, and low-income women have higher STD rates. Intravenous drug use is also a risk factor. But most of the women in these groups do not have STDs, and about 40 per cent of the people who do have STDs don't belong to any of these groups.

Should you be tested for STDs? If you are high risk, you will probably answer "yes." But what if you are in a low-risk group? It's still possible for you to have an infection that could harm your baby, yet if all low-risk pregnant women go for testing, the costs will be very high and the benefits few.

Hepatitis B

Hepatitis B is a virus that affects the liver. It is passed from person to person through direct

RISK FACTORS FOR SEXUALLY TRANSMITTED DISEASES

- multiple sexual partners
- if one sexually transmitted disease is present, the risk of others also being present is higher
- intravenous drug use

contact with blood, saliva, vaginal secretions, or semen, or it can be transmitted at birth from a mother carrying hepatitis B virus to her infant.

Ninety per cent of the adults who are infected with hepatitis B will recover completely and are then immune to the disease. Ten per cent develop chronic hepatitis—they continue to carry the hepatitis B virus in their blood. These people can go on to develop cirrhosis or liver cancer. As well, they are infectious to people with whom they have sexual relations, or with whom they share needles.

Routine testing of large groups of women shows a positive test for hepatitis B in almost 1 per cent. About 20 per cent of the babies born to infected mothers will catch the virus and develop chronic hepatitis. Infection usually happens during the birth when the baby comes in contact with the mother's vaginal secretions.

TREATING THE BABY EXPOSED TO HEPATITIS B

Even if a mother is carrying hepatitis B, her baby's risk of infection can be reduced from 20 per cent to almost zero by an injection of **hepatitis B immune globulin** given to the baby as soon as he is born. This globulin contains antibodies from the blood of people who are already immune to hepatitis B. At the same time, the baby is given an injection of the hepatitis B vaccine, to stimulate him to make his own antibodies. Two more doses of hepatitis B vaccine are given when the baby is two months old and four months old to make the baby completely immune to hepatitis B.

The Evidence About...
Hepatitis B

Hepatitis B immune globulin can protect babies born to mothers with hepatitis B from infection. A mother can't give her baby the benefits of the hepatitis B immune globulin at birth unless she knows she is carrying the virus, so it seems reasonable for all pregnant women to get tested for hepatitis B.

If everyone was vaccinated against hepatitis B it would protect future babies from this disease.

Herpes Simplex

Herpes simplex is a virus that can be transmitted from one person to another by touch or by kissing. There are two types:

- **Type 1** is responsible for the common cold sore or "fever blister" around the mouth. It can occasionally cause sores around the genitals as well.
- **Type 2** is often called genital herpes because it is usually found on the genitals. It is most often caught during sexual contact. This virus is of most concern to pregnant women, because it can be passed on to the baby at birth.

Herpes is very difficult to diagnose, but it is estimated that about 20 per cent of women may have the herpes Type 2 virus. Although this virus is very common, only a few babies will catch the infection from their mothers. While we don't know exactly how many—estimates vary between 1 in 2,500 and 1 in 10,000.

MATERNAL HERPES TYPE 2 INFECTIONS

Many women who have herpes are not aware of it. A woman's first attack or outbreak of genital herpes is usually the most severe. Often she will have a fever, aching and tiredness, plus small painful sores in the vaginal area. There are exceptions—some women with their first outbreak will have only small sores and no other symptoms of illness. The initial attack usually ends within one to three weeks and the sores heal without leaving any sign that they were ever there.

However, the herpes virus is not gone. It can continue to live in the body for long periods of time without causing any symptoms—this is called latent or dormant herpes. After the first attack, some women will never again have the painful open sores. Others have recurrent attacks, usually milder than the first.

During these attacks, and for some days afterwards, live herpes virus is present in the vaginal area. There may also be live herpes virus present at times when the woman is not having an obvious attack, but this is rare.

There is no cure for herpes.

The baby is at the highest risk of infection if the mother has her first (primary) outbreak of herpes right at the time of labour and delivery. At this point her body has not had time to develop any antibodies that would protect the baby from the infection.

When there is a primary outbreak of herpes at the beginning of labour, a Caesarean section may prevent the baby from catching the herpes virus, especially if the membranes have not ruptured. (If they have, there is a small possibility that the baby may have already picked up the virus, but usually herpes is caught as the baby passes through the birth canal.)

If the mother has had recurrent attacks of herpes, she already has antibodies that have been passed on to the baby through the placenta, so the risk to the baby is less. Studies of women with recurrent genital herpes found that only 1.4 per cent had live virus present during labour. If there are no open sores, the baby is at minimal risk of infection during a vaginal birth.

While herpes infections of newborn babies are not common, they are potentially serious. Since there is no cure, researchers have concentrated on ways to prevent babies from catching herpes.

Tests can be done to see if live herpes virus is present when women are in labour, but the results come back too late to be useful. Testing during late pregnancy has not been able to predict which mothers would be infectious at the time the baby was born.

One study compared pregnant women with recurrent herpes who were treated with an antiviral drug to a similar group of pregnant women who did not receive the drug. The drug did significantly reduce the risk of live virus being present in the vagina at the time of delivery. Because of the rareness of the infection, though, neither group had any cases of herpes infection of the newborn.

Some physicians and hospitals have recommended Caesarean sections for all women with a history of genital herpes, but there is absolutely no research to support this. The Society of Obstetricians and Gynaecologists of Canada currently recommends that, when labour begins, *"Delivery by Caesarean section is only indicated in the presence of clinically active lesions (open sores) in the lower genital tract.*" Even this recommendation is not strongly supported by research.

Alana was very pleased when she heard about this new recommendation during her second pregnancy. "I had a Caesarean with my first pregnancy because my doctor recommended it for all women with herpes. I was dreading the surgery and recovery when I got pregnant again, but this time I was able to have a VBAC."

CARE OF THE NEWBORN

If your baby is born when you have an outbreak of genital herpes, the baby should be isolated from other newborns—*but not from you!* Breastfeeding will benefit the baby just as it does any other baby. You will need to wash your hands carefully before touching the baby and make sure he or she doesn't come in contact with any of the herpes sores. The baby will be carefully watched, and can be treated with anti-herpes virus drugs if a fever, rash, or other signs of illness develop.

Babies can also catch herpes Type 1—the common cold sore—so anyone who has a cold sore should not kiss or touch the baby without thoroughly washed hands.

HIV/AIDS

AIDS (acquired immunodeficiency syndrome) is a widely publicized disease caused by HIV (human immunodeficiency virus). It has become the third leading cause of death of American women between the ages of 25 and 44—the years during which most women have babies.

The Evidence About…
Herpes

While genital herpes is very common (about 20 per cent of women may have it), herpes infecions of newborn babies are very rare (between 1 in 2,500 and 1 in 10,000).

Caesarean section is currently recommended for women with active herpes outbreaks at the time they go into labour, although this is not supported by strong evidence.

There is a huge amount of research presently underway on various treatments for people with AIDS. Still, at present there is no cure and the death rate is high.

No one knows exactly how many pregnant women are HIV-positive. The U.S. Center for Disease Control has estimated an overall rate of 1 to 2 per 1,000, but in some communities the rate is much higher.

If a woman infected with the HIV virus becomes pregnant, she has a 13 to 40 per cent chance of infecting her baby; the average rate based on the studies done is about 30 per cent. *This rate can be dramatically reduced by treatment with the antiviral drug* **zidovudine**. If given to the HIV-positive mother during pregnancy, and to the infant for the first six weeks after birth, it reduces the rate of transmission of HIV from 30 to 8 per cent.

Breastfeeding can transmit HIV from mother to baby, although the risk seems small. Recent research has found that when babies of HIV-positive mothers are *exclusively* breastfed—no other liquids or solid foods—their risk is the same as babies who are formula-fed. In developing countries, the World Health Organization

HOW HIV IS TRANSMITTED

- through sexual contact with an infected person's body fluids
- through blood transfusions of infected blood
- through sharing needles contaminated with infected blood
- during pregnancy, from an infected mother to her child

The Evidence About…
AIDS

Treatment of the HIV-positive mother and her baby with zidovudine greatly reduces the rate of HIV transmission to the baby.

If testing for HIV is only offered to high-risk groups, many women who are HIV-positive will be missed, and their babies will not get the benefit of treatment. Letting pregnant women know about this beneficial drug may encourage them to be tested.

(WHO) suggests that breastfeeding is still recommended even if the mother is HIV-positive, as the advantages of breastfeeding when clean, safe water is rarely available would outweigh the small risk of HIV transmission.

Other Sexually Transmitted Infections

Gonorrhea is a sexually transmitted disease caused by a bacteria called the **gonococcus**. Some women with gonorrhea have a greenish vaginal discharge, fever, and pain in the pelvic area. During pregnancy, women with gonorrhea are more likely to feel very ill, with hot, painful joints as well as fever and pelvic pain. However, many women who have gonorrhea have no symptoms from it at all.

Women with gonorrhea are more likely to give birth prematurely. After a miscarriage or after the birth of her baby, the mother who has gonorrhea can get a bad uterine infection that needs to be treated with antibiotics.

Gonorrhea can be tested for during a prenatal visit. If it is present, the mother can take antibiotics that are safe during pregnancy to cure the infection. The baby doesn't catch gonorrhea while it is in the uterus, but picks up the germ while he is passing through the birth canal. So if the mother has been treated with antibiotics, the baby is also protected.

A baby born to a mother with gonorrhea is at risk of developing a serious eye infection that can cause blindness if not treated. The infection usually develops two to five days after birth. In many countries, treatment of all newborns with **silver nitrate eye drops** or, more recently, with **antibiotic eye ointments**, to kill any gonorrhea germs, is required by law. The ointments are more effective in preventing eye infections from both gonorrhea and chlamydia, and are less irritating to the baby's eyes.

Researchers have compared treating all babies with these ointments soon after birth against watching to see if the infection develops and promptly treating only the infected babies. The results were equally good with both methods. However, it is difficult to observe and treat only infected babies because of the trend to shorter hospital stays after birth, and routine treatment is the law in most places.

The Evidence About...
Gonorrhea

Routine treatment—drops or ointment in the baby's eyes shortly after birth—has been carried out to successfully prevent eye infections and blindness for more than 100 years. Undiagnosed and untreated gonorrhea can cause serious infections in the mother's uterus.

The Evidence About...
Chlamydia

There is a lot of uncertainty about how common chlamydia infections are. What is certain is that the bacteria can be dangerous to newborns.

If you are at risk of having chlamydia, you could ask to be tested. Treatment with antibiotics while you are pregnant will significantly reduce the risk to your baby.

Chlamydia trachomatis is the most common sexually transmitted bacteria in women of child-bearing age. Various studies have found that between 2 and 25 per cent of pregnant women (this is a hard germ to diagnose!) have chlamydia.

Chlamydia can cause a yellow-green vaginal discharge, and can make women ill with fever and pelvic pain. However, in most women (and men), the infection causes no symptoms at all. Chlamydia is only caught during sexual intercourse, so women who have many sexual partners are more likely to come in contact with it.

How does chlamydia affect pregnancy and birth? It is suspected that chlamydia may cause premature rupture of the membranes and premature birth of the baby, but the studies on this have been contradictory.

But the risk of infection to the baby is clear from the research.

Between 20 and 50 per cent of babies born to mothers infected with chlamydia will develop an eye infection, and if this condition is not treated, it can lead to blindness. The standard eye ointment given to babies to prevent gonorrhea (silver nitrate, **erythromycin ointment**, or **tetracycline ointment**) will prevent about 80 per cent of

chlamydia eye infections. If the infection does develop, the baby will need to be treated with antibiotics.

Between 3 and 18 per cent of babies born to infected mothers will develop **chlamydia pneumonia**. This can also be treated with antibiotics.

Can we prevent chlamydia infection in babies? It is difficult to diagnose chlamydia in pregnant women: the tests are expensive and are not completely accurate. Treatment during pregnancy is also challenging, because the most effective drug (tetracycline) should not be used during pregnancy. A slightly less effective drug (erythromycin) tends to give women stomach aches and make them vomit, but erythromycin is considered safe during pregnancy.

One study compared women who took the antibiotics for chlamydia during pregnancy with another group who chose not to be treated. The babies of the women who were treated did have significantly lower rates of infection.

Syphilis is a sexually transmitted disease that can be passed from an infected mother to her baby through the placenta. In Canada and the United States, the law requires all pregnant women to be tested for syphilis at their first pre-natal visit. (Remember having all that blood taken then? Some of it was used to test for syphilis.) This test does have some false positives, but further testing will confirm whether or not the mother is actually infected or not.

However, women who have just caught syphilis within the past four to six weeks will test negative, even though they actually have the disease. This false-negative test could be picked up if women who are at higher risk of having syphilis are tested again later in the pregnancy. Once it is diagnosed, syphilis is easily treated with penicillin.

Syphilis starts with a painless "pimple" (usu-ally in the area of sexual contact where the infection was passed on such as the vagina, mouth, or anus), which heals, then causes rash and flu-like symptoms, and then remains dor-mant for years before causing multiple problems. During this whole time, the woman is infectious for syphilis.

If a mother has syphilis, and it is left untreated, her baby has an almost 100 per cent chance of catching syphilis before birth. About 20 to 40 per cent of these babies will die before birth. If the baby is born with congenital syphilis, it may be very ill, with permanent damage to the heart, lungs, and liver. Other babies are born looking well but have syphilis germs present in the bloodstream and nervous system. All of these babies can be treated with penicillin, but while the drug will kill the germs it can't heal the dam-age that is already done.

If the mother is treated with penicillin, the cure rate for her is virtually 100 per cent. The cure rate for her unborn baby depends on how long the baby was infected. Usually the fetus

The Evidence About...
Syphilis

A woman with syphilis may look and feel well, but the disease she is carrying, if left untreated, will be tragic for her baby. This is the reason the law requiring every pregnant woman to be tested was passed. Early treatment when syphilis is present can prevent serious problems for the baby as well as curing the mother.

does not pick up the infection until after the 18th week of pregnancy, so early treatment means the baby is likely to be healthy. Later in the preg-nancy, penicillin may cure the mother but not prevent harm to the baby. About 20 per cent of the babies born to mothers treated for syphilis towards the end of pregnancy will have been damaged by syphilis.

Talking to Your Doctor about Infections during Pregnancy

If you feel you are at risk for a sexually transmit-ted disease, because of multiple sexual partners, for example, you may feel uncomfortable talking to your doctor about this issue. But the test results and treatment may make a huge differ-ence to your baby, so it is well worth overcoming your anxiety.

Andrea struggled with asking about testing. "I'd been with quite a few men before I settled down with Quentin, and I have to confess we didn't always use condoms. Okay, I was young and foolish. I figured I could just put my past behind me—until I got pregnant."

Andrea decided she wanted the testing done, but dreaded making the request. "I couldn't sleep all night before my doctor's appointment. What if it turned out I had AIDS? How would I tell Quentin? And I wondered how my doctor would react."

As it turned out, though, her doctor was very understanding. "I started off saying I wanted to be tested for STDs, and then I was stumbling around trying to explain why, and my doctor told me I didn't have to explain my reasons, he'd be happy to arrange for the tests to be done." To Andrea's relief, they came back negative.

"I'm glad I did it," she says. "Even if it turned out I had an infection, I think it's better to know—especially when there's a baby involved."

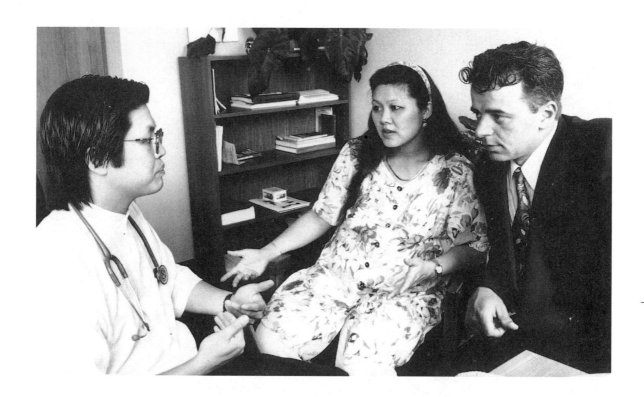

Six Months
❧ *Twenty-two to Twenty-five Weeks* ❧

You're getting used to the feeling of your baby moving inside you now, and probably enjoy having people notice that you're visibly pregnant. This is a good time to think about the kind of support you would like to have during labour and birth. Most women will have their partners with them, but having a doula or another support person as well has real benefits. Your caregiver may also recommend some more testing as you get closer to your baby's birth day, so here's some information to help you make decisions on these issues.

-26-

The Discomforts of Late Pregnancy

You probably think your belly is already pretty big, but over the next few months your uterus will grow bigger than you ever thought possible. Your growing baby will be putting pressure on your internal organs, and you may find that this last trimester brings some new discomforts. (This could be nature's plan to make you actually look forward to labour!) Here are some of the more common symptoms you might experience.

Heartburn

Heartburn is a common problem for pregnant women. It can be reduced to a certain extent by avoiding high-fat or spicy foods and by not lying down right after eating. If those measures don't help enough, any of the antacids available in drugstores can be tried, as research has found no harm to the baby from these. Lemon juice or acidic lemonade can also be tried; they were both found to be helpful.

Elevating the head of the bed to sleep can also reduce heartburn. This does not mean sleeping on more pillows, which can actually make heartburn worse. Instead, put blocks under the head of the bed (or insert a wedge between the mattress and box spring) to put the whole bed on a slight slant.

Leg Cramps

Leg cramps (sometimes called **charley horses**) are more common during pregnancy. Brenda remembers, "I woke up in the night with this terrible, really painful cramp in my leg, and I starting pounding on Marc's chest to get him to help me. He massaged my leg for a few minutes and it went away, but it happened again the next night."

Almost 50 per cent of women experience these severe cramps in their leg muscles, usually at night, at some point in their pregnancy. The muscle spasm can usually be stopped by jumping quickly out of bed and standing on the leg. (Of course, this requires you to roll yourself and your pregnant belly out of bed and stand up while in considerable pain.) Massaging also seems to help.

The most effective treatment appears to be taking **magnesium lactate** or **magnesium citrate**. These are over-the-counter supplements that you can buy as pills or as a drink (milk of magnesia). Diarrhea is occasionally a side effect if you take magnesium on an empty stomach. If your diet is normally low in salt, adding some salt may also help.

Swelling of the Legs

Swelling (**edema**) of the feet and legs is a common and normal symptom, which at least half of women notice by the end of their pregnancy. It is caused by the normal retention of fluid by the body during pregnancy to increase the circulating blood volume. A lot of the fluid accumulates in the legs because of gravity, and the pressure of the uterus slows down the return of fluid to the upper body. Often women will notice that when they get up in the morning, their hands and face may be puffy but their ankles are better, and then by the end of the day the fluid has collected in their feet and ankles.

Swelling during pregnancy requires no treatment, and there does not seem to be any treatment that is very helpful. Bed rest reduces swelling, but is rarely very practical. Keeping your feet up as much as possible can help—some women who are working at desks all day may be able to rest their feet on another chair, at least some of the time. If your job requires you to be on your feet most of the day, see if you can sit or lie with your feet elevated during breaks.

You will feel more comfortable if you have loose-fitting shoes—perhaps a pair in a larger size for wearing at the end of the day would be useful.

Swelling also seems to be made worse by heat. Tanya noticed that she had much more swelling during her two summer pregnancies than when she was pregnant during the winter. "I also found that being in air-conditioning really helped," she says.

Women worry about swelling because they know that it can be a symptom of pre-eclampsia, a serious disease sometimes seen in late pregnancy. Pre-eclampsia, though, also includes high blood pressure and protein in the urine—this is *not* normal and does require careful attention. But swelling by itself is a normal, though unpleasant, symptom of pregnancy.

Hemorrhoids and Varicose Veins

The fluid retention, which is normal in pregnancy, can also cause or make worse **hemorrhoids** (swollen veins around the anus) and **varicose veins** (usually in the legs, but sometimes seen in the vagina or vulva). Hemorrhoids are also made worse by constipation. There also seems to be an inherited tendency to both hemorrhoids and varicose veins.

Because the fluid retention and pressure caused by the growing uterus are normal events, there is no particular prevention for them. Special therapeutic elastic stockings may give some relief from the aching caused by fluid retention and varicose veins in the legs, but this has never been actually studied.

If hemorrhoids cause no symptoms, there is no reason to treat them. If they are itchy or sore, over-the-counter hemorrhoid creams or witch hazel are soothing and will not harm the mother or baby. Avoiding constipation is essential to keep hemorrhoids from getting worse.

Stretch Marks

Many women get these "stripes" on their bellies, breasts, and thighs during pregnancy. While they are a dark reddish purple colour at first, they fade to a silvery-white colour over time but never completely disappear.

The research suggests that massaging any cream into the skin on a daily basis will help to slightly reduce the incidence of stretch marks. The actual cream used doesn't seem to be as important as the daily massaging.

Stress Incontinence

During the last three months of pregnancy, many women (about 12 to 15 per cent) find that when they laugh, sneeze, or exert themselves (for example, by picking up a toddler) they will involuntary release a small amount of urine. Women who are overweight or obese are more likely to experience this problem. It usually improves after the baby is born, although childbirth is another risk factor for stress incontinence.

Special exercises for the muscles of the pelvic floor, often known as Kegel exercises, done frequently and fairly intensively, can prevent stress incontinence in pregnancy and after the baby is born, and can significantly improve it once it develops. Most prenatal class teachers will cover the basic techniques.

-27-
Hospital Routines

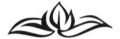

Your due date may still be some months away, but that doesn't mean it's too early to be thinking about the hospital procedures and routines. It's a good idea to go on a hospital tour—often included as part of a prenatal class—so that you're familiar with where to go and what to expect.

The weeks will go by quickly, and soon this could be you:

"Okay, honey, we're here." Your husband scoots around the car and opens the door and you climb out awkwardly. (It's at least nice to think that the next time you get out of the car your big belly won't be in the way.) Before you can walk into the hospital, another contraction hits and you lean on your husband as he gently rubs your back.

As the hospital doors slide open, you walk through. What happens next will depend a great deal on which hospital you have chosen to give birth in. Each hospital has its own policies and routines, and the variations can be quite dramatic even within the same geographic area.

What are some routines that you may encounter, and what steps can you take if you want to avoid some of them? Remember that just because something is routine at your particular hospital, that doesn't make it mandatory. You can always say no. Consider adding your preferences to your birth plan discussed in Chapter 1, page 25.

Admissions Procedures

In most hospitals, you will have to stop at the admitting department and register before going to labour and delivery. Some hospitals arrange for you to send in pre-registration forms ahead of time (or you can arrange this for yourself by checking with your hospital), but there is still a stop at the admitting department to let them know you have arrived and to pick up forms to take to labour and delivery. Sometimes the mother can go straight to labour and delivery and her partner can take care of the admission routines (be sure to have her birth date, insurance information, etc.).

When you arrive at labour and delivery, the nurse will start to make out your chart. She will

WHAT POSITION IS BETTER?

The Society of Obstetricians and Gynaecologists of Canada recommends that women be allowed to walk freely at all times during labour, to use baths or showers as they like, and to choose their own positions for giving birth.

want to hear about when the contractions started and how close together they are. She'll ask if there has been any bloody show or if the membranes have ruptured yet. She'll also ask some questions about your past health, your previous pregnancies, and how this pregnancy has gone, particularly about any special tests you may have had. All this will be written down on your chart.

Then the nurse will take your blood pressure, your temperature and your pulse, and ask you to pee into a bottle. She may do a vaginal examination as well. If you are in a teaching hospital, the intern or resident may come to see you, ask some of the same questions the nurse just asked, and may be the one to do the vaginal exam rather than the nurse.

Sometimes your partner and/or labour support people will be asked to leave during this initial examination; you can ask for them to stay with you. You will be offered a hospital gown to wear but you can bring a comfortable nightgown from home instead, if you prefer. A bathrobe can also be useful so that you won't feel as exposed as you walk around.

None of this admission procedure will be much of a problem if you are in early labour. If you've come in during very hard labour, responding to the nurse will be more difficult, and can break the concentration you are using to deal with your contractions. From the hospital's point of view, though, the paperwork is very important and has to be done. You (or your partner) can certainly ask them to wait until a contraction has ended.

Many hospitals ask all mothers to have the electronic fetal monitor attached for 20 minutes or so after admission, to provide a paper printout of the baby's heart rate to assess the baby's condition. The theory is that babies who need more intensive monitoring can be identified during this period of time. This has not been researched, so we do not know if it has any value. We do know that routine fetal monitoring throughout labour is linked to more unnecessary interventions. You are entitled to decide not to have the 20-minute strip done—just say you don't want to do it.

Patricia says, "When I arrived at the hospital in labour, the nurse said I had to have a 20-minute strip done. Well, I guess she was busy because she didn't come back to take me off the machine for over an hour. I was really uncomfortable lying there, my back hurt so much. But that wasn't the worst part. The worst was that Jeff was paying more attention to the machine than to me. He'd watch the graph and tell me when a contraction was coming—as if I couldn't feel it myself. Then he'd stare at the numbers, while I was trying to cope with the pain. I was so glad when she finally took it off and we could get up and walk around. Next time, I'm going to refuse to have it put on at all."

Enemas and shaving pubic hair were once common routines but since studies showed both had more negative effects than positive ones, they have been discontinued almost everywhere.

Hospital Routines for Labour and Delivery

Should you eat and drink during labour? Hospitals frequently have restrictions on whether women can eat or drink. In one survey, none of the hospitals studied allowed women to eat and drink as they wanted. Most allowed ice chips or sips of clear fluids, but no solid foods at all.

Why are these restrictions in place? The concern is that some emergency situation will arise that requires a Caesarean section under a general anaesthetic, and that the mother will vomit and inhale some of the food into her lungs while she is unconscious from the anaesthetic. The hope is that restricting food and drink during labour will guarantee an empty stomach in the rare situation that emergency general anaesthesia is needed.

However, not eating or drinking after admission to the hospital during labour does not guarantee an empty stomach, because labour slows down the digestion of food—so food that you ate four hours before you arrived at the hospital could still be sitting in your stomach. Even if the mother's stomach has no food in it, it is still possible for the stomach acid to be inhaled during general anaesthesia, causing burns to the lining of the lungs. This is a rare but serious problem. Taking antacids before you have the general anaesthetic will reduce the acidity but not prevent all cases of aspiration pneumonia.

In hospitals where mothers are not allowed to eat or drink, the policy may recommend giving the mother fluids and sugar intravenously instead. However, large volumes of sugar and water intravenously can result in both low blood sugar and low blood sodium in the newborn baby. This is because when the baby gets extra

sugar and salt from the mother before it is born, its body then begins to produce extra insulin (to counteract the sugar) and extra fluid (to counteract the sodium). Once the baby is born, the extra sugar and salt it was getting are suddenly no longer flowing in, but the insulin and fluid levels are still high, so the baby's blood sugar and sodium level will drop abruptly.

HOSPITAL ROUTINES TO AVOID

Research shows that some kinds of care women in labour may receive are *not* beneficial when used routinely (although some of these can be useful in specific situations).

During labour:

- routine continuous electronic fetal monitoring
- routinely withholding food and drink
- routine use of IV fluids
- regularly scheduled vaginal examinations
- keeping women in bed
- having a 20-minute session of continuous electronic fetal monitoring

During the pushing stage and birth:

- having the woman lying on her back with her legs up in stirrups to push the baby out
- routine or liberal use of episiotomy
- routine directed pushing
- pushing with the mother holding her breath and sustained bearing down
- encouraging bearing down or pushing as soon as the cervix is fully dilated
- routine use of vacuum extractor or forceps to shorten the pushing stage

Most women are not hungry during active labour. A reasonable approach might be to allow women to eat and drink as they choose during their whole labour. Most women will choose easy-to-digest, small meals and will stop eating as labour becomes more intense. Continuing to drink fluids during labour avoids dehydration, avoids the possible complications of intravenous fluids, and contributes only minimally to the risk of aspiration pneumonia in the rare situation in which general anaesthesia is needed.

Position during labour and for delivery is sometimes dictated by hospital routine: some hospitals still encourage labouring women to stay in bed during their labour, either as a general policy or because they frequently use electronic fetal monitors. Lying in bed on your back, even if the head of the bed is raised, is probably the worst position for labour. The pressure of the uterus on the blood vessels when you are lying on your back means that there is less blood flow to the uterus. Contractions are not as strong or as effective in this position. Several studies have found that the baby is more likely to show signs of distress (a slow or irregular heartbeat), and labour progresses more slowly, when mothers lie on their backs.

So what position is better? Women who stand, walk, or sit upright have shorter labours, on average, than women who are lying in bed. Walking seems to be especially helpful in encouraging effective contractions. Women who walked or stayed upright were less likely to use pain-relieving drugs, including epidurals. One study also found that babies born to mothers who were walking around during labour had fewer abnormal heart rate recordings and higher Apgar scores (see page 15), but other studies found no differences.

The Evidence About...
Hospital Routines

The benefits or hazards of using an electronic fetal monitor for 20 minutes on every woman when she arrives at the hospital have not yet been researched.

Not allowing women to eat or drink during labour does not guarantee protection against inhaling food or stomach acid in the event of surgery, and can have negative effects.

When women can choose to be upright and walking during labour, their labours are shorter and less painful.

Hilary was in labour for about 30 hours and says, "I walked almost the whole time. At first, we walked around the neighbourhood. Then when we got to the hospital, my contractions slowed down. I put my bathrobe on over the hospital gown and we went walking again. We walked all around the hospital, outside in the courtyard, into the parking lot and down the sidewalk. Every now and then I'd go back to the labour and delivery ward so the nurse could listen to the baby's heart."

Hilary tried sitting in the whirlpool, but her contractions slowed right down. "I had to get out and start walking again, it was the only way to keep my labour moving," she says.

Some labour and delivery units discourage women from leaving the department once they are admitted. This may mean there is literally no place to walk. You may be able to negotiate this, or if labour is still in the early stages you might prefer to go home and return when you are closer to giving birth.

-28-
Do You Want a Doula?

Almost all hospitals now permit the woman's partner to stay with her throughout labour and birth, and many will allow other labour support people to be there as well. Some hospitals allow only one person, but women sometimes want to have more than one. As Nazreen says, "I had a long, tough labour, and I don't know if I could have gotten through it without my husband, my mother, and my sister all with me. They took turns resting or napping and I always had someone to walk with me and rub my back."

A recent study looked at labour support given by people with specific training and experience, commonly known as doulas. It found that mothers who had labour support from other women who had learned techniques for coping with the pain of labour used less medication and fewer epidurals than mothers who had labour partners simply providing reassurance and emotional support.

Perhaps the best situation is when a woman has both the loving support of her partner and the expertise of a trained labour support woman.

What Does a Doula Do?

As well as a person to provide medical care, you might consider arranging for a doula or another support person to help you through labour. A doula is not a doctor or midwife, but a trained labour support person who usually meets with the woman and her partner during pregnancy, then stays with her throughout labour and birth. The doula doesn't provide medical care, but simply supports the mother and her partner. She could be a childbirth educator or student midwife; other doulas may be members of DONA (Doulas of North America).

A doula isn't just a good choice for someone with no other support people. Alisa, for example, had her family doctor, her husband, and her mother (also a doctor) with her when her baby was born, but she says, "I would testify to the *necessity* of professional labour support in addition to the presence of loved ones and family members." She laboured at home with her two doulas until about two hours before her daughter was born. "This arrangement was perfect for me. With the indispensable help of our doulas, we

> **The Evidence About...**
> **Doulas**
>
> One-on-one labour support from a trained support person can lead to shorter labours requiring less pain-relieving medication and fewer Caesareans.

had a peaceful, unmedicated (though very intense) birth."

If you are a single mother, or have a partner who is not planning to be part of labour and birth, a doula can be even more important. Lisa, a single mother, says that finding a doula "was the best decision I made." She met with this support person during her pregnancy and says that "by the time I was ready to give birth, I felt empowered. Even though my labour took 36 hours, I don't consider my birthing experience one of the hardest things I have done, but one of the best and certainly the most rewarding." She spent most of her labour at home, but went to the hospital seven hours before her son was born. Lisa delivered in a squatting position and had no medication. "The whole experience was so positive."

Isn't labour support the father or partner's role? Will the doula come between the husband and wife? Susan Martensen, president of DONA, says, "The doula doesn't replace the partner but helps him. He knows more about his wife, and can provide the love and closeness, but the doula knows more about labour and birth, and techniques that are helpful. Fathers often tell us how glad they were that the doula was there."

Research on doulas and having a support person during labour has been positive. In the research studies, the women who had doulas with them tended to have shorter labours, less medication, fewer forceps deliveries, and fewer Caesarean sections. However, these studies were done in hospital settings where the stress and anxiety levels were quite high, and the results may not apply to all labouring women.

However, it's natural for people to want support and companionship during any stressful or challenging experience. The women quoted above were less concerned about whether having doulas shortened their labours, and more interested in the added confidence and comfort they felt because of the support they received.

-29-
Gestational Diabetes

Karen's first baby, Michael, weighed 10 pounds (4,535 g) at birth. This didn't surprise her, since Karen and her husband are both tall and solidly built. Her labour with Michael was quite long, but the birth was straightforward, and he was a healthy, normal baby.

When Karen became pregnant again, her physician recommended that she be tested for gestational diabetes because her first child had been bigger than average.

"You mean I might have diabetes?" she asked.

"Gestational diabetes isn't the same as regular diabetes," her doctor explained. "It's diabetes caused by being pregnant, and it usually goes away as soon as you have the baby. But it might be a sign that you're likely to develop diabetes later."

Big babies can be a sign of gestational diabetes, he continued. Karen was overweight, and the doctor suggested this also might be a factor. He warned her that the babies of mothers with gestational diabetes, if the condition goes untreated, are at risk.

Worried, Karen went through the glucose tolerance test her physician recommended, and the test came up positive. She did have gestational diabetes. The doctor prescribed a strict calorie-reduced diet which she tried hard to follow.

Two months later, the doctor met with Karen to discuss the results of the ultrasound she had had the day before, to check the size of the baby.

"Have you been following the diet I gave you?"

"Most of the time," Karen said, feeling guilty about the times she had "cheated" a little and indulged in some forbidden treats.

"Well, the ultrasound shows that this is going to be another big baby."

"Bigger than Michael?"

"That depends on whether or not you stick to the diet. I think we should plan to induce labour about two weeks before your due date. I'll book the date at the hospital."

Karen was worried about being induced. "Is that really necessary? I've heard that induced labours are harder than regular ones—and won't the baby be premature?"

Her doctor waved the ultrasound report at her. "Look how big this baby is already. It'll weigh more than 9 pounds (4,080 g) even two weeks early."

LABORATORY TESTING FOR GESTATIONAL DIABETES

Usually, a blood sugar test is done first when the mother has had nothing to eat (this is called a **fasting blood sugar**). Then the **screening test** is given—a drink containing 50 grams of sugar is taken, and the blood sugar is tested one hour later. If this result is 7.8 mmol/l (140.4 mg/dl) or higher, the screen is considered positive. If a woman has a positive screen, then a more formal test—called a **glucose tolerance test**—is performed. This involves drinking 100 grams of sugar and having the blood sugar tested after one, two, and three hours. Upper limits of normal are 10.5 mmol/l (189 mg/dl) after one hour, 9 mmol/l (162 mg/dl) after two hours and 8 mmol/l (144 mg/dl) after three hours. If the woman's results meet or are higher than any two of these three limits, the diagnosis of gestational diabetes is made.

Two weeks before her due date, Karen's labour was induced. Amanda weighed 9 pounds, 8 ounces (4,309 g). Karen found the labour difficult and used more painkillers than she had for Michael; she was also worried about her baby's health because of the diabetes. She and her husband were very relieved when the pediatrician told them Amanda was fine.

When Karen became pregnant again, the doctor recommended that she take insulin as well as following the diet he recommended, since the diet alone clearly "hadn't worked." So Karen took insulin injections and ate according to the doctor's instructions. She used a glucometer at home to measure her blood sugar. Even though it was usually in the normal range, she worried a lot

about it. Again, the doctor's measurements and ultrasound examinations showed a larger-than-average baby so Karen was induced two weeks before her due date. Thomas weighed 9 pounds, 10 ounces (4,366 g) and was also very healthy.

Karen has three healthy children. During her first pregnancy she considered herself to be normal, but through the next two she thought of herself as "high risk" because of her gestational diabetes. Worrying about this made her last two pregnancies very stressful. She felt guilty every time she ate anything sweet or not listed on her diet sheet. She had several ultrasounds during each of her last two pregnancies to check on the size of the babies. In her third pregnancy, she used insulin injections every day from 28 weeks until she was induced at 38 weeks.

What really were the risks to Karen's babies, and were these risks reduced by the treatment she received?

Gestational diabetes is **glucose intolerance** appearing during pregnancy. The mother feels perfectly well and healthy. The "intolerance" is not like an allergy or food intolerance that might make someone feel ill—it means that the blood sugar level measured during the test is higher than average. The diagnosis is made by the laboratory, based on a **glucose tolerance test** (see sidebar) which is done between 24 and 28 weeks of pregnancy. Some doctors recommend this test routinely for all pregnant women.

About 15 per cent of women who are given this test will screen positive, and of those, about 15 per cent will have a positive glucose tolerance test and be diagnosed with gestational diabetes. Unfortunately, this test is not very reliable. If Karen had done the test over again, it might well have come up normal the second time. That happens to between 50 and 70 per cent of the women who are retested.

The primary risk of gestational diabetes is having a larger-than-average baby. Up to 30 per cent of mothers with positive glucose tolerance tests have babies weighing more than 8 pounds, 12 ounces (4,000 g). With bigger babies, there are more Caesarean sections, and more cases where the baby's shoulders are "stuck" in the birth canal, making for a more difficult delivery. There may also be a small increased risk of the baby dying at the time of birth because of this.

In Karen's case, her chance of having a bigger than average baby could have been easily predicted from some other factors: her above-average weight before she got pregnant, the amount of weight that she gained during each pregnancy, and the fact that her first baby, Michael, had been 10 pounds (4,535 g) at birth. The test didn't really tell her doctor anything he didn't already know. The test isn't even all that good at predicting who will have a larger than average baby: 70 per cent of the mothers who test positive will have babies weighing less than 8 pounds, 12 ounces (4,000 g) even with no treatment, while the majority of larger-than-average babies are born to mothers with a normal glucose test.

A recent Australian study divided 1,000 pregnant women who had gestational diabetes into two groups. Half were not treated, and the other half were put on diabetic diets, encouraged to exercise and test their blood, and given insulin if their blood sugars remained high.

The treated group had more induced labours than the untreated group and more planned Caesarean births (although the total Caesarean rate was similar in both groups). More of the

DIABETES AND GESTATIONAL DIABETES

Diabetes is a disease of high blood sugar, which develops when either the pancreas does not produce any or enough insulin or the cells in the body stop responding to insulin.

Type 1 diabetes, an autoimmune disease, is also called insulin-dependent diabetes. It usually comes on fairly rapidly in young people, and requires insulin treatment.

Type 2 diabetes is sometimes called adult-onset diabetes (although more and more children are being diagnosed with it). This type of diabetes is strongly associated with older age, obesity, and lack of physical exercise. It often comes on gradually; many people with Type 2 diabetes don't know they have it. It can sometimes be treated with a combination of nutritional changes and exercise and does not always require insulin.

Gestational diabetes or pregnancy diabetes is high blood sugar first occurring in pregnancy, which goes away after the baby is born. It is associated with obesity, and is associated with developing Type 2 diabetes in later life

babies in the treated group were admitted to the special care nursery after birth than in the untreated group.

However, the rate of significant complications for the baby (dying during the birth or soon after, having the baby's shoulder "stuck" in the birth canal, and being injured during the birth) was higher in the untreated group—4 per cent of those babies had difficulties, compared to 1.4 per cent of the babies in the treated group. And 21.9 per cent of the babies were larger than average,

> *The Evidence About...*
> **GESTATIONAL DIABETES**
>
> Good research has not shown clear benefits in screening for and diagnosing gestational diabetes.
>
> There is real potential for doing more harm than good by performing a glucose tolerance test. When the test is positive, the pregnancy is likely to be considered "high risk" and the mother may be started on an expensive and extensive program of tests and treatments with no proven benefits. The anxiety that is produced is completely out of proportion to any benefit from making the diagnosis.
>
> Diagnosing and treating gestational diabetes *may* reduce the risk of the mother developing Type 2 diabetes in the future, but research is needed to demonstrate this.

compared to 13.4 per cent of the babies in the treated group.

The authors of the study, while recommending testing for and treating gestational diabetes, also speculate that some if not all of the difference in the outcomes between the two groups may be due to the higher rate of induction and planned Caesarean births, since both of these interventions were usually done at least two weeks prior to the due date. This would explain why the babies were smaller and less likely to be injured during the birth, and could possibly also explain the higher rate of admission to the special care nursery in the treated group. If this speculation is correct, the other interventions (special diets and insulin) may have had little effect on the outcomes.

Concerns for the Mother

Women who test positive for gestational diabetes are six times more likely to develop Type 2 diabetes later. Having high levels of blood sugar, even just for the duration of a pregnancy, can cause some harmful side effects, and if a mother has repeated pregnancies her risk of diabetic complications could become significant. Some doctors feel that future risk is a good reason to screen for diabetes as it gives the mother the opportunity to make intensive changes to her eating and exercise habits in the hopes of preventing future Type 2 diabetes.

Should I Be Tested for Gestational Diabetes?

The expert researchers who analyze the research for the Cochrane database continue to recommend against routine testing for gestational diabetes, since treatment with diet and/or insulin has not been shown to improve the outcome for the mother or the baby and a positive test for gestational diabetes is likely to increase the mother's stress and anxiety level.

There may be some benefits in terms of identifying women who are at risk for developing Type 2 diabetes in the future so that they can take steps to reduce this risk, but this has not been demonstrated.

What about Regular Diabetes?

It's important to understand that gestational diabetes is *not* the same as regular or **overt diabetes**. Overt diabetes, with high fasting blood sugar and high blood sugar after meals, is a disease which can start in childhood or adolescence and which does cause significant complications during pregnancy.

Occasionally, overt diabetes will be diagnosed for the first time during pregnancy; the symptoms are intense thirst and unusual hunger, weight loss, passing large amounts of urine, and high blood sugar, both fasting and after meals. Overt diabetes requires treatment involving special diet, exercise, and usually insulin therapy. This treatment must be continued after the baby is born as well. Pregnancy complications are higher for women with overt diabetes than for non-diabetic women; this complication rate can be improved by careful attention to blood sugar control before and during pregnancy.

-30-
Bleeding in the Third Trimester of Pregnancy

"Normal show" or "bloody show" is the name given to the slight vaginal bleeding that often is the first sign that labour is starting. The blood is usually mixed with thick mucus and may be more pink than red when you see it. *Any other bleeding in the latter half of pregnancy is not normal, and should be reported to your caregiver right away.*

About half the women who have bleeding in the second half of their pregnancy are found to have either an abruption of the placenta or a placenta previa. For the other half, the cause of the bleeding is not known.

Abruption of the Placenta

This is the separation of part of the placenta from the wall of the uterus before the delivery of the baby. It can range from a minor bit of bleeding, which does no harm, to a very dangerous situation for both mother and baby.

If you have a **placental abruption**, you will usually see some bleeding and feel abdominal pain. The baby may be in distress as well.

Separation at the edge of the placenta causes the most bleeding, but because it is not near the umbilical cord, it may be less risky to the fetus. If the central part of the placenta separates, there may be hardly any vaginal bleeding, but the fetus is at great risk. In other words, you can't judge how serious this is by the amount of bleeding you experience.

Often an ultrasound can identify an abruption, but sometimes it is hard to recognize. Significant abruptions usually make labour start. Big abruptions, as well as threatening the life of the fetus, can cause abnormalities in the clotting of the mother's blood.

Treatment of abruption depends completely on its severity. If it is minor, the bleeding may stop on its own, the baby will be fine, and the pregnancy can continue to term. If it is severe, though, the mother may need intravenous fluids and blood transfusions to treat her shock and clotting problems, and delivery of the baby is urgent. Each woman with a severe abruption must be assessed individually to decide if vaginal delivery or Caesarean section is a better choice.

Placenta Previa

A placenta previa is a placenta which is either partially or completely covering the cervix. This occurs in about 1 out of 200 births, and can be diagnosed by ultrasound.

Placenta previa causes painless vaginal bleeding, almost always before the onset of labour (only 2 per cent of women with this condition have no bleeding until labour starts). If labour proceeds, this is a very dangerous situation because as the cervix opens the placenta will bleed very heavily. Caesarean section is the treatment, and is life-saving for the mother.

The risk to the baby depends on how premature it is when the Caesarean section has to be performed because of bleeding. If the baby is at term, both mother and baby should do well.

A pelvic examination should never be performed when placenta previa is suspected, as even touching the cervix when the placenta is implanted right over it can start heavy bleeding.

-31-

Group B Streptococcus

It might surprise you to know that all of us, even when we're perfectly healthy, have bacteria living in our bodies. We tend to think of bacteria as causing diseases, but many exist in our bodies without causing any harm to us. These bacteria are called the **normal flora** and parts of our bodies (such as the throat, bowel, and vagina) will have (or "be colonized with") these normal flora most of the time.

One of these common and normal bacteria, which is particularly significant for pregnant women, is the Group B streptococcus bacteria, also called **beta strep**. The normal flora of a woman's vagina and rectum can include Group B streptococcus. At the time of delivery, about 15 to 20 per cent of women will have Group B strep colonizing their vaginas.

Group B strep usually causes no symptoms in the mother. Occasionally, it can cause urinary tract infections, or in rare cases, an infection of the placenta, which can cause premature rupture of the membranes and premature labour.

The main reason health care professionals are concerned about this bacteria, though, is that Group B strep can make newborn babies very ill.

It is the most common infection in newborns. The bacteria can infect the baby during labour or at delivery as the baby passes through the vagina.

As mentioned earlier, 15 to 20 per cent of mothers are carrying Group B strep in their vaginas during labour. Between 40 and 70 per cent of the babies born to these women will be colonized with Group B strep at birth—the research figures vary widely. Of those "colonized" babies, only 1 to 2 per cent will actually develop an infection. When you calculate all these numbers, the rate of Group B streptococcus infection in newborns is about 2 cases per 1,000 babies. So even though about 20 per cent of women carry these strep bacteria in their vaginas at the time of delivery, very few of the babies will be sick.

Those numbers are low, but because the infection is very serious, it is still a cause for concern.

Group B strep disease in the newborn can be obvious at birth, or can develop during the first week of life. (There is also a "late onset" Group B strep disease which begins within the first three months of life and is probably caused by bacteria passed on to the baby after the birth. It can best be prevented by having people wash their hands thoroughly before they touch the baby.)

It is the early onset form of this disease that has generated the most attempts at prevention.

When the disease was first recognized in the 1970s, death rates were as high as 50 per cent. Today the death rate is down to 10 per cent. This improvement may be because the bacteria has become weaker over time, or because of earlier and more aggressive treatment. But a 10 per cent death rate is still very frightening to parents with a sick baby.

When one or more risk factors are present (see sidebar), the baby may be labelled "high risk" for having a strep infection.

Remember that "high risk," in medical and statistical terms, means a risk significantly above the usual or normal risk. A chance of infection of 20 per 1,000 when the usual rate is only 2 per 1,000 would be called high risk. But this is still only an infection rate of 2 per cent; 98 per cent of these babies are *not* going to be infected.

So even in a group of babies labelled "high risk," the majority are still not going to have a strep infection.

This is important to know because often women who are told their babies are at high risk of this infection think it means the baby is almost certain to be sick.

Tina's second baby had been sick with a beta strep infection but recovered and was fine. "When I got pregnant this time," she says, "I was told that this baby was at high risk for beta strep. I remembered how terrible it was when Zachary was sick, and I didn't know how I would go through it again. Then I went into labour prematurely—another risk factor. Mario and I were so worried. The doctor recommended having intravenous antibiotics, which I did. Chloe weighed 4 pounds, 6 ounces (1,984 g), but she never came down with beta strep. It seemed like a miracle the day we took our healthy daughter home from the hospital."

Strategies to Prevent Group B Strep

Can Group B strep infections in newborns be prevented? No single strategy has been completely successful, and some treatments which have been tried have been shown in clinical trials to be ineffective.

WHO IS MORE LIKELY TO GET GROUP B STREP?

Which babies are at the greatest risk of getting Group B strep infection? Major risk factors include:

- baby was premature and had a low birth weight
- membranes were ruptured for more than 18 hours before the baby was born
- labour was long, with many interventions and frequent vaginal examinations
- tests of mother's vagina showed heavy colonization of Group B strep
- during labour, the mother had a fever or the baby had an unusually fast heart rate
- baby needed resuscitation at birth
- mother has had a previous baby with a Group B strep infection

SCREENING DURING PREGNANCY

The first approach was to test all pregnant women to find out if they had the Group B strep in their vaginas. Doing the test is easy and painless; the opening of the vagina is wiped with a swab which is put into culture medium in a tube and sent to the lab. It takes 24 hours to get the results.

However, colonization of the vagina by strep occurs intermittently during the nine months of pregnancy. Sometimes it's there, sometimes it's not. Seventy per cent of women who tested positive for Group B strep in their vaginas at 28 weeks of pregnancy did not have strep bacteria present when they were retested during labour.

Positive test results after 34 weeks of pregnancy are much more likely to also be positive at delivery. Testing later in pregnancy, then, sounds like a better approach. But remember the list of risk factors? A premature baby was first on the list. Waiting until after 34 weeks to do the culture means that women who go into premature labour (when the risk of infection is higher) will not have been tested, and so they will not know if they have Group B strep in their vagina.

PREVENTIVE TREATMENT DURING PREGNANCY

Once women with Group B strep in their vaginas were identified, researchers hoped that giving these women antibiotics during pregnancy would reduce the number of babies with the infection. Unfortunately, the studies found that it didn't work.

If, however, the mother has a bladder infection caused by Group B strep, giving antibiotics

can be useful, as studies have shown that this reduces the chance of premature rupture of the membranes and premature labour.

PREVENTIVE TREATMENT DURING LABOUR

Although antibiotics given during pregnancy were not effective, treatment of the mother during labour with intravenous antibiotics has been shown by studies to reduce infection rates in newborns. This is very encouraging, but leads to another question: Which women should be given the antibiotics?

The obvious solution would be to test women for strep during labour. However, since testing for Group B strep takes at least 24 hours (longer if a lab is not constantly available), the results of tests done during labour are not available quickly enough to be useful.

Several different approaches have been suggested and are used by various caregivers:

- Testing all women for the strep bacteria at 28 weeks of pregnancy, and treating all strep carriers who have any other risks (e.g., prematurity, fever during labour, prolonged rupture of membranes) with intravenous antibiotics during labour.
- Treating all women in premature labour with IV antibiotics; and testing everyone else at 36 weeks of pregnancy and treating only those women who tested positive with intravenous antibiotics during labour.
- Treating all women who have one or more risk factors for strep infection, without doing any tests for strep.

Each one of these approaches has been shown to reduce the risk of newborn strep infection.

Unfortunately, though, each of these approaches also means giving antibiotics to many, many women whose babies would never have developed an infection anyway.

TREATING THE BABY AFTER BIRTH

Newborns with Group B strep infections are born with the illness already present, or become ill in the first few hours after birth. But the symptoms are not very obvious.

If your baby is born infected with Group B strep, his early symptoms will be vague: he could be lethargic, irritable, and not feeding well. He may have a fast heart and respiration rate. Cultures of the baby's blood and spinal fluid are the definitive way to make the diagnosis, but it takes 24 to 48 hours to get results. It's important to diagnose this infection quickly, because the earlier the baby is treated with antibiotics, the better the outcome.

This puts the doctor, and the parents, in a difficult position. Is newborn baby Adam lethargic, or just a relaxed and quiet baby? Is baby Benjamin jittery and irritable because of illness or because he has a sensitive and fussy temperament? How long should we wait before starting treatment? Most pediatricians feel "it's better to be safe than sorry," so many infants who do not have infections are treated with antibiotics to be sure that the few who are infected are treated early.

Some infants will be born who do look perfectly well, but are considered to be at risk for infection because of one or more risk factors during labour, such as a mother colonized by strep, prolonged rupture of the membranes, or prematurity. There are no good studies to suggest the best way to take care of these babies. Routines for their care will vary from hospital to hospital, and even among individual pediatricians at the same hospital. These routines can be one of the following:

- the usual care given to every baby, with no special tests or antibiotics;
- doing blood counts and cultures for strep, and then observing the baby while waiting for these results;
- giving preventive intravenous antibiotics without waiting for the results of tests or observations, for varying lengths of time.

There are no studies to suggest which of these approaches is the best care for babies who look well but are identified as being at risk. Similarly, there are no studies to suggest the best care for babies whose mothers have received antibiotics during labour because of risk factors, but who are born looking perfectly well.

Since there isn't any conclusive research, you and your caregiver should evaluate your individual situation and make a decision together about the best approach.

Overuse of Antibiotics: Why the Concern?

Does it matter that antibiotics are being given to many mothers and babies who would never develop this disease?

The Evidence About...

Group B Strep

This is a rare (2 cases per 1,000 babies), but serious infection for newborn babies.

While some risk factors are known, we can't predict very accurately which babies will develop the problem. Any treatment to reduce the number of infected babies will mean giving antibiotics to large numbers of mothers and babies who don't need them, and will miss some babies who really do need treatment.

The side effects of this treatment may seem minor for the individual mother and baby, but the consequences of increasingly resistant bacteria are serious for society as a whole.

Yes, because there are side effects and complications from antibiotics that are significant. The most important complication of unnecessary antibiotic use is the development of resistant bacteria—bacteria that do not die when the sick person is given antibiotics. (It is the bacteria that becomes resistant, not the person.) This is an increasingly serious problem in our society, but it does not affect, in any way we can measure, the individual mother and her baby at the time she is given the antibiotics.

For individual mothers and babies, antibiotics can cause side effects like diarrhea and yeast infections. There is also an effect, difficult to measure, of labelling babies as "high risk," and separating them from their mothers to treat them with IV antibiotics. This creates anxiety in the mother, may make it difficult to establish breastfeeding, and may affect the relationship she develops with her baby.

Regina's premature baby was considered to be at high risk of infection and was treated with antibiotics in the intensive care nursery. Regina was discharged from the hospital and had to leave her newborn behind, although she visited every day. Regina remembers: "I think it was worse for my husband, Alec, than it was for me. I spent more time with the baby, and I thought he looked pretty good. But my husband focused on the IV and the monitoring equipment and how small our son was, and he was convinced he was going to die."

Even when the baby came home, Alec felt nervous handling the baby and Regina says it took him some time to believe that this child would survive.

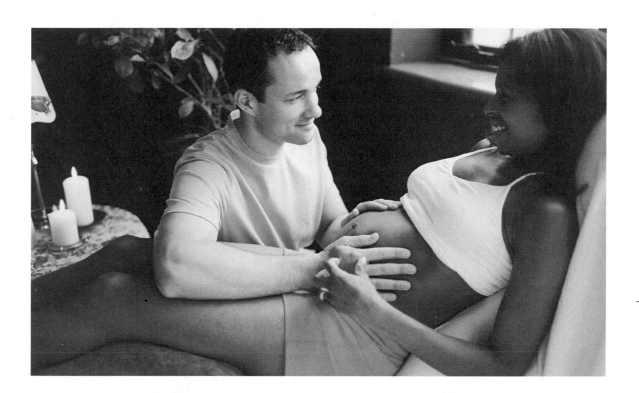

Seven Months
❧ *Twenty-six to Twenty-nine Weeks* ❧

Sometimes when your baby kicks or moves, you may think to yourself, "Oh, that's a foot" or "this part has got to be the baby's head." Babies take many different positions inside the uterus, and it can be important to know how your baby is positioned when it's time to give birth.

At this point it's also important to be aware of the possibility of a premature birth. While most babies born at this stage will survive, they will need extra medical care as their bodies are not really ready for life outside the womb. This section will tell you more about premature birth and premature babies.

-32-
Your Baby's Position in the Uterus

Your doctor presses her hands against your very pregnant belly, slides them down towards your pelvis, and announces: "Feels like a vertex presentation, probably anterior."

It might sound like a foreign language, but all your doctor means is that your baby is in the most common position: head down, with its face towards your backbone. The word **presentation** means the baby's position inside the uterus; the part of the baby's body which comes out of your vagina first is called the **presenting part**.

About 95 per cent of babies are head-down at the time of birth—this is called a **cephalic**, or a **vertex** presentation. Earlier in pregnancy, when the baby is smaller, her position will change frequently as she moves around inside the uterus. The baby will be head-down sometimes and feet-down at other times. Probably because the baby's head is normally the heaviest part of her body,

The most common presentation: the baby is head-down and baby's face, angled slightly to one side, is towards the mother's spine.

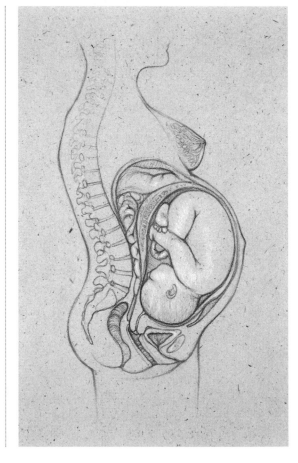

she will usually settle into a head-down position a few weeks before birth.

Even with head-down babies, though, there are some variations.

Posterior Position

About one in four babies will be in a posterior position during labour. This means that the baby is head-down but the baby's face is towards the mother's stomach. Often the baby will rotate around to the more common **anterior** position (with the face towards the mother's back) either during labour or at the time of birth, but as long as the baby is in the posterior position, labour is likely to be longer and more painful.

Susan's third child was posterior, and the intense back pain she felt during this labour took her by surprise. "With Zoe, my posterior baby, when the contractions went away, the pain didn't stop. It wasn't as intense as when I was having a contraction, but it was a strong ache in my back. And the labour went on and on—18 hours altogether."

Susan found that having steady pressure on her back right at the centre of the pain was the most helpful. She also spent a good part of her labour kneeling on the bed. "I walked around with the other two but walking made me feel worse with Zoe. So I knelt on the bed and rocked."

After 18 hours, Susan says, "I felt something move. I didn't know what it was, but I yelled to Steve—who was still patiently rubbing my back—to call the nurse. Zoe had finally turned, and she was born within a couple of minutes. The doctor just barely made it."

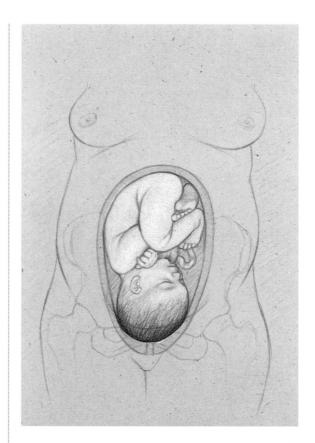

In the posterior position, the baby is again head-down and slightly to one side, but the back of the head is towards the mother's spine. The increased pressure against the spine frequently causes backache during labour.

Most babies in a posterior position, like Zoe, will turn spontaneously at some time during the labour and be born in the usual position, with their faces looking down. Some babies will stay in a posterior position and will be born face-up. This is unusual and usually causes some comment in the delivery room—these babies are referred to as being "sunny-side up."

When a baby stays in the posterior position, it is more difficult to push out, and some women

A FACE-FIRST BABY

Elizabeth was in hard labour with her second baby. "How much longer do you think it will be?" she asked her doctor.

The doctor did a pelvic exam and looked puzzled. "Well, Elizabeth, I'm not feeling what I'm expecting to find," she said. "The cervix is well over half dilated, but the presenting part of the baby doesn't feel like a head; it feels soft."

"Does that mean something's wrong with the baby?" Elizabeth asked in a panic. Suddenly the pain of the contractions felt like nothing compared to this new worry.

"I don't know. I just can't tell what I'm feeling. I'll get the radiologist to come and do an ultrasound. That should tell us what's what."

The radiologist, called out of bed at 3 a.m., showed up 10 minutes later in shorts and sandals. He could see how worried Elizabeth and her doctor were, and the ultrasound was quickly arranged. It showed that the baby was in a face presentation.

"The soft, squishy things I was feeling are the baby's lips and cheeks—I'm glad I was gentle!" laughed the doctor.

"But can I get the baby out in this position? I almost feel like I have to push already," asked Elizabeth.

She had had an easy labour with her first baby, who was over 8 pounds (3,625 g). The doctor was obviously not worried, now that she knew what she had been feeling in the vagina. "Your labour seems to be going fast. I'm sure you'll be able to deliver this baby. But be prepared for the face to look really swollen and bruised."

Elizabeth says: "The actual birth was amazing. The pushing felt just like with my first baby but it went a lot faster. After just a couple of big pushes, I could feel the burning at the opening. The doctor had set a mirror up so I could watch. The first things we saw were these swollen purple things. As the baby came further out, we realized they were his lips! Then came the cheeks, then the whole rest of the head and body. He started crying right away, so I knew he was fine, but did he ever look funny. His lips and cheeks were so swollen, his face looked like a little piggy. That disappeared within a few days, and he was as handsome as his dad."

will push for a long period of time without making much progress. In these cases, the doctor will usually suggest helping to get the baby out with a vacuum extractor or forceps. The mother will usually be given an epidural, and then the doctor will either try to turn the baby into an anterior position so that it can be pushed out more easily, or will simply deliver the baby in the posterior position.

Sometimes it becomes clear that the posterior baby is not going to turn, and is not going to fit through the mother's pelvis in this position.

Then a Caesarean section may be the safest course for both mother and baby. Each situation must be evaluated individually.

Face or Brow Presentation

In less than 1 per cent of pregnancies, the baby will be head-down but have his or her neck arched, so that either the baby's face or forehead is coming through the vagina first. Usually, the labour contractions will gradually change this

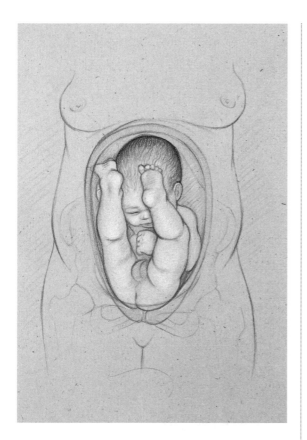

A frank breech presentation, with the baby's legs folded up against his body. Some breech babies "sit" in the pelvis with their legs crossed (complete breech) or even extend one or both legs straight down (footling breech).

position to the more common chin tucked-in position. If the baby remains with the forehead first (called a brow presentation), a Caesarean section is usually necessary, as this presentation of the baby's head just does not fit through the birth canal. If the baby's neck really arches so that the face actually presents, the baby can often be born vaginally.

Compound Presentation

Lesley's first child was a compound presentation. She says, "My water broke several days after Melissa was due, and I went into labour right away. Labour was pretty intense, but short and I didn't need much medication. But the pushing stage was really hard and long and more painful than I had expected."

The reason for that unexpectedly difficult pushing stage was clear as soon as baby Melissa emerged. Her left arm was extended up beside her head; the pressure of the birth left an imprint of her hand on the side of her face that lasted several days.

A compound presentation means that more than one part of the baby is trying to get through the birth canal at once. In some cases, like Lesley's, it can just make the birth more difficult; in other cases, vaginal birth is impossible and a Caesarean section is necessary. Compound presentation cannot be diagnosed before labour, as babies move around in the uterus, and even during labour the baby's position can shift.

Breech Presentation

Some babies take a completely opposite approach to birth—they want to come out bottom or feet first. This is known as a breech presentation. About 15 per cent of babies are breech at 29 to 32 weeks, and between 3 to 4 per cent will still be breech when labour begins. Once labour is active, it is unlikely that the baby will turn by itself because of the tightness of the uterus—however, some do "flip over" during labour.

Turning Breech Babies

Linda, whose son Joshua is now two years old, was told by her midwife that Joshua was in a breech position when she was 32 weeks pregnant. The midwife suggested she try some positioning exercises—"basically having my bum stuck up in the air"—two or three times a day to see if the baby would turn head-down, but it didn't work. She also visited another midwife who attempted an **external version**. This is a technique to turn the baby into a head-down position by manipulating the baby through the mother's abdomen. This was also unsuccessful.

At 37 weeks, Linda went to an obstetrician and a second attempt at external version was made. This time she had an intravenous started and was given **ritodrine**, a drug to relax her uterus. Linda had both the obstetrician and an intern working together to move her baby and "it felt like the baby was going to come out of my mouth while they were doing it." Twenty minutes later, her baby was head-down, and three weeks later her healthy baby boy was born vaginally. "Yes," she says, "it was well worth the trouble to get him turned around."

Strategies to turn a breech baby into the more favourable head-down position include exercises for the mother, such as the ones Linda tried, and a technique called external version of the baby.

USING THE MOTHER'S POSITION

Midwives have often suggested exercises for women to do to turn breech babies. One is for the mother to lie on her back, flexing her hips

and knees, and to roll from side to side for five or ten minutes. Another is for the mother to go on her hands and knees on the floor and have someone else actually shake the uterus for a few minutes.

The third, and the only one to have been studied at all, is for the mother to kneel on the floor with her hips flexed a bit but not pressing on her abdomen, and her head and shoulders on the floor, for 15 minutes three times a day. The single uncontrolled study that was done found no difference in outcome that could not have been caused by chance.

EXTERNAL VERSION OF BREECH BABIES

External version, when done by a doctor, is usually performed in hospital. Usually a recording of the baby's heart rate is done first for 15 or 20 minutes. An ultrasound is used to locate the placenta and the umbilical cord and to identify the exact position of the baby's legs. The physician puts his hands on the mother's abdomen and tries to rotate the baby around, watching the ultrasound to make sure that the heart rate remains normal.

Some breech positions will turn more easily than others. If the baby has its hips and knees bent so it is all curled up, the version is most likely to succeed. If the baby's legs are sticking straight up, or if they are dangling down into the pelvis, version is less likely to work.

External version has some risks. It is safest if it is performed with continuous ultrasound, so that the position of the placenta can be seen, and the fetal heart rate can be continuously monitored. Moving the baby can occasionally cause the placenta to be separated from the wall of the uterus, resulting in bleeding and fetal distress. (Rh-negative mothers who are having versions should be given Rh immune globulin—see Chapter 12.) Being turned can also cause slowing of the baby's heart rate, presumably because of tangling or compression of the umbilical cord. If fetal distress occurs, the doctor will stop trying to turn the baby, and if the heart rate does not improve promptly, a Caesarean section may be needed.

Lisa was about 34 weeks pregnant with her second child when the doctor told her the baby was in a breech position. "I knew something was different from my first pregnancy. I could feel a hard bump under my ribs that wasn't there when I was pregnant with Olivia."

Her doctor scheduled an ultrasound when Lisa was 37 weeks pregnant and the baby's position hadn't changed. "I have to admit I was scared. My doctor offered us the option of trying a version. We went into the hospital, and the doctor explained that if the version caused fetal distress, he would need to do an immediate Caesarean section. I also knew that it could bring on labour, so I had Gary and my labour support person with me as well."

Lisa was settled in bed and attached to an ultrasound machine and a fetal monitor. "The baby's heart rate was great, and we could all see her little head right up under my ribs." After a few minutes to be sure the heart rate was stable, the obstetrician placed his hand behind the bump on Lisa's stomach that showed where her baby's head was, and pushed. "It was a bit uncomfortable but not as bad as I had thought it might be. And it was over much faster than I had expected."

Watching the ultrasound while he manoeuvred the baby into position, Lisa's doctor made sure that the baby wasn't tangled in the umbilical cord or showing signs of distress. Within a few minutes, her baby was head-down. Lisa stayed sitting up in her hospital bed for another hour while nurses monitored the baby's heart rate, but the actual procedure had taken only five minutes. That evening she walked around a lot, hoping it would help the baby's head settle deeper into her pelvis.

"I worried that the baby would flip back, but she didn't," Lisa says. And five weeks later, she delivered a 9-pound (4,080-g) baby girl—head first—after a short, straightforward labour.

What Is the Best Timing for an External Version?

While it's easier to turn the baby early in pregnancy (because baby is smaller and there is more amniotic fluid), waiting until you are 37 weeks pregnant is usually a better choice. If you turn the baby earlier, there is still enough room that the baby may move back into the breech position. By waiting, the baby may flip into a head-down position on its own. It also allows enough time for complications like **placenta previa**—which will require a Caesarean delivery anyway—to show up. As well, at 37 weeks, the baby is mature enough to be born, so that if the version does cause a separation of the placenta or fetal distress from tangling the cord, the baby can be promptly delivered by Caesarean section without running the risks of prematurity.

External version after 37 weeks reduces by 80 per cent the chance of the baby being breech at delivery.

EXTERNAL VERSION IN EARLY LABOUR

Turning of breech in early labour has been reported to be successful in 75 per cent of cases, but the studies have been very small. Using drugs to relax the uterus may increase the success rate of the procedure and reduce the amount of force needed.

Complications of Vaginal Breech Delivery

The reason that so much attention has been paid to turning breech babies into a head-down position is that the breech position is associated with a higher death rate for the baby. Breech babies do tend to have a higher rate of congenital abnormalities, so not all of the risk is due to the delivery itself.

The actual delivery of a breech baby is more difficult than a head-down baby. With a head-down baby, the vagina is gradually stretched as the large head descends. When the baby is breech, the relatively small and soft buttocks and legs deliver first and the perineum does not get very stretched. Then the larger shoulders and head have to manoeuvre through quickly so the baby can start breathing. For this reason, episiotomy in a breech delivery is often done to speed up the birth.

If the baby is coming feet-first rather than buttocks first, there is a 15 per cent risk of **cord prolapse**—the umbilical cord slipping through the cervix ahead of the baby. This is dangerous because the cord will be compressed and cut off the baby's oxygen supply. An emergency Caesarean section is the treatment.

Breech birth is riskier for premature babies, because their tiny legs and buttocks may deliver before the cervix is fully dilated; then the relatively large head may be trapped. This can lead to a very difficult delivery with possible injury to the baby's brain.

Caesarean Section versus Vaginal Breech Delivery

Recent studies found that planned Caesarean sections reduced the risk of breech babies dying or suffering serious injury during the birth, although there was increased morbidity (infection or injury) for the mother in the Caesarean groups. The experts who reviewed the research for the Cochrane database point out that external version should be attempted first, and that the results would not apply to "methods of breech delivery that differ from the clinical delivery protocols used in the trials reviewed." About 45 per cent of the mothers in the "planned vaginal birth" part of the studies ended up having Caesarean births, which could suggest that the doctors were not skilled or entirely comfortable doing vaginal breech births. The Cochrane reviewers add that decision making about breech delivery should still be made on an individual basis, and that research on strategies to improve the safety of breech birth is needed.

As a result of this research, most North American doctors recommend a planned Caesarean birth for any baby in a breech position. However, some other countries, such as Norway and Sweden, continue to have a significant number of vaginal breech births and are

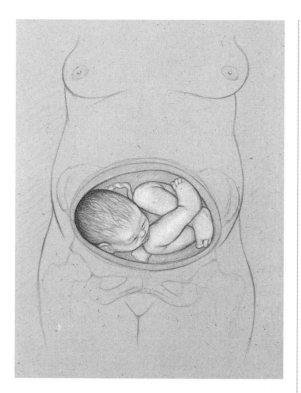

A transverse lie. If the baby can't be turned by external version, a Caesarean delivery will be required.

actively researching ways to make these births safer for both mother and babies.

Transverse Lie

Approximately 1 in 500 babies will be in a transverse position—lying at right angles to the birth canal with perhaps a shoulder or arm as the pre-

The Evidence About...
Your Baby's Position

Using external version to turn breech babies after 37 weeks substantially reduces the chance of the baby being breech in labour. This reduces the risk of Caesarean section.

When a baby is in a breech position and can't be turned by external version, a planned Caesarean birth may reduce the risk of the baby dying or being injured during the birth.

senting part. (This is completely different from the *head* being in a transverse position in the birth canal, which means it is rotated half-way between anterior and posterior.)

About 80 per cent of babies in a transverse lie at 37 weeks will move to a normal head-down position before delivery, so usually the physician or midwife will simply wait and see.

In early labour, if the baby is still in a transverse position, it is worth trying external version—pushing the baby into a head-down position by manipulating through the mother's belly. The success rate for this isn't very high, but if the baby doesn't move, a Caesarean section will be needed.

-33-
Hypertension (High Blood Pressure) and Pre-eclampsia

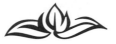

You've probably noticed that every prenatal appointment includes a check of your blood pressure. What exactly is being measured?

There are two numbers in every blood pressure reading: one, called the **systolic blood pressure** (usually given as the first or top number) measures the height of the pumping action from the heart to the artery; and another called the **diastolic blood pressure** (usually given as the bottom number) measures the resting pressure in the artery. These are the numbers that will be written on your chart.

Hypertension, or high blood pressure, means that the blood pressure is above a certain level which has been designated as the top of normal.

Normal blood pressure isn't a single number; it's a range. Normal systolic blood pressure ranges from 90 to 140; normal diastolic blood pressure ranges from 60 to 90. A blood pressure of anywhere from 90/60 to 140/90 is considered within the normal range; higher than 140/90 will cause concern.

Why Is It Important to Have Your Blood Pressure Checked When You're Pregnant?

Between 5 and 10 per cent of pregnant women will develop high blood pressure during their pregnancy. This **pregnancy-induced hypertension** (PIH) can cause serious problems for both mother and baby, and it's most likely to show up in the third trimester.

If a pregnant woman has PIH, plus protein in her urine, plus **fluid retention** (swelling and puffiness), the condition is called pre-eclampsia (or **toxemia**, although this term is rarely used now). Pre-eclampsia rarely occurs before the third trimester. That is one reason the visits become more frequent at the end of pregnancy—to detect pre-eclampsia in its early stages, before it makes the mother sick.

Some women have high blood pressure before they ever get pregnant. These women's high blood pressure may improve somewhat in early pregnancy, but they are at higher risk of developing pre-eclampsia in the third trimester.

What are the Risks of Pre-eclampsia?

In North America, 7 out of every 1,000 babies will die before birth. When mothers have moderate pre-eclampsia (with a diastolic pressure of 94 to 105), the risk of the baby dying triples to 21 per 1,000. If the woman's blood pressure is higher than that, the risk to the baby also increases. Most of these babies die because the placenta separates from the wall of the uterus, or because the placenta stops nourishing the baby.

The baby's growth may also be restricted because of these placental problems caused by high blood pressure. While in the womb, the baby gets all its nutrients through the placenta (via the umbilical cord), and a placenta with circulation problems won't provide enough nutrition for proper growth. That means the baby will be smaller than it should be for the length of time it has been growing inside the uterus, a condition called **intrauterine growth restriction**. This baby is more likely to have health problems after it is born.

Pre-eclampsia can also be dangerous for the mother. She may have seizures (this is then called **eclampsia**) and this can be accompanied by bleeding into the brain. The mother may even go into a coma. This condition can be fatal.

The seizures can happen during pregnancy, during labour, or in the 48 hours after the baby is born. Fortunately, they only happen in about 1 out of every 2,000 births.

Women with severe high blood pressure can also develop kidney failure, bleeding from the liver, and abnormalities of their blood clotting mechanisms. All of these complications to the mother have been reduced with modern treatment.

What Causes Pre-eclampsia?

The cause of pre-eclampsia is unknown. It appears to be a disease which starts in the tiny blood vessels in the kidney. The underlying process probably starts months before the actual signs of elevated blood pressure and protein in the urine (**proteinuria)** appear.

However, there are factors that make women more likely to develop pre-eclampsia.

- first pregnancy
- multiple pregnancy (twins, triplets, etc.)
- mother's age at pregnancy is under 18 years or over 35 years
- mother has diabetes before becoming pregnant
- mother has high blood pressure before becoming pregnant

How do you know if you have pre-eclampsia? In the early stages, there are no symptoms. This is one reason that prenatal visits to your doctor or midwife are so important. Your caregiver will check your blood pressure and test your urine for protein at every visit. Towards the end of your pregnancy (when the chances of developing hypertension are higher) you will see your caregiver more frequently, so that the condition can be quickly caught if it does develop.

Many pregnant women worry about swelling or fluid retention (also called **edema**) because they know it is a symptom associated with pre-eclampsia. But more than half of all pregnant women will have some swelling during pregnancy, and it is perfectly normal. Unless your caregiver also finds protein in your urine and high blood pressure, you do not need to be concerned.

However, swelling occurring suddenly during pregnancy should prompt more frequent visits to check the blood pressure and urine for protein. Swelling is only abnormal when high blood pressure and proteinuria are also present.

When pre-eclampsia begins, the expectant mother feels fine, and by the time she starts to feel ill, the disease is usually severe. Some signs that the situation is very serious include: headaches, pain in the upper abdomen, vomiting, blurred vision, or seeing flashing lights. Any of these mean she should seek immediate medical care.

One of the frightening things about pre-eclampsia is that it is unpredictable and can progress very rapidly. Some women with mild pre-eclampsia will not get worse, and will reach the end of the pregnancy with no problems for mother or baby. In other cases, a woman will have slightly elevated blood pressure and a small amount of protein in her urine one day (and be wondering what her caregiver is fussing about since she feels great). Three days later she may be feeling terrible, with severe headache, extreme swelling, and dangerously high blood pressure. At present, we can't predict which cases will end up being a minor blip in an otherwise normal pregnancy, and which will become very serious.

Can Pre-eclampsia Be Prevented?

Because pre-eclampsia is a relatively common and potentially serious problem, there is great interest in methods which might prevent its development.

DIET

Many attempts have been made to reduce pre-eclampsia by modifying the diets of pregnant women. Unfortunately, nothing diet-related, including reducing salt intake or weight gain, increasing calcium or protein, or overall good nutrition, has been shown to reduce the risk of pre-eclampsia.

DRUGS

Various medications have also been tried, with the hope that they might keep pre-eclampsia from occurring. Again, none have proven effective.

How Is Pre-eclampsia Treated?

Once pre-eclampsia develops, delivery of the baby is the only cure.

All other treatments are just buying time. Of course, sometimes buying time is an important and valuable goal. If the baby is very premature, a little longer time inside the uterus will give it a better chance for survival. If pre-eclampsia is mild and the pregnancy is full term, the extra time might allow labour to start spontaneously, avoiding induction. When a woman is very ill with severe pre-eclampsia, the treatments described below can possibly reduce the risk of other complications and help her feel better while arrangements are made to get her baby delivered.

COMMON TREATMENTS FOR PRE-ECLAMPSIA

Bed rest has traditionally been ordered for the mother who has pre-eclampsia. Often the mother is admitted to hospital. There is no evidence to suggest that strict bed rest, either at home or in hospital, improves any of the complications of pre-eclampsia.

However, being admitted to hospital can be useful. It allows the medical caregivers to closely monitor the mother's blood pressure and the protein levels in her urine, to perform blood tests and to assess the condition of the baby in a disease which can change rapidly. If the mother or baby is thought to be getting worse, delivery can be arranged quickly.

Melanie thought her pregnancy was going fine until, at her 32-week visit, her doctor found that her blood pressure was high and there was some protein in her urine. On his advice, she took a leave of absence from her job and rested at home. But when her blood pressure was even higher a week later, she was admitted to the hospital.

Melanie says, "I wasn't very pleased about being in the hospital, especially because I didn't feel too bad at first. Things got rapidly worse, though, and within a week I was feeling awful. I couldn't believe how swollen I was, I woke up every morning with a headache, and I was having stomach aches as well. My husband and I were really worried about the baby—I was having a **non-stress test** every day (a recording of the baby's heart rate for 20 minutes). I realized that I was going to be giving birth sooner rather than later."

Soon after that Melanie's doctor recommended inducing labour. Although her baby girl weighed only 3 pounds (1,360 g) when she was born, she was healthy and gained weight rapidly after her birth. Melanie also recovered rapidly once the baby was born, and is pleased that she has been able to successfully breastfeed her daughter despite their challenging beginning.

Antihypertensive drugs (drugs that lower blood pressure) given to the mother with pre-eclampsia can substantially reduce the risk of her already high blood pressure becoming higher. Keeping the blood pressure under control benefits the *mother* by reducing her risk of kidney damage, liver damage, and brain hemorrhage. It may also reduce her chances of being induced and of having a Caesarean section.

Unfortunately, there is no good evidence that these antihypertensive drugs directly benefit the baby. They don't seem to reduce the number of stillborn babies or the number of babies with **intrauterine growth restriction**. The results of these studies may mean one of three things: that there really is no benefit; that the studies done so far have been too small to show any benefits; or that the benefits to some babies are outweighed by the risks of the treatment to others.

Medications known as **corticosteroids** are sometimes given to mothers with **HELLP syndrome** (page 185) to prevent or reduce some of the complications, but further research is still needed on the effectiveness of this treatment.

Anticonvulsants are drugs that are used to prevent seizures. Once a seizure occurs, further seizures must be prevented as quickly as possible. Treatment with a medication, **magnesium sulphate**, has been shown to be both safe and the most effective.

HOLLY'S EXPERIENCE WITH PREGNANCY-INDUCED HYPERTENSION

"The first six months of my pregnancy were medically uneventful. At the start of my last trimester my blood pressure started to rise a little bit. My doctor advised me that it wasn't anything to worry about, as long as it didn't get any higher and no other symptoms developed. By my 32nd week, my blood pressure was a little higher and the swelling started.

By week 33, my blood pressure and weight were still climbing and my fingers and toes looked like little pork sausages. I took a leave from work and rested a lot; my blood pressure didn't improve much, but at least it didn't get worse. My 36-week visit to the doctor's office was spent talking about the possible need to be induced. I gained 40 pounds (18 kg) in the last few weeks of pregnancy due to edema, my blood pressure stayed up at about 150/90, but I didn't have any protein in my urine.

Sunday morning—the day before we had finally decided to induce—I woke up with labour pains. By afternoon they were about five minutes apart so we went to the hospital. My blood pressure had risen even higher, and I was quickly attached to a blood pressure gauge, an IV, and a **catheter** (to measure my urine). By midnight I'd been given an epidural and **oxytocin** to speed up the labour. I wasn't scared because my baby's heart rate was always good. I'll never forget the nurse who held the hand my husband wasn't holding and reassured and comforted us through a very long night. She even stayed past the shift change to see my baby born.

Because of the risk of seizures, the doctor didn't want me to push for too long. First I tried pushing myself, but I was pretty frozen from the epidural and it didn't do much. They decided to try the vacuum extractor. When it was in place, the doctor pulling on it helped me get the feeling of where to push. I pushed as hard as I could and our son, Jack, weighing 6 pounds 6 ounces (2,892 g), was born.

My husband was in tears. He held Jack first, and I was so happy, so tired, and so relieved that I couldn't stop crying."

If the mother has severe pre-eclampsia, but has not yet had a seizure, doctors will often suggest one of these **anticonvulsants** to prevent seizures from starting.

In these cases it is difficult to weigh the benefits to the mother against the risk to the baby. How severe should the pre-eclampsia be before anticonvulsants are given? How soon after this will the baby be born, and how will the drug affect the baby?

DELIVERING THE BABY

With severe pre-eclampsia and eclampsia, the best treatment is to deliver the baby.

Usually, labour is induced and the mother kept on medication to lower her blood pressure and prevent seizures during the labour. The medications will be continued for 48 hours after the baby is born. By that point, her blood pressure should be returning to normal and the risk of seizures is almost zero.

If the attempts to induce labour fail, or if the woman's cervix has not begun to thin out or show any signs of readiness for labour, then a Caesarean section will probably be recommended.

With less severe pre-eclampsia, deciding when to induce labour is a difficult clinical judgment that worries even experienced obstetricians. This condition is fairly unpredictable and each case has to be considered individually. Even if medical treatment has produced some improvement in the blood pressure readings, the baby is still at risk. The doctor must try to decide when the risks to the baby of being premature are outweighed by the risks of the pre-eclampsia getting worse. If the cervix seems not ready for induction or if the induction doesn't work, the doctor must consider whether the risks of a Caesarean section are outweighed by the risks of the mother developing eclampsia.

HELLP Syndrome

A severe form of pre-eclampsia is known as HELLP syndrome. The letters in the name stand for **hemolysis** (which means red blood cells

breaking down more rapidly than normal), **elevated liver enzymes** and **low platelets**. It is a rare but very serious condition. The mother will have high blood pressure and protein in her urine, and may experience abdominal pain, nausea, severe headaches, and vision problems. This severe pre-eclampsia threatens the life of both mother and baby. The treatment is admission to hospital, stabilizing the mother's condition, and delivering the baby.

-34-
Premature Labour and Birth

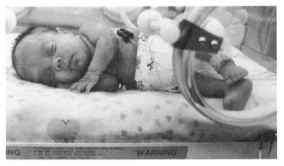

Brenda was at home alone when she noticed that the cramps she'd been feeling all day were getting stronger and more regular. Finally she called her sister-in-law, who already had two children, and described the odd pains she was feeling.

"I hate to say this, Brenda," her sister-in-law said, "but I think you're in labour."

"I can't be in labour," said Brenda. "I'm not even seven months pregnant!"

But Brenda was, in fact, in labour and she gave birth to a 3-pound (1,360-g) baby girl later that night. Her daughter spent nearly eight weeks in the special care nursery of the hospital. Complications of her prematurity continue to affect her walking and her speech.

Not all babies born prematurely will be disabled as Brenda's daughter is, of course, but many are. Premature birth is a major cause of death among babies, and a major cause of disability among children who survive being born too early.

Premature or Just Small?

The premature baby is born before 37 complete weeks of pregnancy. The length of time inside the uterus is more important here than the baby's weight, as some premature babies are considerably larger than others.

Shannon, for example, gave birth to her son when she was 34 weeks pregnant. He weighed 5 pounds, 9 ounces (2,523 g). Even though he had arrived early, he was large for his gestational age. Despite his bigger-than-average size, he did have some of the other problems common in premature babies: he developed **respiratory distress syndrome** (breathing problems) and occasional spells of **apnea** (when he would stop breathing altogether). However, he soon overcame these problems and was able to go home with his family after three weeks in a special care nursery.

Babies who are born between 34 and 37 weeks are premature, but they are almost as likely to survive and be healthy as full-term babies. They usually only need some extra help in staying warm, in getting enough calories to grow, and in learning to nurse in the first few weeks. There isn't much point, then, in trying to stop labour if the mother is more than 34 weeks pregnant. Research on premature labour and birth, therefore, has concentrated on situations where the mother is less than 34 weeks pregnant.

Lots of research has been done on premature babies between 26 and 34 weeks, and the survival rates for this group have increased tremendously. Newborn intensive care has also made possible survival of some infants of less than 26 weeks gestation and very low birth weights—below 36 ounces (1,000 g).

"When I first saw John, I couldn't imagine that he would survive," says Marjorie. "I remember that he was so small that my husband Jack could cradle his whole body in the palm of his hand. But the nurses said he was a fighter, and he made it."

But while Jack and Marjorie were thrilled that John survived his very premature birth, they also had to contend with the complications. John needed surgery before he was a month old, and had two more operations before he was a year. He is deaf and developmentally delayed. Disabilities and various health problems are more common in these very small babies.

Can We Prevent Premature Labour Before It Starts?

There has been great interest in trying to predict early in pregnancy the 10 per cent of women who will go into premature labour, with the hope that a treatment can be discovered to prevent it.

The risk factors listed in the sidebar are sometimes used as a scoring system to predict women who will deliver prematurely, but it hasn't turned out to be very reliable. At least half of the women who give birth prematurely will not have any of the risk factors on the list.

However, women with high scores on this list *are* more likely to have premature births, and this has given researchers a group to work with.

SOME FACTORS THAT MAKE PREMATURE BIRTH MORE LIKELY

- mother has already had a premature baby
- mother is less than 20 years old
- family is poor and food is inadequate
- mother smokes
- mother drinks or uses recreational drugs heavily
- mother has a chronic disease such as hypertension or diabetes
- mother is carrying twins, triplets, or other multiples
- the baby has serious birth defects
- mother's blood pressure has become high during this pregnancy
- the placenta has separated from the uterus, or is covering the cervix
- the baby has intrauterine growth restriction
- there is an infection in the uterus

Several treatments have been studied to prevent premature labour and birth.

SOCIAL INTERVENTIONS

When women live in poverty and don't get enough food, they have a higher chance of giving birth prematurely. Several programs have tried to improve the situations of these pregnant women by providing additional food or improved living conditions, but none have reduced the number of premature births. It may be that this support must start long before pregnancy to be helpful.

SUTURING THE CERVIX CLOSED

Suturing the cervix closed (called **cervical cerclage**) in early pregnancy and releasing it at term has been used to attempt to prevent premature birth. The mother needs an anaesthetic for this procedure. For most women considered to be at risk of premature birth, the procedure did not make any difference. The only benefit seen from cervical cerclage was in a very small group of women who have already had three premature births.

OTHER APPROACHES

Other approaches that have not been successful in improving outcomes include: bed rest, checking the cervix frequently during pregnancy, having the mother monitor uterine activity at home, and giving the mother various medications during pregnancy.

Can We Stop Premature Labour Once It Starts?

It sounds simple: stop premature labour and you'll prevent premature births. But the situation isn't quite that black-and-white.

Not all premature labour does lead to premature birth. You might be 30 weeks pregnant and experience painful contractions for six hours; then they stop and your pregnancy continues until you are full term. Yes, you experienced premature labour, but it was a **false labour** that was going to stop anyway. If you had gone to the hospital and been treated with medication, you might have given the drug the credit for stopping your labour and preventing the premature birth of your baby.

Also, stopping premature labour does not necessarily prevent premature birth. You might go into labour at 28 weeks, have it stopped with drugs, and then give birth to a premature baby a week later. The treatment worked at the time, but you still had a premature baby.

For these reasons, randomized controlled studies are exceedingly important in assessing interventions to stop premature *labour*, to see if they actually prevent premature *birth*. To assess any treatment proposed for the prevention of premature labour, it is essential to have a control group of untreated women with the same symptoms and signs of labour.

The first challenge researchers face is deciding whether or not a woman is actually in labour. The earlier in labour that an intervention is started, the better the chances of stopping labour. But it is in the earliest stages that it is hardest to know whether you are actually in labour or not; contractions come and go, with some being strong and some weak.

Most researchers have arbitrarily defined pre-term labour as regular contractions (at least every five to eight minutes) which have produced 80 per cent effacement or 2 centimetres dilation of the cervix.

Many different methods of stopping premature labour have been tested in clinical trials. None of them have proven effective at actually preventing premature births. Either they don't work at all, or they don't improve the overall outcome, or there are serious harmful side effects.

The most useful drugs appear to be the **betamimetic drugs** (ritodrine and terbutaline). These drugs relax the uterus and have been shown in studies to reduce the numbers of babies born 24 and 48 hours after starting treatment. But the drugs don't reduce the number of infant deaths or the number of babies with respiratory distress syndrome. There are several possible reasons for this. The drugs do have some side effects, which may balance out the benefits. And they appear to only stop labour temporarily, so that the baby may still be born prematurely. *This temporary delay, though, can be very valuable when the time gained is used to arrange the best possible conditions for the baby's birth.* Read on....

Helping the Baby's Lungs to Mature

The most serious risk to premature babies is **respiratory distress syndrome** (RDS). Fifty per cent of the babies born before 34 weeks will have this problem. Babies with RDS breathe very hard and fast, and often, despite their struggles, they can't get enough oxygen. Then they are either given extra oxygen to breathe or, in serious cases, attached to a machine called a **ventilator**, which breathes for them.

Corticosteroid drugs, *given to the mother in premature labour, can cut her baby's risk of RDS in half.* The maximum benefit to the baby's lungs is achieved if the baby is born within one to seven days after the treatment is completed, but there are still benefits if the baby is born sooner or later than that.

Corticosteroid treatment to the mother also reduces the risk of two other complications of the first week of life of premature babies: bleeding into the brain and a serious inflammation of the bowel.

In pregnancies where the only complication is prematurity, corticosteroid drugs don't cause any side effects. In premature labours when there are other complications as well, the situation is less clear-cut. Particularly in pregnancies with high blood pressure, intrauterine growth restriction, or diabetes, the risks and benefits of corticosteroids appear about equal.

When Should Premature Labour Be Allowed to Continue?

Stopping premature labour is not always the best thing. In some cases, doctors have suggested that the premature labour is nature's way of removing the baby from a uterus that is no longer nourishing it adequately. There are some situations where it may be best for the mother and/or the baby for premature birth to occur.

For example, if there is a severe infection of the uterus, mother and baby will be better off if the baby is born quickly and they are both treated with antibiotics. When the mother has hypertension and/or a growth-restricted infant, premature labour may be welcomed, as there is concern about the safety of the baby inside the uterus.

In fact, in pregnancies complicated by conditions such as hypertension, diabetes, or Rh problems, premature labour may be deliberately planned and induced. Planned, elective pre-term deliveries represent about one-quarter of all premature births. In these situations, it is felt that the risk of being born prematurely is less than the risk of more time in the uterus exposed to the complicating disease.

Pre-term Pre-labour Rupture of the Membranes

If your water breaks before labour starts, the medical term for this is **pre-labour rupture of the membranes**, or PROM (see Chapter 42). When this happens before you are 37 weeks pregnant, it is pre-term **PROM**. Most women will give birth within a week of the membranes rupturing, so your risk of having a premature baby at this point is high.

There is also a risk that bacteria will get into the uterus from the vagina and the baby will become infected. This risk is greater the more premature the baby is. As well, there is increased risk of **prolapse of the umbilical cord** out the cervix, either at the time of the rupture or at the time of the start of labour. Separation of the placenta from the wall of the uterus is also more common, because of the sudden decrease in size of the uterus as the amniotic fluid flows out.

Several different methods of treatment of the woman with pre-labour rupture of the membranes pre-term have been studied:

PREVENTIVE ANTIBIOTICS

Antibiotics given to the mother, either before labour starts or during labour, will reduce the infection rate for both mother and baby—but, in the studies done so far, don't change the number of babies who do not survive. This is hard to explain, unless the studies simply have not been big enough to show an effect on a rare event like death.

CORTICOSTEROIDS

Giving corticosteroids to improve lung maturity has the same benefit with ruptured membranes as without, a 50 per cent decrease in the incidence of respiratory distress syndrome in the newborn. There is no increased risk of infection.

INDUCTION OF LABOUR

Studies comparing induction of labour with waiting to see what happens after pre-labour rupture of the membranes pre-term showed no benefit from induction of labour.

WAITING

Waiting to see what happens, while carefully observing the mother and baby, seems to be a safe approach with pre-term PROM. If labour starts, as it usually does, there is no benefit in trying to stop it. Sometimes labour does not start, the membranes seal themselves again, the fluid will re-accumulate, and the pregnancy continues to term.

That's what happened to Elaine. "At seven months, I thought I'd lost control of my bladder. When I went to the doctor, she told me that my membranes had ruptured and I'd better get to the hospital because I was probably going to have a premature baby.

"I was surprisingly calm as we headed to the hospital. I think it was because I wasn't having any contractions, so the possibility of giving birth soon didn't seem real to me. After discussing different options with my doctor and my husband, we decided to just wait.

"Within 48 hours, the dripping had stopped. My doctor told me that the membranes seemed to have re-sealed, and sent me home the next day. I ended up going past my due date and we were starting to talk about induction! I thought that was pretty funny when two months earlier we'd been worried about a premature baby."

Place of Birth

The safest place for the very premature infant to be delivered is in a specialized centre with a newborn intensive care nursery. This centre will have expertise caring for any complications in the mother, as well as the availability of **neonatologists** (pediatricians who specialize in premature infants) around the clock to attend the birth and subsequently care for the baby in the nursery.

If you go into labour prematurely, decisions will need to be made about the best place to deliver your baby. Your community hospital may have the equipment and expertise to take care of your baby if you are 35 weeks pregnant, but if you are only 31 weeks pregnant you might need to be transferred to a specialized centre. You'll have to factor in how far along you are in labour and how far away the other hospital is.

But here is where some of the treatments for premature labour can come in. The betamimetic drugs that seem to temporarily stop labour can buy you some time to get to a hospital with a special-care nursery, and to take the corticosteroids which will help your baby's lungs mature.

Preventing the Complications of Premature Birth

When prevention hasn't worked, and it is obvious that the labour is going to continue and you are going to deliver a premature baby, there are more things to think about.

If you are in premature labour, an ultrasound examination can be helpful. Ultrasound shows your doctor the position of the baby. Because premature babies haven't had time to settle into the normal head-down position of the full-term baby, your baby is more likely to be lying crosswise or in a **breech** (bottom-first) position. An ultrasound will also check to see if the placenta is overlapping the cervix.

With the ultrasound information to help you, you can discuss the best approach to your baby's birth with your doctor.

You will probably be offered corticosteroids to help prevent respiratory distress syndrome.

Your baby's risk of infection may also be decreased if you are given antibiotics while you are in labour.

Many premature babies have bleeding into their brain. The more premature the baby is, the more common and serious this is. Some studies have found that giving the drug **phenobarbital** or **vitamin K** to the mother during labour has reduced this risk, but more research on this is needed.

Slowing down of the fetal heart rate is frequently seen during premature labour, especially when the membranes have ruptured before labour begins. This is possibly due to the umbilical cord being compressed once there is less amniotic fluid to provide a cushioning effect. If a small tube is inserted through the cervix into the uterus, fluid can be infused into the uterus. This is called **amnio-infusion**. No definite conclusions about whether this is helpful in premature labours can be made based on the current evidence.

WILL A CAESAREAN SECTION PREVENT COMPLICATIONS?

Should your premature baby be delivered vaginally or by Caesarean section? We don't have good evidence to say that delivery by Caesarean is safer for all premature babies or for specific groups of premature babies (such as those in a breech position, or those who are very small). Since Caesarean sections have significant risks for the mother, the decision should not be made lightly.

While some studies have found a higher survival rate for premature babies by Caesarean section when compared to those delivered vaginally, the two groups compared were not the same. Some of the mothers who delivered vaginally had babies who were considered too small or ill to be delivered by Caesarean section. Others were too far along in labour to arrange for a Caesarean. These mothers in advanced labour also didn't have time to be given corticosteroid drugs, or to arrange for a neonatologist to be present at the delivery.

CAN INTERVENTIONS IN VAGINAL BIRTHS PREVENT COMPLICATIONS?

A number of interventions have commonly been recommended when premature babies are born vaginally, and are routine in many places. Considering how many babies are born prematurely, it is surprising that these interventions have not been more extensively studied. However, the small studies that have been done find absolutely no benefit to these widely used interventions.

Epidural anaesthesia is often advised for every woman in premature labour. The theory is that this will relax her muscles, reduce her urge to push, and make the birth gentler for the baby. The research has produced no evidence that this can help the baby. For similar reasons, forceps are often used to deliver premature babies, with the goal of protecting the baby's head at birth. Research again does not support this. It is also very common to routinely do episiotomies on women who are giving birth to premature babies, once again with the intention of protecting the baby's head from pressure. As with the other interventions, there is no evidence that this is beneficial.

KANGAROO CARE

Research beginning in 1983 by Dr. Anthony Hadeed and Dr. Humberto Rey, both working in Colombia, South America, has found that parents may hold the key to helping their premature babies. Their studies, confirmed by others, discovered the value of skin-to-skin contact for even very tiny babies.

The Kangaroo Care parent (both mothers and fathers can participate) carries the premature baby, who is wearing a diaper and usually a hat, chest-to-chest and skin-to-skin. A blanket covers the baby and holds in the warmth provided by the parent's body.

Research shows that the benefits to the baby include:

- a stable heart rate
- more regular breathing
- longer periods of sleep
- better temperature
- decreased crying
- longer periods of alertness
- more opportunities to breastfeed

Parents also benefit from Kangaroo Care because the experience helps them feel more confident and prepared for the day when baby comes home.

Kangaroo Care has succeeded with babies as small as 28 ounces (800 g). IVs and monitors don't interfere with Kangaroo Care. Generally, the baby needs to be stable and not on a ventilator, although recent research has shown that babies stabilize more quickly in Kangaroo Care than in an incubator.

Being held close to a parent this way duplicates many of the experiences the premature baby would have in the womb. It is a relaxing, safe environment for any newborn but is even more important for the fragile premature baby.

Of course when you are worried about having a premature baby, you want to do all you can to make the birth easier for him or her. However, these interventions all carry some risks and, since they have not been shown to be helpful, you may want to ask your doctor about avoiding them.

CARING FOR THE PREMATURE BABY

A premature baby needs special care from the minute it is born. You may have a neonatologist waiting in the delivery room to begin caring for the baby from the moment of birth, especially if the baby is very small.

As previously mentioned, premature babies are at high risk of developing respiratory distress syndrome. A drug called **surfactant**, put into the baby's lungs shortly after birth, reduces the risk of respiratory distress syndrome significantly. The evidence for this treatment is so good that the use of surfactant can be recommended routinely in the care of all very premature infants.

Rebeka, who had premature triplets by Caesarean section, says, "I couldn't believe the crowd of people in the room. Each baby had a team assigned to him, and as the doctor lifted each baby out, he'd pass it on to the right person and everyone would rush into action. I only got little glimpses of them as they went by."

The Evidence About…
Premature Labour and Birth

About 1 out of every 10 babies will be born prematurely—before 37 weeks of pregnancy. In most
cases, we don't know what caused a particular
premature labour; in fact, half of the mothers
who give birth prematurely do not even have any
identified risk factors.

Drugs are available which can stop premature
labour, but they don't seem to improve the outcomes for the babies. Often labour starts again
and the baby is still born prematurely. These drugs
can buy some valuable time so that treatment can
be given to help the baby's lungs mature or the
mother can be transferred to a hospital with a
neonatal intensive care unit.

The most successful treatment in premature
labour is to give the mother corticosteroids. This
reduces the risk of her baby developing respiratory distress syndrome by 50 per cent. Treating
the very premature baby with surfactant immediately after birth also significantly reduces the risk
of respiratory distress syndrome.

The safest place for the very premature infant
to be born is in a specialized centre with a neonatal intensive care unit.

Decisions about vaginal births and Caesarean
delivery must be made on an individual basis.
There is no evidence that routine use of epidural
anaesthetic, forceps delivery, episiotomy, or continuous fetal monitoring during labour produce a
better outcome for the premature baby.

Having a premature baby can be a frightening
experience. Your baby may look unbelievably
tiny and fragile, and seeing him hooked up to
monitors and respirators is alarming. You may
not be able to touch or hold your baby right
away, and even when you can, you might be
afraid of hurting him because he's so small.

It helps to know that your touch is extremely
important to your baby. We now have a solid
body of evidence (see sidebar on Kangaroo Care,
page 193) about how much better babies do if
they are in skin-to-skin contact with their mothers as much as possible. While this is not routine
at many North American hospitals, it is very
important.

Most premature babies can't breastfeed right
away, and you may have to pump your milk for
weeks. However, your milk is valuable for your
baby, and several studies have shown significant
health benefits for premature babies who were
given their mothers' milk. All efforts and support
should be given to help mothers of premature
babies pump milk and breastfeed as soon as
possible.

At one time, it was believed that breastfeeding was more difficult for the premature baby
than bottle feeding, so these babies were given
bottles first. Only after the baby was used to the
bottle were the mothers allowed to try breastfeeding, and often by then the baby had a hard
time learning to nurse properly at the breast. But
researchers discovered that, in fact, breastfeeding is easier and less stressful for the premature
baby.

Emily's son Carl was born at 30 weeks and
weighed 3 pounds (1,360 g). She pumped milk
for him and spent every day at the hospital,
watching him grow slowly. "When he began to
suck at the feeding tube, they told me I could try
nursing him," she says. "He still looked so tiny,
but he took my nipple right away. It was the
most wonderful feeling! I'd breastfeed him every
few hours during the day and they'd top him up

by tube-feeding my expressed milk. Eventually he was getting all his milk at the breast, and we started to make plans to bring him home."

Carl weighed 5 pounds (2,270 g) the day he came home, nearly two months after his birth. "It was great to have him home, but it was a shock, too," Emily says. "I'd gotten used to sleeping through the night while he was in the hospital, but he'd wake up to nurse every two hours. It took a couple of days to build up my milk supply at night. But we all managed."

You and your baby have some challenges to face, but there is help available. Ask about support groups for parents of premature babies which may be connected with your hospital. Just knowing how other parents coped can make a big difference.

-35-
Sex during Late Pregnancy

"One night I said to Jack, 'Do you want to do it?' and I guess he could tell from my voice that I was feeling pretty tired," recalls Emily. "He looked at my big belly with a doubtful expression and then we both just started laughing and laughing. There's a point where sex can seem so awkward that it's just ridiculous. But after we'd laughed about it, we actually started feeling kind of amorous."

Sex in late pregnancy is like that. When your uterus is so large that it's hard to find a reasonably comfortable position to sleep in, finding a position that makes sex fun and enjoyable can seem pretty daunting. You may find your interest in sex is unpredictable, too. Some women are much more interested towards the end of pregnancy, others much less so. Men also vary in their responses to their partner's changing body—some love it, some don't—and some men worry about injuring the baby during intercourse.

In most pregnancies, sex is perfectly safe. The baby continues to be well-protected, and the contractions you experience during orgasm will not trigger labour in a normal pregnancy. You can have intercourse or other sexual activity at any point during the pregnancy—even in labour, if you want to.

However, sex may be risky if:

- you have placenta previa (the placenta is across the bottom of the uterus overlapping or covering the cervix)
- you have unexplained vaginal bleeding
- you are leaking amniotic fluid
- you have a history of premature labour and births (in this case, the doctor may recommend that you avoid nipple stimulation, intercourse, and orgasms)

Women who feel interested in sex during pregnancy often report that the increased blood flow to the pelvis and the increased vaginal secretions actually make it more enjoyable. Pregnant women often have orgasms more easily and may have multiple orgasms (although they may not get the same sense of relief and resolution afterwards).

Of course, the sheer logistics of sex with a close-to-full-term pregnant belly can be a challenge. It's best to look for positions that don't involve having the pregnant woman lying on her back—try having the woman on top, on her hands and knees, or use spooning or side-lying positions. You may want to change positions a few times while making love, as most will soon become uncomfortable for the expectant mother.

This can be a time to experiment with new positions and techniques, and also a time to show a little extra love and consideration for each other.

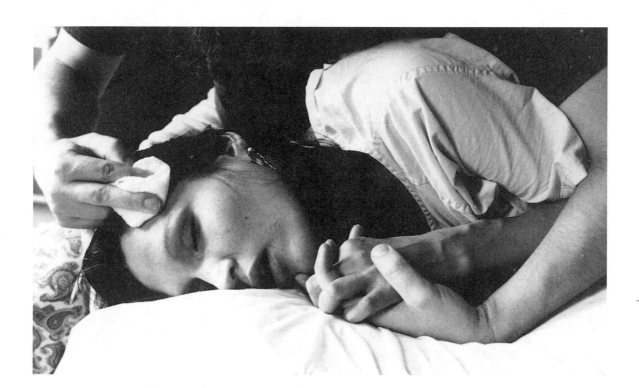

Eight Months
❧ *Thirty to Thirty-three Weeks* ❧

If you could see your baby right now, you'd think she was ready to be born—right down to her tiny eyelashes and fingernails. But much is still happening. Her lungs still need a little time to be ready to breathe air, her brain is still growing, and the extra weight she'll gain in these last few weeks will make her transition to the outside world an easier one.

You may be anticipating your baby's birth with both excitement and a little anxiety. Often by this time expectant parents find themselves ready to create a nest for their new arrival—buying tiny clothes, stocking up on diapers and baby items so that everything will be ready when the big day comes. It gets harder to think about anything other than your pregnancy and the new baby, as your belly gets bigger, your baby gets more active, and your bladder needs to be emptied with increasing frequency. People may be asking, "Aren't you due soon?" Not yet, but it is getting close.

-36-
Labour and Its Variations: False Labour, Long Labour, Precipitate Labour

The day after her due date Cindy and her husband Rob were watching TV when she began to feel a cramping feeling in her abdomen. "It hurt," she says. "It wasn't like a menstrual cramp." When Rob put his hand on her belly, he could feel it getting tight, so he began to write down the times. After an hour, he noted that the contractions were pretty regular and about 10 minutes apart. They waited another hour, still recording the times, and decided to go to the hospital.

Cindy was very disappointed when the nurse who examined her found that her cervix was still firm and not dilated at all. The hospital staff suggested she go home and wait until the contractions got stronger and closer together. Within an hour after getting home, the contractions stopped. Her doctor explained, at her next prenatal visit, that she'd simply had a bout of false labour. A week later, her water broke and her baby was born after an easy seven-hour labour.

Diane was two days before her due date with her third child when she woke up feeling "crampy—like having menstrual cramps." Her previous two births had involved a lot of back labour, so she didn't at first identify the cramps in her lower abdomen as contractions. "I thought maybe I had a bladder infection or something," she says. "Because I didn't feel anything in my back this time, I didn't think it could be labour."

The cramps continued throughout the day. "I had lots of things to do, but every now and then I'd have to sit down and catch my breath," says Diane. "Finally, I decided to call my doctor because I was concerned. It didn't really feel like my usual labour, but it wasn't going away."

Her doctor told Diane to come to the hospital to be examined, and found she was well along in labour—7 centimetres dilated. Diane's baby boy was born two hours later.

When Esther was expecting her third child, she had three episodes of false labour before the real thing arrived. "You'd think I'd know, after two previous babies," she says. Each time she called her midwife and had her support people gathered at her home, only to have the contractions fade away. "It was very embarrassing," she confesses.

When she woke up a few nights later with strong contractions, she decided to wait until she was absolutely certain it was "the real thing" before making any calls. By the time she was sure enough to wake up her husband, Brian labour was so strong she could barely talk and he had to make the calls to the others. When the midwife and Esther's friends arrived, the baby was already born. "Brian did a wonderful job catching the baby," Esther says, "but he did say I have to wake him up sooner next time."

As these stories demonstrate, it isn't easy to determine whether or not labour has really begun. Sometimes there will be strong contractions, but no apparent change in the cervix. Occasionally, the contractions will seem irregular or mild and yet the cervix is dilating quickly.

Other signs of labour are also unreliable. The membranes containing the amniotic fluid may break before labour starts or in early labour, but sometimes they don't break until the baby is actually being born. The **mucous plug**, which is in the centre of the cervix, often comes away in early labour. The mother usually sees this as blood-tinged mucous on her underwear or in the toilet after she goes to the bathroom. Sometimes, though, pink-tinged mucus will be seen several days before labour starts.

Contractions may be regular and strong from the beginning, or they may take several hours to settle into a clear pattern. Sometimes the contractions stay quite far apart all through labour; in other cases they quickly become very close together, with little chance for a break or rest in between.

Because of these wide variations, women are often puzzled about when they should either go to the hospital or call the midwife if they are giving birth at home. Deciding when to go to the hospital can be important, because research has found that women who go to the hospital early in labour are more likely to be diagnosed with "abnormal labour," to receive more interventions, and to have a Caesarean section than women who arrive at the hospital further along in labour.

So when should you go to the hospital or call your midwife? Your own feelings are the best guide. Would you really like to have your midwife with you to provide some reassurance and let you know what's happening? Are you feeling anxious about being at home and wanting to get into the hospital, or does the labour feel manageable at this point? Is the weather bad, so that it's best to leave extra time?

For women who have a long drive to the hospital, deciding when to go is difficult. Perhaps you can go to the home of a friend who lives near the hospital, or stop in a park or the hospital grounds to walk for awhile. (Of course, if it turns out to be false labour, you might end up going home again.)

How Labour Progresses

Labour progresses in two ways. First the **cervix** (which is like a thick, small doughnut with a tiny hole in the middle before labour starts) must thin out, or **efface**. Then the cervix must open up, or **dilate**. The contractions of labour move it

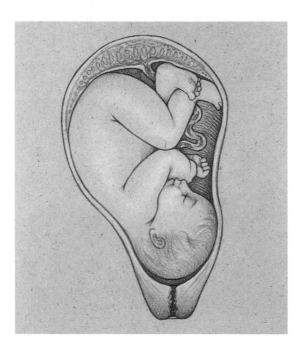
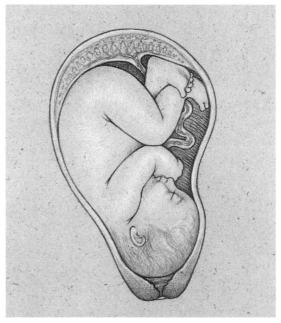

The first stage of labour: Before the onset of labour, the cervix is like a thick donut with a very small hole in the middle (top left). As labour progresses, the cervix first thins (top right), then opens (bottom left) to allow the baby to pass out of the uterus and into the vagina (bottom right).

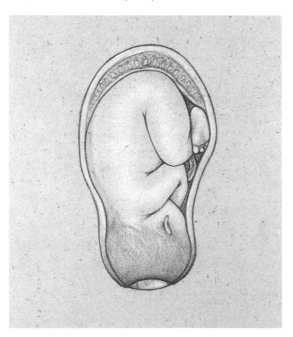
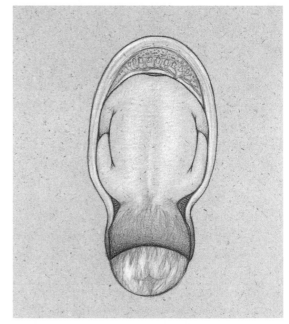

from completely closed (0 centimetres dilated) to completely open (10 centimetres dilated)—at this point the baby's head can come through and into the vagina to be born.

To check on the progress of your labour, the doctor, midwife, or nurse will insert one hand into your vagina to feel the cervix and estimate how many centimetres it has opened. No studies have been done to see how precise these examinations are, but often different caregivers examining the same woman will give different numbers—a difference that could be important if there are concerns about how labour is progressing.

Long Latent Labour

Early or latent labour is the time from the first contraction to the point where the cervix is 4 centimetres dilated and 80 per cent effaced. How long does this take? Some women have contractions for several days or even weeks and the cervix changes very slowly during this stage. Other women are not even aware of it—when they first notice contractions, they are already 4 or 5 centimetres dilated. It can be very discouraging to the mother who has felt strong contractions for 12 hours or more to learn that she is only 2 centimetres dilated and not even in active labour.

What does it mean if this latent labour stage is longer than average? The studies tend to contradict themselves. Some see no higher complication rate with a long latent stage; others find that if it takes the mother a long time to dilate to 4 centimetres she is more likely to have a forceps delivery or a Caesarean section. It's pos-

sible that the increased numbers of forceps or Caesarean births were caused by attempts to speed up the labour, rather than by the slow labour itself—the research doesn't make this clear.

Claire's labour with her second child started on a Friday evening. "I called my doula and she came over right away. The contractions were pretty solid ones, and I was glad to have both her and Glenn to help me get through them. We laboured all night and then Saturday morning I had some bloody show, so we went to the hospital."

To Claire's disappointment, the nurse who examined her found that she was only about 1 centimetre dilated. "I couldn't believe it. I'd been in labour something like 11 hours by then." Her doula reminded her that she was about 50 per cent effaced, so the contractions were working. They went back home and tried to rest.

Labour continued, though, and nobody got much rest. By Saturday night Claire was sure she must be further along, but another visit to the hospital found she was only 2 centimetres dilated. This time she decided to stay, and wandered the hospital corridors with Glenn and the doula. It wasn't until very late Sunday night that she reached 4 centimetres dilation and then her labour got going; Claire's baby boy was born at 6 a.m. on Monday morning. "And then," she says, "I fell asleep."

Labour does not proceed at an even speed from beginning to end. In early labour, it may take several hours of contractions to dilate the cervix 1 centimetre, while at the end of labour the cervix may dilate 3 centimetres in 45 minutes.

A long latent phase of labour, and a longer labour overall, are both more common when the first baby is being born. Usually subsequent labours are shorter—but not always.

Prolonged Labour

Measuring the rate of dilation of the cervix is only useful once the mother is in active labour. Once active labour is established, a rate of dilation of 0.5 to 1 centimetre per hour is considered average. Sometimes doctors are concerned when labour is moving more slowly than average—if, for example, a mother who is 5 centimetres dilated takes three hours to get to 6 centimetres. However, many women with slower rates of dilation have normal births.

Other factors should also be looked at before labour is considered to be progressing too slowly and in need of being "speeded up." Is the baby doing well, or showing signs of distress? Is the mother comfortable, walking around, and coping with the contractions, or is she exhausted and overwhelmed? If mother and baby are both handling the slower labour well, there is probably little need for concern or intervention.

Maria's contractions were about six or seven minutes apart and it had taken her nearly 20 hours to get to 7 centimetre dilation. If she sat down or lay down, her contractions would slow down to 10 or 12 minutes apart, so she kept walking even though she was feeling tired. Periodic checks on the baby's heartbeat showed that he was doing well, and labour simply continued slowly but steadily. Four hours later, Maria's baby was born with the help of a vacuum extractor.

Women often find their contractions slow down or stop temporarily when they arrive at the hospital. For most of us, a hospital is a fairly stressful environment, and stress significantly affects labour. Other sources of stress may also prolong labour—like worrying about child care for your older children. Walking around has been clearly shown to speed up labour, and having a support person of your choosing present can also contribute to a shorter labour.

When active labour is going slowly, it may be labelled **failure to progress**, also known as **dystocia**. Attempts to speed up the labour are called **augmenting** labour.

One common treatment is to rupture the membranes (called **amniotomy**). The doctor uses an instrument like a crochet hook to break the membranes open; the mother will not feel any pain, only the sudden gush of warm fluid. When this is done routinely fairly early in labour, studies have shown it can shorten the time until the baby is born by one or two hours. No adverse effects have been demonstrated in the research studies. However, there are concerns that if the labour turns out to be false—in other words, contractions stop—that the ruptured membranes may increase the risk of infection. For that reason, this should only be used when labour is clearly underway.

Unfortunately, when amniotomy is specifically used to speed up labours which are progressing slowly, it is less effective.

Another very common way to augment the labour is to give a synthetic form of the hormone **oxytocin** intravenously. This is usually done if spontaneous or artificial rupture of the membranes has not made the labour speed up.

Is oxytocin effective to speed up labour? The studies have found that women given oxytocin

LABOUR THAT DOESN'T PROGRESS: MARINA'S STORY

Some labours just don't progress to the normal, vaginal birth of a baby, no matter how patient the mother or skilled the caregiver. Marina and John vividly remember their two long and unproductive labours.

John says, "With our first baby, Marina finally started to have contractions at six o'clock on Saturday morning—two weeks after her due date. The contractions seemed to come and go. Some were really hard and painful, some just made her stop walking for a minute. That night, the midwife came to check Marina. Even though she'd been having contractions all day, her cervix hadn't dilated at all.

"We tried to get some sleep, but Marina was too uncomfortable. On Sunday we tried everything we could think of to make the contractions stronger and closer. We walked for miles. We danced. We sang that Bob Dylan song: 'Ooowee, ride me high, tomorrow's the day my baby's gonna come.' But the baby didn't come. By Sunday night, we were both exhausted. The midwife checked again and Marina was just 2 centimetres dilated.

"We decided to go to the hospital."

The doctor suggested breaking Marina's water, and that did bring on stronger and more painful contractions. By Monday morning, Marina was finding the pain just about unbearable. But after all those contractions, she'd only dilated one more centimetre.

John continues, "Marina decided to have an epidural for the pain, and as soon as it took effect she fell asleep. Four hours later, though, she still hadn't dilated any more. The decision was easy—this baby would be born by Caesarean section. I was so exhausted that the masks and lights in the operating room were almost surreal. Jesse cried right away as soon as he was lifted out of Marina's belly."

Two years later, John and Marina conceived a second child. Marina says, "I still wanted to have a vaginal labour and birth. I talked to my doctor a lot, and decided not to think too much about the first Caesarean, but just to go into labour and see what happened."

Once again, Marina went past her due date. "My contractions were fairly regular and got quite strong after a few hours. Then my water broke, and they got really painful and close together. We went to the hospital, and the nurse was sure I'd be delivering soon because I was in such hard labour. But when my doctor examined me, I was hardly dilated at all."

Marina walked around for the next eight hours, groaning through intense contractions, but when her doctor examined her she was only 2 centimetres dilated. "I could see that this was going the same way as Jesse's birth, and we decided—after 22 hours of labour to have another Caesarean."

Marina says, "I'm still disappointed that I couldn't give birth vaginally. My doctor couldn't tell me why it happened this way—she says we just don't know why some cervixes don't dilate. I'm not happy that I had Caesareans, but I am glad they were available when I needed them."

---

will dilate more quickly when compared with women who are kept in bed during labour, but more slowly than those who are walking around during labour. There did not seem to be any more complications or problems for the babies when oxytocin was given than when it was not.

However, most of the mothers who had been given oxytocin in the hopes of speeding up labour said it made the contractions more painful and they found the treatment unpleasant. Only a small percentage of the mothers who walked during labour said they found the contractions more painful when they walked.

In general, studies suggest that in most cases walking around is as effective as giving oxytocin in labour, and more comfortable for the mother. If the mother is feeling too tired to walk, or if she is unable to walk because of painkilling drugs or epidural, however, oxytocin is helpful in augmenting labour and making it go faster. Since women vary in how sensitive they are to oxytocin, the best method is to give small doses initially, increasing the amount every 30 minutes while watching the contractions carefully.

Fast Labour

What about labour that goes too fast? A **precipitate labour**—one that is very intense and quick—sounds ideal to many pregnant women, but mothers who have experienced them are less enthusiastic. The intensity of the contractions can be overwhelming, and often the mother is frightened about giving birth unexpectedly without the opportunity to get to the hospital. Also, there is a higher risk of heavy bleeding after the baby is born with an unusually fast labour.

Colleen's labour started very abruptly late on a Saturday night. "The contractions just hit me all of a sudden, and they were really strong and close together. I knew the baby was going to come soon, so I told my husband we'd better get moving."

They drove to the hospital, and Colleen felt the contractions getting even stronger. "The hos-

---

The Evidence About…
Labour and Its Variations

The variations in labour can be pretty dramatic—from very slow to very fast—and yet all fall within the range of "normal." It's these variations that make it hard to plan for labour and birth, because each experience is unique.

Artificial rupture of the membranes in early labour makes the labour shorter by an average of one to two hours, without causing any other complications. It is, however, less effective when used in slowly-progressing labours.

If labour is progressing slowly, walking is as effective as oxytocin to speed it up and more comfortable for the mother. If walking is impossible because of fatigue or drugs, oxytocin is an effective way of augmenting labour.

---

pital's only about 15 minutes from our house, but it seemed like the longest drive I ever did." They parked the car, and as they began to walk towards the hospital entrance, Colleen's water broke.

"That did it," she says. "I knew the baby was coming *now*. All I could think was that I didn't want to have the baby on the pavement, so I made my way to the grass, pulled my shorts off, and lay down on the grass just in time for the baby to come out."

As Colleen lay on the grass, holding her newborn daughter, her husband ran into the hospital. He shouted that his wife had just had a baby "on the grass" and rushed back out to be with her. Unfortunately, he ran back out again so quickly that the nurses couldn't see which way he had gone in the dark. Several nurses fanned out and began searching the area around the hospital. It wasn't long before they discovered Colleen and her newborn, and the new family was ushered into the hospital to get cleaned up.

Colleen can laugh about it now. "I know what story we'll be telling at her wedding," she says. But at the time it was pretty frightening, and she worried that the baby would be injured by the rapid birth.

-37-
Problems with the Amniotic Fluid

Your baby floats in your uterus in a pool of amniotic fluid contained in a sac or membrane. Amniotic fluid is normally clear or very pale yellow. The average amount of amniotic fluid by term is about 1 litre, but volume ranges tremendously in normal pregnancies with healthy babies. A very large amount or a very small amount of amniotic fluid can be associated with bad outcomes, but there is a large overlap between normal and abnormal fluid volumes. You will have the most amniotic fluid at about 36 weeks; the amount gradually decreases over the final few weeks.

When there is an unusually large amount of amniotic fluid, it is called **polyhydramnios**—defined as two litres or more of amniotic fluid. About 1 woman out of a 100 has polyhydramnios and most of the time there is no known cause. Polyhydramnios is associated with a higher than average rate of premature labour, premature separation of the placenta, and postpartum hemorrhage. As well as these serious complications, it can be extremely uncomfortable for the mother.

"People kept asking me if I was having twins," Caroline remembers. "I knew I wasn't, but it was obvious that I was much larger than the other women in my prenatal class. When labour started and my water broke, the reason became obvious—it was like Niagara Falls!"

Too little amniotic fluid is called **oligohydramnios**. This is a difficult diagnosis to make, as small volumes of fluid are hard to measure, even with ultrasound. From 15 to 25 per cent of cases of low fluid volume are caused by abnormal fetuses. If you have very little amniotic fluid, your baby is more likely to show signs of distress in labour. Fetal heart rate abnormalities during labour frequently occur with oligohydramnios, because the lack of cushioning from the fluid makes it easier for the umbilical cord to be compressed, cutting down the oxygen supply to the baby.

Meconium in the Amniotic Fluid

Meconium is the baby's first bowel movement. About 80 per cent of babies do not pass meconium until after they are born. That leaves 20 per cent who will have this first bowel movement while they are still inside the uterus, either before or during labour.

When there is meconium in the amniotic fluid, the baby is at a greater risk of potentially serious complications. The baby may inhale some of the meconium either before labour, during labour, or as he is being born, and this can cause pneumonia.

If your membranes rupture in labour (or are deliberately broken by your caregiver) you may see the fluid looking yellowish, medium green, or dark green, depending on how much of the stool the baby has passed and how long ago he passed it.

If there is lots of meconium and little amniotic fluid at the beginning of labour, the risk to the baby is significant. On the other hand, if you have a normal amount of amniotic fluid, and you see a slight yellow staining, there is probably little risk to your baby. It is unusual for a baby to pass meconium for the first time in labour (unless the baby is breech), and this may mean he is in distress.

Considering how often meconium is seen in the amniotic fluid (20 per cent of the time), there have been very few studies to test different methods of management of these labours.

Unless the membranes have ruptured, you won't even know if you have meconium in the amniotic fluid. Some physicians have suggested that every labouring woman should have her membranes ruptured as soon as she arrives at the hospital, so that the doctor can check for meconium. Alternatively, the doctor or nurse could use an **amnioscope** (a tube with a light) to look through the vagina and cervix and assess the amniotic fluid without breaking the membranes. Neither of these suggestions has ever been

researched, so it is impossible to say whether they would improve outcomes for the baby or not.

Treatment Options

AMNIO-INFUSION

Some small research studies have tested amnio-infusion on mothers in labour. Amnio-infusion is a technique of adding intravenous fluids to the uterus to increase the volume of amniotic fluid and dilute the meconium.

In several studies, this treatment did seem to reduce the number of babies who developed problems from inhaling meconium.

Amnio-infusion has also been studied in cases where the mother has very small amounts of amniotic fluid. Babies in this situation often have heart rate abnormalities during labour. Amnio-infusion did decrease the heart rate abnormalities; more importantly, it also decreased Caesarean section rates, the number of babies asphyxiated at birth, low Apgar scores, and low umbilical artery pH at birth.

It must be noted that these trials have been performed on small numbers of women, and that they have been carried out at major teaching institutions by researchers skilled in the techniques. However, if you are having your baby at a large teaching hospital, and are concerned because you have little amniotic fluid, it would be worth asking your doctor if this treatment is available to you.

SUCTIONING THE BABY

When there is meconium in the amniotic fluid, the risk of the baby breathing in the meconium at birth and getting pneumonia can possibly be reduced by suctioning the baby's mouth and nose immediately after birth. This is virtually routinely done, even though its usefulness in preventing aspiration pneumonia is unproven. Too vigorous suctioning deep in the baby's throat can cause slow heart rate and impair the baby's breathing.

Suctioning of the **trachea** (windpipe) for infants who have passed meconium before birth is a much more difficult and dangerous procedure, requiring a small tube to be inserted into the trachea. Risks include injury to the throat or windpipe, slow heart rate, reduced oxygen supply to the baby, collapse of the lung, and infection. It has not been tested in randomized studies. This procedure may be beneficial if it is used *only* for babies who are born with very thick meconium present and who are showing signs of distress.

The Evidence About…
Amniotic Fluid

When the amount of amniotic fluid is very high or very low, the baby is more likely to have problems. In most cases, though, these problems are not preventable. Amnio-infusion may help when there is too little fluid.

If **meconium** (the baby's first bowel movement) is present in the amniotic fluid, it may be a sign that the baby has been stressed in the uterus. There is also a danger that the baby may also inhale some of the meconium at birth and become seriously ill as a result. Suctioning the baby as it is born is the usual treatment for this; although it has not been studied, it seems to be safe.

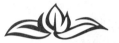

-38-
Coping with Pain in Labour

How Much Does Labour Hurt?

As soon as you knew you were pregnant, you probably started to wonder what labour would be like and how you would cope with the pain. Reading books and seeing videos doesn't really tell you what it will feel like, and as you talk to other women you will discover that everyone's experience is unique.

Sylvia's labour, which took about eight hours, she remembers as being "easy." "Except for the last 20 minutes or so, I would describe the contractions as being like strong menstrual cramps. It wasn't as bad as I had expected, and it really fooled the nurse because she thought I was a long way from delivering."

Pam remembers being absolutely terrified of the pain of labour all through her pregnancy. "When labour started, I kept telling myself not to get too upset, because I knew it was going to get worse. I paced around the house saying, 'Keep calm, it's going to get worse.' Finally I went to the hospital. The nurse told me I was 8 centimetres dilated. I asked her when it was going to get really bad. She laughed and said it was as just

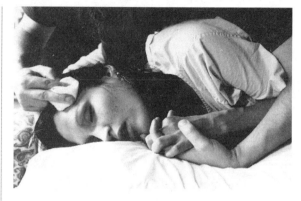

about as bad as it was going to get right now, and just to keep doing what I was doing. I walked and muttered 'Keep calm, keep calm' . . . right up until I pushed the baby out."

Angela had a three-hour labour and says that almost from the first contraction "the pain was unbearable. The first pains were so awful that I woke my husband and we went to the hospital right away. The contractions became even more intense in the car. I was crying uncontrollably by the time we got to the hospital."

"We had to wait in the admitting department for the clerk to find my form, before we went to the birthing suite. In the birthing suite, as soon as the nurse heard that my contractions had started not even an hour ago, she obviously just thought I was hysterical—which I was! The department was really busy—people kept popping in to do things and then leaving again. The nurse went through this whole questionnaire. After a while, an intern came and saw me and of course asked most of the same questions. The lab came and took my blood. During it all, I was crying in between the contractions and just about screaming during them. My back never stopped aching, and during the contractions I felt like I was being ripped apart."

"Then I started to feel like I had to go to the bathroom. I knew women sometimes got diarrhea in labour, and I thought that was coming. I went into the bathroom and I could hear this grunting noise. It was me. Then the nurse rushed in—I guess she heard me—and before I knew what was happening I was on the bed and my own doctor was there and the baby was born."

Even though people were with Angela to do particular procedures, she felt alone most of the time. She thinks now her panic was not just from the pain itself. "All the stories I had heard said a first labour takes about 12 hours. I was only two hours into labour and I couldn't stand it. It never occurred to me I was going to be quicker than average, I just kept thinking, 'I can't bear this pain for 10 more hours.' My husband didn't have a clue what to do—he was as frantic as I was."

Were Angela and Sylvia and Pam all feeling the same thing? Why is one labour more painful than another? Why is one labour longer than another? And why does one treatment to relieve pain work well for one woman and do nothing for the next person? There are more questions about pain in labour than there are answers.

The pain of labour is different from most pain, in that it does not result from an injury or disease, or signal that something is wrong. It's a "working" pain, pain that occurs normally as the uterus does its job of opening the cervix and getting the baby out. But how *much* pain is "normal" or tolerable is not something that can be measured.

Individual women have different experiences of labour, and they also have different expectations and attitudes. Some women take for granted that labour will be painful. Alice says, "All those muscles that had to hold the baby in for nine months had to open up completely in a few hours. It hurt about as much as I figured it should." Other women are equally clear that they are not willing to go through a painful labour. Lisa told her doctor at her first prenatal appointment, "I want an epidural as early as I can have it. I have no intention of suffering."

Do women who believe that pain in labour is normal find it easier to put up with? Do women who believe that pain in labour is something that needs to be controlled or relieved actually find the pain worse? These are questions that don't have any answers, and it is hard to imagine designing research that would answer them.

Research on Pain Relief

The perfect pain reliever in labour would need to have many qualities:

- It shouldn't cause any negative effects in the mother (such as vomiting, dizziness, being unable to empty her bladder, or feeling as though she is "watching" her labour but not participating).

- It shouldn't have any negative effects on the labour, such as making it take longer, or taking away the urge to push, or making it more likely that the woman will bleed too much. It shouldn't make it more likely that the woman will need forceps or a Caesarean section.
- It shouldn't have any bad effects on the baby, such as making his heartbeat slow, or causing breathing problems after the birth.
- And, of course, it should relieve the pain!

Unfortunately, most of the pain-relieving techniques that really take pain away can affect the labour, the mother, and the baby.

Pain-relieving techniques are generally divided into two big groups: those that involve the use of drugs and those that don't.

Drug-Free Approaches to Easing Labour Pain

BREATHING TECHNIQUES

What about breathing? Using specific patterns of breathing in and out is probably the first technique that comes to mind when we talk about non-medication ways of coping with pain in labour. It was the central focus of most of the earlier prenatal classes, and some childbirth educators have written entire books about different types of breathing for different stages of labour.

Using breathing patterns is intended to help you focus your concentration on something other than the pain of the contractions. This distraction, it is hoped, will help you relax and be

less aware of painful sensations. Does it work? Some women find the breathing techniques extremely helpful, while others find they don't help at all.

While breathing patterns themselves have not been researched, studies have been done to see if prenatal classes reduce the need for pain-relieving drugs during labour. When these studies were done, prenatal classes spent a great deal of time teaching breathing techniques, and the studies did find that the classes reduced the need for medications to relieve pain in labour.

Melanie felt that the breathing techniques she learned helped her: "I just used the basic, slow breathing almost all the way through. It helped me relax and gave me something to concentrate on during contractions, and I know it made the contractions more bearable."

Suzanne, on the other hand, didn't find them helpful at all: "I did the breathing in the beginning, but after awhile it all fell apart. Instead, I just groaned really deeply during the contractions. My husband didn't like it; the noises I was making scared him, but it really helped me."

VISUALIZATION

Women who use visualization during labour might create mental images of a relaxing setting or peaceful memory, and usually practise this in advance with their partners. Other images used during visualization are those that remind the mother of the cervix dilating and the baby coming out, such as a flower opening.

Visualization has not been researched in the context of labour, but has proven useful in some other areas, such as sports.

PRENATAL CLASSES

Attendance at any prenatal classes (no matter what the content) has been consistently shown to reduce the amount of pain-killing drugs that are used during labour.

Does this mean that the pain was less; or does it mean that education about labour helped women to accept pain as normal? Does it mean that learning about the complications of drugs made women more ready to tolerate pain rather than use drugs; or does it mean that women who decide to take prenatal classes are less likely to use drugs anyway? We don't know.

FREEDOM OF MOVEMENT IN LABOUR

When women are given the freedom to move and choose any positions they want for labour, most prefer to be sitting, standing, or walking most of the time. When women choose to lie down, it's usually during very early labour (when **resting up** is a good idea), or at the very end of labour. Women who are experiencing **back labour** (feeling most of the pain and pressure on their lower backs) will often get down on their hands and knees, lean against a chair or the bed, or sit on the toilet.

Deanna danced through much of her labour. "I felt it really helped me to keep moving. I played the tape I had prepared when I was pregnant, and walked around the room, swaying to the music. I'd hum loudly—okay, sometimes it was moaning—during the contractions. It all helped."

Ann gave birth to her son on a beautiful spring day in May. "We dropped the older two children off at my sister's and then went to walk in the park. I spent about four hours there, walking along the pathways and enjoying the sunshine. I was surprised at how relaxed I felt. Eventually the contractions got strong enough that we decided to go to the hospital. Even now, every time I drive past that park, I remember walking there on that gorgeous day and waiting for my son to be born."

Norah spent a lot of her labour on the toilet. "It worked best if I sat backwards so I could rest my arms and head on the tank. Plus I liked that it was cool, because I was really sweating at that point. Afterwards my midwife said she was a bit worried that I was going to give birth right on the toilet, but I did move onto the bed when I felt like pushing."

There are a number of studies which show that walking during labour is linked to shorter labour, less medication for pain, and less fetal distress. Yet, women in labour in hospital have often been kept in bed for no particular reason. The introduction of continuous fetal monitoring and IVs made it more difficult for the mother to move around or get out of bed. Skimpy hospital gowns embarrass some women and discourage them from walking around, so bring a generous bathrobe, your own nightgown, or an oversized T-shirt from home to wear.

Sometimes women have been so conditioned by years of movies and TV shows that showed women lying in bed as they laboured, or are so intimidated by the hospital environment, that they find it difficult to know what positions or ways of moving would be most comfortable for them. Caregivers and support people can help with suggestions ("Let's go for a walk down the hall" or "Why don't you sit up for a while?")

As labour progresses and the baby moves down into the pelvis, a position that was helpful and comfortable may quickly become painful and the mother will need to move again. The mother is the best judge of what feels the most comfortable to her at any particular point in her labour.

TOUCH

Touch reminds the labouring woman that she is not alone, that there are people here who care for her, and that she has support and help close by. No wonder a gentle touch can be so relaxing! A hot water bottle on the back, or a cold cloth pressed to a sweaty forehead give not just physical relief, but a sense of being cared for.

The variations of touch are infinite. It can be as simple as holding hands or letting her lean against you during a contraction. Suzanne describes walking around her apartment with her husband David in early labour: "We were just strolling around, and then when the contraction would hit, I stopped walking. I didn't even have to say anything. David would put his arms around me and I'd rest my head on his shoulder and stay in that position until the contraction went away."

Massage is another form of touch that can be helpful in labour. It can be used to relax tense shoulders, arms, or legs. Some women like to have their abdomens massaged lightly during contractions. If the mother is experiencing a lot of back pain, she may like very firm massaging of her lower back and buttocks, or **counterpressure** (firm, direct pressure) against her lower back. Since a long labour can mean many hours of massaging, it's a good idea to bring powder or lotion to use on the mother's skin to prevent irritation.

Mariana had both her husband and a doula walking with her in labour. When a contraction arrived, she'd lean against her husband and he would massage her shoulders. The doula would rub her lower back, where she was feeling increasing pressure. "The massaging helped so much," Mariana says.

Rita says, "I think the most important thing is for your husband to pay attention to you. I could hardly talk once the contractions got strong, and I remember one time saying 'Back!' to John so he would rub my back, but he wasn't paying attention so he didn't do anything. When the contraction finally went away I yelled at him."

Partners and support people also need to be aware that massaging or other touch that has been helpful at one point in labour may suddenly become annoying and uncomfortable. The mother may only be able to say "Stop" or "No" at that point, so the partner needs to be alert.

Massage and other forms of touch have not been systematically researched, but it is difficult to see how they could have any risks. Since women almost universally speak positively about it, touch will continue to be an important part of pain relief in labour.

IMMERSION IN WATER

During the "walking-around" process, many labouring women find themselves—like divining rods—heading for water. Baths, whirlpools, and showers are often comforting and relaxing during labour, and increasing numbers of hospitals are adding these to their labour and delivery units. Women with back labour sometimes like to stand with the shower aimed at their lower backs. Other women find sitting or lying in warm water, in either an ordinary bath or pool or a whirlpool, is very relaxing and reduces their awareness of pain.

"One reason I chose this hospital," says Inez "was the Jacuzzi. I loved feeling the water swirling over me. It was like being massaged by several people at once, and it got me through the worst part of labour."

Some mothers end up giving birth in the bath or pool (either intentionally or because the mother finds it too difficult to get out of the water when the moment of birth arrives), and while this has not been extensively researched, no higher complication rates have been noted so far. A few individual case reports suggest that it is safest to keep the water at around body temperature, so the woman does not get overheated, and that the baby should be lifted from the water as soon as it is born.

ACUPUNCTURE

Acupuncture consists of the placement of needles in specific points, and then stimulation through these needles either by twirling them, or sometimes through an electric current. No controlled trials of acupuncture for pain relief during labour have been published, although it is used effectively for more chronic pain.

Acupressure is "acupuncture without needles." It consists of deep pressure on specific acupuncture points. No trials of its effectiveness in labour have been published.

INJECTION OF STERILE WATER

Controlled trials have shown dramatic relief from back pain in labour by injecting 0.1 millilitres of sterile water just under the skin of the low back at four specific spots around the **sacrum** (the very bottom bone in the spine). This simple measure has no known complications. The reason it relieves the pain is not known, but it might be the same mechanism that makes acupuncture work for pain relief.

Since sterile water is normally available in hospitals, you could ask your doctor about this if you are interested in trying it.

HYPNOSIS

When people have been hypnotized, they are temporarily more relaxed, more open to suggestion, and more able to change the perception of pain. Theoretically, hypnosis would be an ideal painkiller during labour.

It can be used in either of two ways: the woman can be hypnotized during her pregnancy, and left with the post-hypnotic suggestion that the sensations of labour will be powerful and intense, but not painful; or the woman can be taught to hypnotize herself and enter a trance during labour to reduce awareness of pain.

However, one clinical trial of hypnosis during labour found no difference in drug use between the hypnotized and the control group. The length of labour in the hypnosis group was much longer. Another study found shorter labours in the hypnosis group.

MUSIC

Music during labour can be a pleasant distraction that can help the mother to picture relaxing surroundings and images. Music can also create a cheerful atmosphere for the companions of the mother, and the staff caring for her. As well, music can block out unpleasant "hospital" sounds (such as the woman screaming in the next room).

The specific use of soothing music between contractions and "white sound" during contractions, at a volume controlled by the mother, has been researched in small clinical trials. The mothers listening to the music reported less pain and also used fewer drugs during labour.

Stephanie brought a tape she and her husband had put together of songs they liked to the hospital. "I think it made us all feel calmer. I will always remember my doctor and my husband singing along to the tape while we waited for me to have another pushing contraction. I don't know if it really relieved pain, but I definitely felt more relaxed."

TENS (TRANSCUTANEOUS ELECTRICAL NERVE STIMULATION)

TENS uses a portable box containing a battery-powered generator of electrical impulses. Electrodes are taped to the back and the electrical impulses are transmitted to the skin of the back via wires attached to the box, resulting in a buzzing or tingling sensation. The woman can adjust the intensity of these impulses during the contractions. The electrical impulses are intended to "block" the pain sensations.

More clinical trials have been done on TENS than any other non-drug method of pain relief. Their results are almost contradictory—results show that women like TENS and report favourably on it, yet report a higher incidence of intense pain. The use of TENS does not reduce the use of drugs during labour.

If a woman plans to use TENS, she must rent the equipment and learn to use it before the start of labour. The women who select this method may be those who anticipate both that the pain of labour will be severe, and that it will need treatment.

How We Think about Pain in Labour

Do non-drug therapies for pain relief "work"? There isn't any objective way of assessing their effectiveness.

If "working" means do women use them and like them, the answer is an emphatic "yes."

If "working" means do women who use them use fewer drugs during labour, the answer is "we don't know for sure, but probably not."

The 1997 edition of *Williams Obstetrics*, a standard textbook, devotes 20 pages to pain relief in labour. Of those 20 pages, only three paragraphs are spent on non-drug methods. One of these paragraphs is interesting: "When motivated women have been prepared for childbirth, pain during labour has been found to be diminished by one-third. The presence of a supportive spouse or other family member, of conscientious labour attendants, and of a considerate obstetrician who instils confidence, contributes greatly to accomplishing this goal of pain relief."

The small space allotted to non-drug techniques in this textbook sends a clear message—that doctors don't really think these methods are important. The textbook gives lip service to the idea that these methods are useful and have been shown to reduce pain, but then doesn't bother to describe the methods or how they might become part of standard care.

This message is often reinforced in hospital. The doctor's last words as he leaves the labouring woman's room are often, "I'll leave an order for a shot of Demerol when you want it." The nurse making her regular blood pressure check often bustles in on the couple who are managing each contraction with back massage and some groaning and says, "Just ring when you want your epidural."

Is this just making sure choices are available, which is a stated goal of family-centred maternity care? Or does this undermine the normalcy of labour? Every time a mother is reminded about the availability of medication during labour, it reinforces the idea that "something should be done" about the pain.

How important is suggestion in pain relief? Even using the phrase pain relief suggests that labour pain—which is, after all, a universal and normal experience—*needs* to be relieved. Perhaps the methods described as non-drug pain relievers don't actually diminish the pain but help the mother cope with it. That's equally valuable.

Medications for Labour Pain

There has been more research about drugs for pain relief in labour than any other pregnancy treatment. However, most of this research has been aimed at discovering which drug works best (with the research being financially supported by the drug company) and comparing one drug to another. They are rarely compared to non-drug methods and there is little attention paid to possible effects on mothers and babies.

The important question to ask is: What method will give good relief without harm to mother or baby?

TRANQUILIZERS

Sedatives, tranquilizers, and sleeping pills have been used either by mouth or injection in early labour to help women relax, to lessen their anxious feelings, and to help them sleep. They have no pain-killing effect at all. They can cross the placenta and cause the baby to be depressed at birth, meaning it will not breathe well, or suck well, and may be limp until the drug has worn off.

NARCOTICS

Narcotics (Demerol is the most common) can provide very good pain relief, but only at doses which can cause side effects in both mother and baby. Lower, safer doses will not noticeably relieve pain. Different narcotics last for different lengths of time, varying from two to four hours. Narcotics are given either by intramuscular injection or intravenously.

Side effects in the mother may include nausea and vomiting, dizziness, and drop in blood pressure. Narcotics usually keep food that is eaten from being digested; instead, the food just sits in the stomach, and may be vomited even hours after it has been eaten. There is no convincing evidence that Demerol makes labour longer.

Narcotics cross the placenta and can cause the baby to not breathe well at birth. If this happens, the baby may need to be given oxygen through a mask, or spend some time on a respirator. The baby can be given an injection of a narcotic antagonist, which will counteract the effect of the narcotic and improve the baby's breathing. The possibility of depressed breathing in the baby is unpredictable—many mothers have had full doses of Demerol close to delivery and their baby has not had any breathing problems at all.

In one study, babies of mothers who received narcotics in labour tended to have lower Apgar scores and to be less responsive to their parents immediately after birth than those who received a placebo.

Another study compared shots of Demerol given by the nurse with an arrangement in which the labouring woman could give herself a dose of Demerol through an intravenous. The results showed that the pain relief was better, and a lower dose of narcotic was used, when the woman gave the drug to herself as she needed it. The usefulness of this method is limited by the need for an intravenous with a special pump.

Amy was given Demerol in labour and remembers it with mixed emotions. "It did help the pain, but I felt like I was going to throw up the whole rest of the labour. The worst part was after the baby was born, because I felt sleepy and completely out of it. The nurse was trying to give me Andrew to hold, but I kept drifting off."

Nancy, on the other hand, felt the short-acting narcotic she was given really helped. "I was 7 centimetres, but the labour was so painful, much more than I was expecting. My doctor sug-

gested a shot and I said yes. In about 10 minutes the pain of the contractions was much less and I was napping in between them. I thought the labour had really slowed down, but my husband said the contractions were still coming about every three minutes. I totally lost track of time. Then I had a really painful contraction and I said, 'This is wearing off,' and the very next contraction I had to push. The pushing didn't hurt at all like the labour pains—that one shot was all I had for the whole labour. It was great."

ANTINAUSEA DRUGS

Labour itself often causes women to feel nauseated and to vomit, and narcotics given for pain in labour cause nausea and vomiting as well. Drugs like Gravol can be given during labour to try to control the nausea, and are often given at the same time as the injection of narcotic. Antinausea drugs can, like narcotics, cause dizziness and sleepiness in the mother.

INHALED PAINKILLERS

Anaesthetic gas (usually **nitrous oxide**) can be inhaled by the mother at a dose that does not put her to sleep but helps to relieve the pain of labour. This can be used during the first stage of labour, or during the pushing stage. It is usually administered by a mask, which the woman holds on her face herself, and breathes in during contractions. The woman is awake and in control of the painkiller, which doesn't last long and is easily stopped by taking the mask away.

Its disadvantage is that the mask must be

tightly on the face while the mother is breathing in for it to have a chance to reach a level which will relieve pain, and this is often a claustrophobic sensation for the labouring woman. It does not give complete pain relief, and its effectiveness varies a lot from one woman to another, at least in part because many women find it difficult to use. It can cause nausea and vomiting.

No obvious side effects on the baby have been noticed.

Donna tried this method and didn't like it: "It was hard for me to focus on getting the mask in the right position and breathing in deeply when I was also trying to relax and get through the contraction. I took about four breaths and then I just barely got the mask out of the way in time to throw up. Since I was feeling pretty queasy anyway, I really didn't need that."

EPIDURAL ANAESTHESIA

The epidural is probably the first thing that most women think of when they are asked about pain relief during labour. Since its introduction in the early 1970s, it has become very widely used, because it can provide complete relief from pain, yet the mother is still conscious and able to see her baby being born.

The drug used is a local anaesthetic, the same local that is injected by the dentist to freeze your mouth for dental work or is injected by the doctor to freeze you before you have stitches. In an epidural, the local anaesthetic is injected into the epidural space, which is in your back, just outside the spinal canal.

The epidural is put in by an **anaesthetist**, a doctor who specializes in administering this kind of medication. First, an intravenous will be started because having extra fluid in the circulation helps to prevent a drop in blood pressure from the epidural. The mother will either lie on her side curled up, or sit up with her chin on her chest so the anaesthetist can get the needle into the **epidural space** near the spinal cord and inject the drug. Usually a tiny tubing is left in place for more drug to be injected as needed—this is called a **continuous epidural**. The drug can be injected periodically, either as the freezing wears off and the mother needs it, or on some regular schedule.

Studies have shown that regularly scheduled doses of freezing (called **top-ups**) give better pain relief than waiting for the freezing to wear off and then topping up.

Another arrangement is a pump, which is attached to the catheter and pumps the anaesthetic continuously into the epidural space.

The epidural gives extremely effective pain relief—in fact, most women feel nothing at all in the area that is "frozen." Eighty-five per cent of

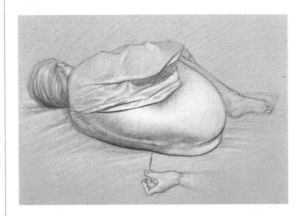

Epidural or spinal injection: The woman is asked to lie with her back rounded to increase the space between the bones of the spine.

women have complete relief of pain and 12 per cent have partial relief. For the 3 per cent who do not get relief, sometimes taking the catheter out and doing the epidural all over again will work.

The epidural can be put in at any stage of labour. It can be given in very early in labour without using any other form of pain relief, or it can be used just for the delivery. It can be used as the next step if narcotics do not provide enough pain relief.

Women in labour are occasionally told that it is "too late" to have an epidural. This is not really true; an epidural can be put in at any time. In practical terms, though, starting the intravenous, getting the anaesthetist to the labour and delivery department, and then the technical aspect of putting in the epidural all take time. If, in the estimation of the nurse or doctor, the woman is going to give birth within the next hour or so anyway, she may be told that "it's too late."

There have been very few studies with only small numbers of women on the effects of epidural on the baby. In these studies, there was no difference in the fetal heart rate, or in passing meconium during labour, with epidural anaesthetic. Epidural is less likely than narcotic painkillers to cause low five-minute Apgar scores, or **low umbilical artery pH**. The pH is a measure of the acidity of the blood in the umbilical cord—if the pH is low, then the baby is not doing well. (Low Apgar and low pH indicate a depressed baby who needs to be resuscitated.) A single report on 18-month-old babies found no difference between epidural and non-epidural babies.

More recent studies, though, have shown that epidurals do have some subtle effects on babies and this shows up in particular with respect to breastfeeding. The unmedicated newborn will crawl to the breast on his own, self-attach, and begin to breastfeed if given the opportunity. But when researchers conducted this same experiment with newborns whose mothers had been given epidurals in labour, the babies were not able to find the breast or latch on. They sometimes made crawling movements but mostly seemed confused and disoriented. Some studies have shown that these effects on breastfeeding can last up to a month. Even with skilled breastfeeding help, babies exposed to epidurals during labour seem to have more difficulty in latching on to the breast and extracting milk. Often this baby will take the mother's nipple into his mouth but then seem confused about what to do next.

With help and persistence, most of these babies will eventually learn to breastfeed, but this difficult start can be a real problem for some.

The epidural does also have effects on the mother, and on the labour.

Studies have found that the first stage of labour tends to be longer with an epidural, and oxytocin tends to be used more frequently to speed up labours when an epidural has been given.

Researchers have also found a tendency for the second stage of labour to be longer, and a substantial increase in forceps or vacuum delivery. There also may be a slight increase in the incidence of Caesarean section with epidural anaesthetic.

Epidural anaesthetic almost always means that the mother will be in bed for the rest of the labour, because it temporarily weakens the muscles in her legs. Some anaesthetists specialize in "walking epidurals," which provide pain relief with less effect on the muscles. However, this is not widely available, and in most hospitals the policy is that women who have an epidural are in bed for the rest of the labour.

CLARIFYING YOUR FEELINGS ABOUT PAIN AND MEDICATIONS IN LABOUR

The Number:	What it Means:	Your Partner, Doula, or Caregiver Can Help You By:
+10	I do not want to feel anything in labour. I want anaesthesia before labour begins.	Explaining to you why this is not possible or safe.
+9	I have great fear of labour pain. I believe I cannot cope. I have to depend on the staff to take away my pain.	Doing the same as for +10 above. Teaching you some simple comfort techniques for early labour. Reassuring you that someone will always be there to help you.
+7	I want anaesthesia as soon in labour as the doctor will allow or before labour becomes painful.	Doing the same as +9 above. Making sure the staff knows you want early anaesthesia. Making sure you know the procedures and the potential risks.
+5	I want epidural anaesthesia in active labour (4–5 cm). I am willing to try to cope until then, perhaps with narcotic medications.	Encouraging you in your breathing and relaxation. Knowing and using other comfort measures. Suggesting medications when you are in active labour.
+3	I want to use some medication but as little as possible. I plan to use self-help comfort measures for part of labour.	Doing the same as +5 above. Committing themselves to helping you reduce medication use. Helping you get medications when you decide you want them. Suggesting half doses of narcotics or a "light and late" epidural.
0	I have no opinion or preference. I will wait and see. (A rare attitude among pregnant women.)	Helping you become informed about labour pain, comfort measures, and medications. Following your wishes during labour.
-3	I would like to avoid pain medication if I can, but if coping becomes difficult I'd feel like a "martyr" if I didn't get them.	Emphasizing coping techniques. Not suggesting that you take pain medications. Not trying to talk you out of them if you request them.

CLARIFYING YOUR FEELINGS ABOUT PAIN AND MEDICATIONS IN LABOUR (CONTINUED)

The Number:	What it Means:	Your Partner, Doula, or Caregiver Can Help You By:
-5	I have a strong desire to avoid pain medications, mainly to avoid the side effects on me, my labour, or my baby. I will accept medication for difficult or long labour.	Preparing for a very active support role. Practising comfort measures with you in class and at home. Not suggesting medications; if you ask, suggesting different comfort measures and more intense emotional support first. Helping you accept pain medications if you become exhausted or cannot benefit from support techniques and comfort measures.
-7	I have a very strong desire for a natural birth, for personal gratification along with the benefits to my baby and my labour. I will be disappointed if I use medication.	Doing the same as -5 above. Encouraging you to enlist the support of your caregiver. Requesting a supportive nurse who can help with natural birth. Planning and rehearsing ways to get through painful or discouraging periods in labour. Prearranging a plan (e.g., a "last resort" code word) for letting them know if you have had enough and truly want medication.
-9	I want medication to be denied by my support team and the staff even if I beg for it.	Exploring with you the reasons for your feelings. Helping you see that they cannot deny you medication. Promising to help all they can but leaving the final decision to you.
-10	I do not want any medication no matter what happens, even a Caesarean.	Helping you to learn about complications that require medication and intervention.

(Used with the permission of Penny Simkin PT and Childbirth Graphics)

Epidural anaesthetic can cause a temporary drop in the mother's blood pressure, which can cause dizziness, nausea, and vomiting. As well, the epidural frequently makes women shiver, occasionally violently, and even though this is not harmful it is extremely unpleasant.

Women who have epidurals often develop a fever after the baby is born. While this fever is not serious, hospital protocols usually require that a mother with a fever be separated from her baby, in case the fever is a sign of an infection that could be dangerous for the baby. This separation may interfere with the establishment of breastfeeding and is stressful for both mother and newborn.

The combination of being in bed and the anaesthetic itself often makes women unable to empty their bladders, so a urinary catheter is frequently used for the rest of the labour. This increases the risk of a bladder infection after delivery. Studies have found that mothers who have epidurals are more likely to have difficulty passing urine after the birth.

When an epidural is given, fluids are also administered intravenously. These extra fluids are important for a number of reasons, including reducing the risks of very low blood pressure, but after the baby is born the mother may experience **edema** (extra fluid) in various parts of her body, including her breasts. Having edema in her breasts can make them painfully hard and make it difficult for the baby to latch on.

When the epidural is being put in, it is possible for the anaesthetist to accidentally puncture the **dura**, the lining of the spinal cord. This means that the epidural anaesthetic cannot be given, and can also lead to severe headache for several days.

Life-threatening complications of epidural are rare, probably from 1 in 5,000 to 1 in 10,000.

For women with lower-back tattoos, there is a small theoretical risk of transferring some of the pigment from the back to the epidural space around the spinal cord, which could cause neurological damage.

Women's feelings about epidurals range from great enthusiasm to disappointment.

Ruth Anne says, "In the small town where I had Cody, epidurals were rare. They had to call in an anaesthetist specially, so they hardly ever did them unless you needed a Caesarean or something. My labour wasn't long, but it really hurt, and the shot the nurse gave me didn't help a bit. Then we moved to Toronto, and I had Jamie. I couldn't believe the difference. As soon as I got to the hospital, they offered me the epidural and I took it. It was like I wasn't even in labour—there was no pain at all, just the excitement of waiting for the baby. A few hours later, Jamie was delivered with forceps, and even when the doctor stitched me up I didn't feel a thing. If I have another baby, I'll definitely get the epidural again."

Daria was also glad she had the epidural, but was unhappy about some parts of it: "Frankly, once I had the epidural, it was boring. I was glad not to feel the pain any more, but it was like I wasn't there. The nurse came in, looked at the monitor, checked my blood pressure, and went out again. My husband was put off by all the tubes—I had the epidural catheter in my back, an intravenous, a catheter in my bladder, and the fetal monitor on my belly—and he spent most of the time in the waiting room watching TV."

For Danielle, the experience of having an epidural was less positive. "I really wanted to have a natural birth. My labour turned out to be very long, and towards the end I was really tired. The nurse kept asking me if I wanted the epidural now. I told her a couple of times that I didn't want it, I would try to keep going a little longer, and finally she said, 'You know, it's going to get worse.' That did it. I said I'd take the epidural.

"But as soon as it was in, I started to cry. It stopped the pain, but I felt so detached from the whole thing, it was more like watching a movie than really having a baby. The next day, I felt really angry at that nurse for pushing the epidural when she knew I didn't want it. I'm sure she was just trying to help, but that was how I felt."

The frequency with which epidurals are used has a lot more to do with how available they are than with variations in the amount of pain women are experiencing. Some hospitals have anaesthetists on hand to provide epidurals for any woman who requests one; in other hospitals, an anaesthetist must be called in and epidurals are reserved for Caesarean sections or forceps deliveries.

One community hospital experienced this when the anaesthesiology staff changed their policy and became much less available. In one year, the rate of epidural use dropped from 75 to 30 per cent. The women didn't change, labour didn't change—epidurals just weren't as easy to get.

Does this mean women are suffering because they can't get epidurals, or that women at this hospital have lost some important choices in childbirth? Generally, when epidurals are less available, the nursing staff offer a wider array of methods for coping with labour pain. Women in hospitals where epidurals are readily available sometimes complain that they felt "pushed into having one." This demonstrates, perhaps, the

challenges hospitals face in meeting the needs of all labouring women, from the mother who wants an epidural as early as possible to the mother who wants no interventions.

Most of the research about epidural has compared one local anaesthetic with another. Considering how frequently epidural is used, it is staggering that there is virtually no data from randomized trials to explore the possible effects of epidural on either mother or baby in the long term. The studies that show the increased incidence of Caesarean section are quite recent, and there have been, so far, no good studies to explore if delaying epidural anaesthetic until labour is well-established would decrease the risk of vacuum or forceps delivery or Caesarean section.

SPINAL ANAESTHESIA

Spinal anaesthesia is similar to epidural in that an intravenous is started first, and local anaesthetic is put in through a needle in the back. The difference is that with a spinal anaesthetic a much smaller needle is used and the **dura** (the lining around the spinal cord) is deliberately punctured so that the local anaesthetic can be put right into the cerebrospinal fluid.

Spinal anaesthetic gives extremely good pain relief for Caesarean section and for forceps deliveries, often better than can be achieved with an epidural.

No catheter is left in place with spinal anaesthesia, so the pain control is not as prolonged or controllable as epidural.

Complications of spinal anaesthesia are similar to those for epidural. The drop in blood pressure after it is administered is even more frequent and severe than with epidural anaesthetic, and pre-treatment with large volumes of intravenous fluid is usual.

About 1 per cent of women after a spinal get a **spinal headache** that lasts three to five days. Mothers have been advised to lie flat, or have been given lots of fluid to prevent this, but these techniques have proven unsuccessful. In recent years, the incidence of spinal headache has been decreased by the use of extremely fine needles to do the spinal. If spinal headache occurs, a treatment called a **blood patch**, in which a very small amount of the mother's blood is injected into the epidural space at the site of the puncture, is usually successful.

Narcotics can be injected into the cerebrospinal fluid as well as local anaesthetic, and can give pain relief for up to 12 hours after a Caesarean section. There is recent interest in this method for pain control during the first stage of labour.

GENERAL ANAESTHESIA

General anaesthesia (going right to sleep) was used for years as pain relief for vaginal deliveries. This practice was discontinued for several reasons. There was a high risk of the baby being sleepy and not breathing properly after birth because the anaesthetic crosses the placenta easily and quickly. There was a small risk of the mother vomiting while asleep and breathing the vomit into her lungs, causing aspiration pneumonia. Even though this was rare, it was an extremely serious complication.

Most importantly, epidural anaesthesia was developed. The epidural was immediately much

---

The Evidence About...
Pain in Labour

Few of the many drug-free approaches to easing labour pain provide dramatic pain relief, but many mothers find that they help them to cope with the pain they are experiencing.

Narcotics reduce pain in labour, but their usefulness is limited by their side effects, particularly their effect on the baby's breathing.

Inhaling nitrous oxide is moderately effective in relieving pain, but can be difficult to use and may make the mother dizzy and nauseated.

Epidurals provide more effective pain relief than any other method, but substantially increase the risk of forceps or vacuum delivery, the need for oxytocin to augment labour, and some other complications. They also make the first stage of labour longer. Epidural anaesthesia seems to be safe for the baby, but can cause breastfeeding difficulties.

---

more popular with women, can be used for labour pain as well as delivery, and eliminates the risk of aspiration pneumonia.

General anaesthesia is still sometimes used for Caesarean sections, especially when a speedy delivery is critical, because a woman can be put to sleep faster than she can be given a spinal or epidural without the same risk of the drop in blood pressure.

For planned Caesarean sections, where the woman is not in labour and has not eaten or drunk for the prescribed amount of time, general anaesthesia or epidural or spinal anaesthetic are all very safe choices. The decision may be offered to the woman, or the anaesthetist or surgeon may have a preference.

-39-
Assessing the Baby during Labour

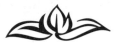

Shirley was relaxing on the couch and watching TV with her husband when labour started. "I couldn't believe how close the contractions were right from the start," she says. "After about 10 contractions, my water broke—right there in the living room—and then things got even more painful."

The intensity of the contractions scared her, but she was also worried about her baby. Was this fast-moving labour as stressful for the baby as it was for her?

Shirley was comforted when her midwife arrived and listened to the baby's heartbeat with a stethoscope. "Baby's doing fine," the midwife reassured her.

When you go into labour, either the midwife who attends you at home or the nurses in the hospital will frequently listen to the baby's heart. The baby's heart rate is the main indicator of his or her well-being during labour. The goal is to detect any problems—signalled by changes in the baby's heart rate patterns—which might indicate that the baby is not getting enough oxygen. The baby who has a problem is often described as being "in distress."

With everything that is going on in labour, keeping an eye on the baby's well-being is important. Ideally, this monitoring process would be selective enough that it won't produce many "false alarms" and subject a lot of babies to interventions they don't need, yet sensitive enough to pick up all the babies who are in distress. We also want to be sure that the interventions done to help those babies in distress are actually improving the outcome.

Heart Rate Monitoring

INTERMITTENT MONITORING: SPOT-CHECKS THROUGHOUT LABOUR

There are several different ways of keeping an eye on the baby's heart rate for signs of stress during labour. The most common method is intermittently listening to the baby's heart either with a special **stethoscope** or with a hand-held ultrasound monitor.

How often should the nurse or other caregiver check the baby? Every hospital will have its own policy, but a common routine is for the nurse to listen for one minute every 30 minutes in early labour, every 15 minutes in active labour, and every five minutes when the mother begins to push the baby out. The nurse will count the number of beats per minute she hears and write that on the mother's chart.

In practice, there are wide variations in how long the nurse listens and how frequently she makes these checks. If the labour and delivery department is very busy, the nurse may need to spend more time with a mother who is having some difficulties, and another mother, where labour is going well, will be checked less frequently.

The baby is considered to be in fetal distress if the heart rate is faster than 160 to 180 beats per minute, or slower than 100 to 120 beats per minute, for any length of time. It is also a concern if the baby's heartbeat is very irregular.

Researchers have assumed that listening to the baby's heartbeat in labour is beneficial, but there have been no studies comparing listening to the baby with not listening. It's unlikely that this research will ever be done, since listening to the baby's heart is now such an accepted part of care during labour.

There have also been no studies to see if there are better outcomes depending on how often these checks of the baby's heart rate are done. (This is why various hospitals will have different routines—no particular schedule has been established as "the best.")

CONTINUOUS MONITORING: THE HIGH-TECH APPROACH

In the 1970s, a new machine was developed that could listen to and record the baby's heartbeat continuously throughout labour: the **electronic fetal monitor** (EFM).

There are two ways of doing continuous monitoring. With external monitoring, a belt is strapped around the mother's abdomen and holds an ultrasound paddle in place to record the baby's heartbeat. A second belt picks up the contractions. For internal monitoring, the membranes must be ruptured. A clip is inserted through the vagina and cervix and attached to the baby's scalp.

With either type, the heart rate is then recorded on a monitor positioned beside the mother's bed and attached by wires to the belt or clip. Usually, the machine beeps each time the baby's heart beats, and shows a constantly-changing number giving the baby's heart rate (you might see 138, 140, 144, 145, 142, and so on). The other belt records the contractions. A continuous record of the baby's heartbeat and the contractions of the uterus is printed out on a long strip of graph paper and in some hospitals it is also transmitted to a computer screen at a central nurse's desk.

Continuous monitoring is technically much more difficult than just having a nurse press a stethoscope against the mother's belly. With external monitoring, whenever the fetus or mother moves the signal may be lost and the paddle must be readjusted. Sometimes it is the mother's heart rate that is being recorded, rather than the baby's, and this can worry everyone because it's normally much slower than the baby's. Once the baby starts to move down into the birth canal, it becomes quite challenging to position the paddle over the baby's heart, especially if the mother is upright or moving around to find a comfortable position for birth.

Elisabeth recalls, "Every time I moved, the monitor's beep of the baby's heart would get really faint. I'd panic, my husband would panic, and I'd try not to move anymore. Then the nurse would calmly readjust the belts and it would be fine—until I moved again. After awhile, my husband asked them to turn off the sound, and that helped."

Noor found the monitor restrictive. "They wanted me in one position and I just wasn't comfortable. I wanted to be able to move around more. Then, at one point, the nurse came in and said, 'Have you stopped having contractions?' I'd somehow moved the belt again so it wasn't recording the contractions at all. She was quite annoyed with me about that."

When internal monitoring is used, there is a risk of the scalp clip coming off the baby's scalp. This can cause a momentary panic because it looks as though the baby's heartbeat has stopped. There is also a higher risk of infection when a scalp clip is used. This may be not just from the clip itself, but from the fact that the clip is often used in long or complicated labours where there have been lots of vaginal exams and other interventions.

WHICH TYPE OF MONITORING IS BETTER?

Even when continuous monitoring is working well, there are concerns. Doctors interpret the patterns they see in different ways, and what one

doctor thinks is a sign of a baby in distress, another doctor may think is perfectly fine. There are no hard and fast rules; the more years that continuous monitoring has been used, the more researchers have realized that what they thought was an abnormal pattern may be normal for many babies.

Many women find continuous monitoring uncomfortable. It makes it impossible for them to walk around and prevents them from moving into positions that might be more comfortable.

But the most important issue is whether or not continuous monitoring can improve outcomes for the baby. Large clinical trials (including 17,000 women) have been reported comparing the outcomes for mothers and babies of using a stethoscope to check on the baby intermittently or continuous monitoring with an EFM during labour.

The results were disappointing for those who had high hopes for EFM: Caesarean section rates and rates of forceps and vacuum deliveries were all significantly higher in the continuously monitored group. Outcomes for the babies, however, were exactly the same in both groups. The number of fetal deaths, low Apgar scores, and admissions to special care nurseries was the same in both the continuously and the intermittently monitored group. Long-term follow-up showed no difference in the rates of cerebral palsy between the two groups.

The inescapable conclusion is that continuous monitoring increases interventions—Caesarean section, forceps, and vacuum delivery—with no benefit to the baby.

If continuous monitoring is used at your hospital, you can refuse it and ask that a nurse check your baby intermittently instead. This will also

The Society of Obstetricians and Gynaecologists of Canada currently recommends intermittent monitoring of the baby during labour rather than routine continuous monitoring.

allow you to walk around and change position during labour more easily.

WHAT ABOUT THE 20-MINUTE INITIAL "STRIP"?

At many hospitals, women who arrive in labour are hooked up to the fetal monitor for a period of time, usually 15 to 20 minutes. After this, the mother may have the belts removed and be permitted to walk around or change position.

This brief use of continuous monitoring has not been studied enough to identify any risks or benefits. There is no reason to believe that it is any more helpful than longer periods of continuous monitoring, which have been shown not to improve outcomes for the baby.

Andrea says: "I was only supposed to be on the monitor for 20 minutes, but then things got busy and nobody came back to take it off. I was having back labour and the position I was in made it worse. I wish I'd had the confidence to just take the belts off myself and get up, but I kept waiting for someone to come and tell me it was okay."

You can decline to have the 20-minute strip done. Just tell the nurse you have decided against it.

Fetal Scalp Sampling

Another method used to assess the baby is fetal scalp sampling.

When the baby is not getting enough oxygen, the **pH** (a measure of the acidity of the baby's blood) decreases. By taking a sample of blood from the baby's scalp, your doctor can measure the pH level and determine if the baby is in distress.

This is a technically tricky procedure. It's most easily done with the mother lying on her back with her legs up in stirrups (a position that can actually *cause* fetal distress). A special speculum is put into the vagina so the doctor can see and feel the cervix and baby's head. The spot to be sampled must be wiped completely clean of all fluid and any of the mother's blood before the scalp is pricked to get the blood sample. Then pressure must be kept on the spot to make sure the baby doesn't keep on bleeding. Since fetal scalp sampling is awkward and time-consuming, it is usually done only if heart rate changes suggest the baby is in distress.

A fetal scalp pH of 7.2 or more suggests that the baby is fine, and that no intervention is necessary. A fetal scalp pH of less than 7.2 suggests that the baby is in distress.

This gives three possible methods of assessing the baby in labour: intermittent monitoring, continuous monitoring, and scalp sampling if the baby's heart rate suggests it might be in distress. When researchers compared these procedures, the results were:

- Caesarean sections, forceps, and vacuum extractors were used most often with continuous monitoring, less often when fetal scalp sampling was added, and least often when the baby was intermittently monitored.

- Babies did equally well in all three groups, with one small exception. When fetal scalp sampling was used, fewer babies had seizures during the newborn period. These seizures were not associated with any long-term problems.

Stimulation of the Fetus to Assess Fetal Heart Rate

If the baby's heart rate speeds up in response to contractions or movement, this is considered to be a positive indicator that baby is doing well.

Some researchers have noted that sound and touch can also cause the baby's heart rate to speed up. Studies have been done comparing the baby's reaction to sound (using a noise-making device placed on the mother's abdomen) and touch (using pressure or gentle pinching of the baby's scalp). The researchers also did fetal scalp sampling on these babies.

They found that if the baby responded to the sound or touch with a faster heartbeat, the fetal scalp sampling result would be good as well.

More research is needed, but this looks like a promising—and much simpler—way to monitor babies in labour. Only those who do not respond to the sound or touch would need scalp sampling to further assess the possibility of distress.

If the Baby Is in Distress, What Then?

When the baby's heart rate drops and stays low, the doctor or midwife will usually do a vaginal examination to see if the umbilical cord has slipped into the vagina and is being compressed by the baby's head. This vaginal exam will also indicate how close the woman is to giving birth.

The simplest step to take when the baby appears to be in distress is to change position. If you are lying on your back, even when the head of the bed is elevated, you are compressing the **aorta** (the major artery) and **vena cava** (major vein of the body) and reducing blood flow to the fetus. You can try lying on your side, which can dramatically increase the circulation to the baby. Changing position may also improve heart rate problems caused by pressure on the umbilical cord.

If the mother is given extra oxygen (in a mask she can hold over her nose and mouth) the baby will get more oxygen as well.

If the mother is receiving oxytocin by IV to stimulate the labour and the baby shows signs of distress, the oxytocin should be immediately discontinued.

If the mother's blood pressure drops, the baby may show signs of distress. This frequently happens when an epidural or spinal anaesthetic is given. The drop in blood pressure can be prevented by giving the mother intravenous fluids to increase her blood volume before administering the epidural or spinal.

Your blood pressure can also drop if you change position suddenly (sitting up or standing up quickly, for example). You are more likely to experience this if you have been given narcotic painkillers such as Demerol. Try not to get up quickly when you are in labour; if you do find yourself feeling faint, lie down on your side. Drinking frequently during labour also helps to reduce this problem. If you are throwing up

---

The Evidence About…

Assessing the Baby during Labour

When continuous monitoring is used during labour, more babies will be delivered by Caesarean section, forceps, or vacuum extractors, with no improvement in outcome.

When fetal scalp sampling is added to this, the intervention rate is lower.

When babies are monitored intermittently, the intervention rate is lowest of all, and the babies do just as well as with the other methods.

While prompt delivery is the usual method for dealing with fetal distress, changing the mother's position or giving her oxygen may also be helpful.

The story of continuous electronic fetal monitoring should serve as a cautionary tale: monitors were readily accepted and quickly pressed into routine use at many hospitals before their value had been tested by research. As a result, many women experienced unnecessary Caesarean sections and other interventions. Any new procedures should be thoroughly researched before being introduced into practice.

This can be a frightening time for parents. Hannah remembers her labour as "overwhelming. I was going too slowly at first, so they gave me oxytocin in an IV to get things moving. But before long the contractions got really strong, and then the baby went into distress. We could all see it on the monitor, his heart rate just dropped, and it was just *beep…beep…beep*. My husband started yelling at the nurse to 'do something.'

"They stopped the oxytocin and got me to roll onto my side. But it didn't help. There was still that ominous, slow beeping. The doctor shook his head and told me we had to do a C-section. They gave me a general anaesthetic because it was faster, and when I came around again I didn't even know if the baby was okay. I was afraid to ask. I think it was even worse for Chad, waiting outside the room to hear the news. But the news was good. Mark's first Apgar score was low, but then he was fine, and he's doing great now."

Other Approaches for Fetal Distress

Clinical trials to assess other methods of managing fetal distress have been too small to allow any conclusions other than that they look promising and need larger trials.

When there is only a small amount of amniotic fluid (called **oligohydramnios**), there is more opportunity for the umbilical cord to be compressed and the oxygen supply to the baby decreased. The volume of fluid can be increased by putting a little tubing through the vagina into the uterus and infusing solution through it into the uterus. Small studies have shown improved

repeatedly and not able to keep liquids down, you might consider having an IV put in to give you more fluids.

If these steps haven't improved the baby's heart rate, the next step is to get the baby born. If labour has progressed far enough, that can mean the use of a vacuum extractor or forceps to deliver the baby quickly. If the cervix is not fully dilated, or if the baby is not low enough in the birth canal to make vacuum or forceps possible, then a Caesarean section will be recommended.

fetal heart rates and healthier babies, without increasing the rate of Caesarean section. (See also Chapter 37.)

Terbutaline is a drug that relaxes smooth muscles and is used to stop premature labour. Intravenous terbutaline has also been used to reduce signs of fetal distress when there is some delay before the baby can be delivered. Studies have shown better outcomes for babies, but these trials have been very small.

Piracetam and **pyridoxine** (vitamin B6) are drugs to "treat" the fetus to prevent damage from fetal distress. Small studies appear promising.

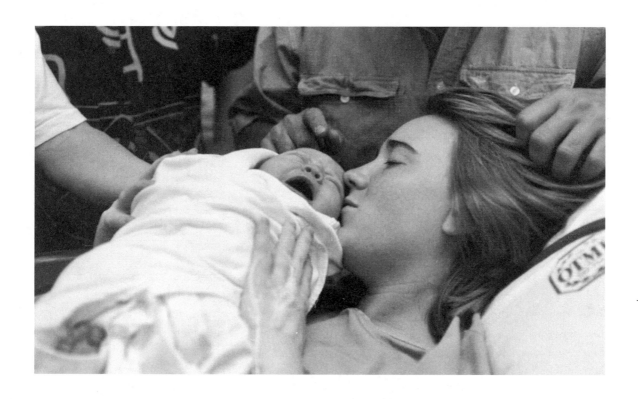

Nine Months
◈◈ *Thirty-four to Thirty-eight Weeks* ◈◈

Have you noticed that everywhere you look, you see other pregnant women? Or mothers with new babies? It's getting to the "home stretch" now and you can't help but be both nervous and excited about the birth and finally holding your new baby in your arms.

-40-
Supporting Your Partner through Labour

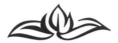

Tracy's husband, John, attended prenatal class and worked at preparing the nursery, but he confesses that impending fatherhood remained an abstract concept through most of the pregnancy. Even when Tracy held his hand against her belly so he could feel the baby's movements, it was hard to connect that sensation with an expected child.

"Actually," John says, "I don't think it really seemed real until we drove up to the hospital with Tracy in labour." But John remembers that he always felt confident about Tracy's ability to carry and give birth to a healthy baby. "I just felt things would go well," he says. That confidence helped Tracy feel positive about the coming birth.

At four-thirty on a Wednesday morning, those weeks of preparation came to an end. "Tracy still says she just tapped me lightly, but I say she shook me awake. And there was her face, her eyes three inches wide and staring at me. I thought the house must be on fire. Then she said, 'I think I'm in labour.'"

Tracy and John tried, unsuccessfully, to get a little more sleep. Within a few hours they were settled into the hospital, and Tracy's labour was really moving. Now John realized how important his presence was to her. "I don't think I really did anything. She didn't even want to be touched, but it was soothing for her just to have me there. I would have done anything she wanted, but all she really needed was to have me there, supporting her," John remembers.

"I was holding the baby less than a minute after he was born," John says, "and that's when I really got emotional. That's when it hit me. I couldn't even talk for about five minutes because I knew if I did I'd start crying."

In retrospect, John would have liked to have been more involved in the actual birth, perhaps cutting the cord or assisting with the actual delivery. He believes that his doctor would have been happy to let him do these things, but he hadn't thought to ask in advance.

Most fathers these days attend the birth of their child and support their partner through labour. You may also have a sister, friend, or other support person with you. This is an exciting role, but it can be worrisome as well. As the pregnant woman's support person, you may wonder if you will really be able to help, and how you will cope with seeing your partner in pain. As Tracy and John's story shows, just your loving presence will be a big help. But there are also practical things you can try to help a woman in labour.

These suggestions may get you started:

- Your love for her and your confidence in her ability to give birth are the most important things you can give her. Try to stay with her throughout labour if at all possible: pack a lunch so you don't have to leave to eat, and take any bathroom breaks immediately after a contraction.
- Providing comfort in labour is always a matter of trial and error. Try gently massaging her stomach, back, arms, legs, or shoulders—but be prepared to stop if she doesn't like it. She may prefer a firm, steady touch, or she might not want to be touched at all. If she's hot, wipe her face and wrists with a cool washcloth. Encourage her to try different positions—walking, sitting backwards on the toilet, squatting, hands and knees—and see what feels best.
- Encourage her to eat lightly in early labour, and offer sips of water, ginger ale, or ice chips in later labour.
- Remind her to pee every hour or so, even if she doesn't feel like she has to.
- Give her something to focus on by talking to her, breathing with her, or holding her. If she seems scared or panicky, ask her to look at you, and breathe with her. Use touch to relax and reassure her, rubbing her legs if they begin to shake, gently holding her if she becomes tense or anxious.

"I COULDN'T HAVE DONE IT WITHOUT HIM"
WHAT WOMEN SAY ABOUT THEIR LABOUR PARTNERS

You can't control the course of her labour, or take away her pain. You might even feel that you really aren't much use. But chances are, you will help her more than you know. Here's what some women remember about their partners' support:

"He timed the contractions so he could warn me when another one was about to start and I'd get into a comfortable position before it hit."

"He really physically supported me. I walked around through much of my labour and every time a contraction hit I'd lean on him. And when the baby was born I was squatting and he held me up under my arms."

"He held the basin for me to throw up in and never said a word."

"When I felt like I couldn't go on he held my face in his hands and made me look at him and said, 'Breathe now, breathe, breathe,' and just kept me going through those really hard contractions."

"He was just there for me. He held my hand and whenever I looked at him he'd smile and nod. That was so important to me."

"I had a Caesarean and a general anaesthetic, but when I opened my eyes again he was standing there holding the baby and tears were running down his face. He said, 'You did it, you did it,' and I felt wonderful despite the surgery."

"I couldn't have done it without him."

- As labour progresses and gets more intense, she may get discouraged. Remind her that it is "almost over," and encourage her to get

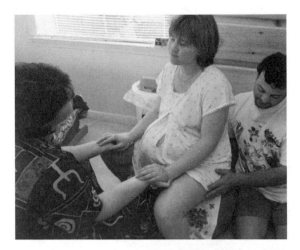

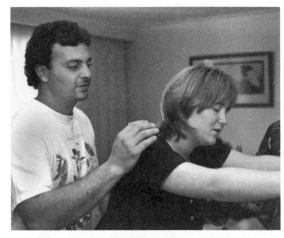

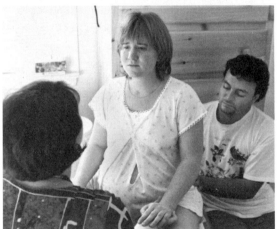

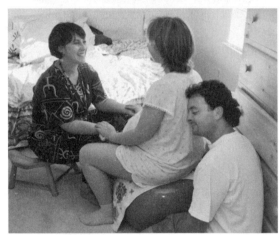

Kieran's Birth Day

Christy and Angelo had planned to have lots of
support for the birth of their first child, and
appreciated all of it when labour turned out to
be long and slow. Christy laboured at home for
17 hours, encouraged by her aunt, her midwives,
and Angelo. She spent some time walking in her
yard, relaxing in the bathtub, and sitting upright
while her support people rubbed her back and
helped her relax. Eventually, they went to the
hospital where Christy had some medication for
pain relief, and baby Kieran was born 7 hours
later, weighing just over 9 pounds.

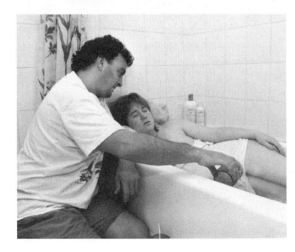

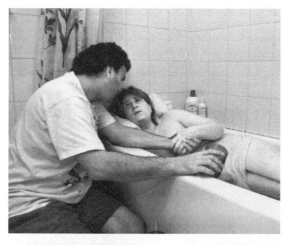

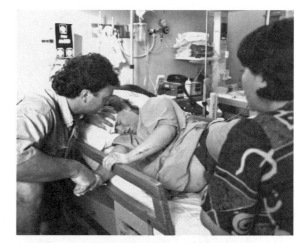

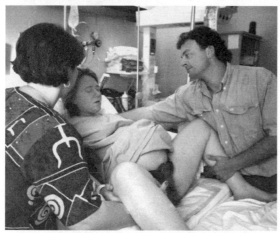

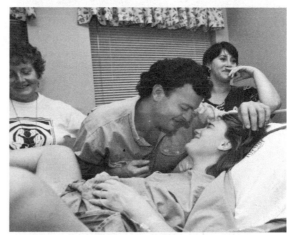

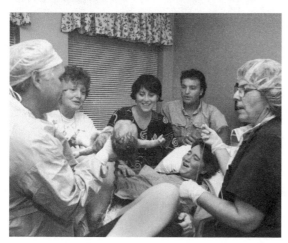

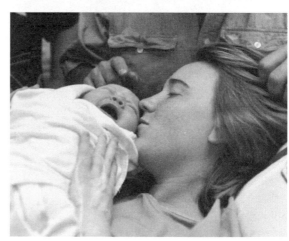

REMINDER LIST: COMFORT TECHNIQUES

What you can do to help your partner through labour:

- massage her face, arms, or legs to help her relax
- gently stroke her belly
- rub or press on her back firmly to ease back pain
- support her in an upright position during contractions
- remind her of relaxing breathing patterns by breathing with her
- help her find comfortable positions in which to labour
- put cold wet cloths on her face, if she feels warm
- give her ice, water, or juice to drink
- help her to develop a contraction "ritual" of breathing, humming, moving, etc.
- remind her to pee every hour or so
- be her advocate and speak up for her as needed

through "just one more contraction." Tell her how well she is doing, how well the labour is going, and that soon she will see her baby.

- It may be hard for her to talk during active labour. You can help her by asking for explanations of things the medical staff say or do. She may also need you to repeat any instructions the doctor gives, because she may only be focusing on your voice.
- You may want to hire a labour support person or midwife. She will help with specific coping measures, provide information, and allow you to concentrate on the special, loving support that only a partner can give.
- You might feel scared or tense, too, especially if the labour is not going the way you expected. Remember that the labour and delivery nurses (and your labour companion, if you have one) are there to support *you* as well as your partner, and let them know your fears and needs.

-41-
Induction of Labour

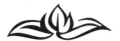

Induction of labour is a deliberate attempt to start labour artificially, rather than waiting for it to start on its own. The most important question about induction of labour is not how the induction will be done, but if it should be done in the first place. As obstetricians have found more effective methods to induce labour, the number of inductions has gone up considerably.

Induction of labour often seems very appealing. We are used to making appointments for important things, scheduling events into our daytimers, and setting aside a certain block of time to do important tasks. We also tend to believe that it is good to "do something" rather than be passive. The unpredictable nature of labour can be frustrating. Labour can start anytime within three weeks before or after the due date, and it can take from a couple of hours to a couple of days. This is not how we handle any other crucial happening in our lives, so planning the date of a baby's birth can seem like a good option. It's a reason mentioned by many women in choosing a repeat Caesarean over a VBAC, for example.

Induction can be helpful in some situations, but it is an intervention in the normal processes of pregnancy and birth and like all interventions can bring its own problems.

The "outcomes" of inductions are not all measured in Caesarean section rates or number of babies needing resuscitation. A woman's confidence in her body's ability to labour and give birth normally is probably lessened if she is told that she "needs" to be induced. This suggests that her body is not working properly, and this lack of confidence may influence the progress of her labour.

Why Induce Labour?

The reasons given for inducing labour range from those that are lifesaving for mother or baby, to those that are minor. You, your partner, and your caregiver will need to decide which reasons make sense to you.

One approach might be to induce labour only when continuing the pregnancy would put the mother or baby at greater risk than the risks of induction or Caesarean section.

At the other end of the spectrum, one might consider inducing labour in any situation where the outcome for the mother and baby is likely to be just as good with induction as with waiting for spontaneous labour. With this approach, as long as induction does not produce more complications than waiting, it is considered reasonable.

Sometimes the need for induction is clear. But when the reasons are not compelling, it is your preference (not your doctor's) that should be the deciding factor.

Reasons to induce labour are discussed below.

ILLNESS IN THE MOTHER

The development or worsening of some disease in the mother completely unrelated to her pregnancy may be a reason for induction. Pregnant women can get cancer, thyroid disease, kidney disease, and other medical conditions which need urgent treatment, but sometimes the treatment can't be started with the baby still in the uterus. Getting the baby born as soon as it can survive outside the uterus can allow the start of essential treatment for the mother.

Pre-eclampsia is an illness in the mother that is caused by pregnancy and threatens the safety of both mother and baby. With severe pre-eclampsia, the research is clear—the only cure is delivery of the baby. (Chapter 33 tells you more about this condition.)

PRE-LABOUR RUPTURE OF THE MEMBRANES

It is fairly common for the membranes containing the amniotic fluid to break before labour contractions start; usually this means that the labour is going to start within the next few hours

and that the baby will be born within the next day or two. Two to 5 per cent of women who have this pre-labour rupture of the membranes, though, will still not have delivered their babies at the end of five days. The main concern when the membranes rupture long before the birth of the baby is an increased risk of infection in the mother and newborn.

Research that compares waiting for labour after pre-labour rupture of the membranes with inducing labour *appears* to indicate that induction reduces the rate of infection in the newborn, but this may not be accurate. The diagnosis of infection in the newborn is difficult to make in the first hours after birth, so many babies are treated preventatively with antibiotics simply because the membranes were ruptured for a long time. When studies are done which look back at cases, these babies would then be classed as having been infected because they were on antibiotics. In reality, though, the babies may have been perfectly healthy.

The studies also found that induction of labour after spontaneous rupture of the membranes causes a longer and more painful labour, and higher rates of Caesarean section. The risk of Caesarean section is less if **prostaglandin** is used for the induction, rather than oxytocin. The methods of inducing labour with these two drugs are described in more detail later.

UNUSUALLY BIG OR SMALL BABIES

The baby who is bigger than average at term will sometimes be induced because of concerns that he will grow too big to deliver vaginally and will need a Caesarean section. Unfortunately, size alone does not predict which babies won't fit—the position of the baby's head in the pelvis is also important, as well as the strength of the labour.

There is no evidence that inducing big babies at term is either beneficial or harmful.

Small babies raise different concerns. With the routine use of ultrasound, the diagnosis of the small-for-dates baby is made much more frequently. If the growth of the baby is seen to be less than average on a series of ultrasounds, induction may be recommended on the basis that the environment inside the uterus is not nourishing the baby and it would grow better on the outside.

Unfortunately, the ultrasound can't always show the difference between babies who are suffering malnutrition in the uterus because of lack of circulation to the placenta, and who would be better out, from babies who are just small and would benefit from more time in the uterus to grow.

PROLONGED PREGNANCY

Being "overdue" probably represents the major reason for induction of labour in North America.

Prolonged pregnancy in most cases is a variation of normal and the baby does well regardless of whether the labour is induced or the mother waits for labour to start.

Very large comparisons of induction versus waiting have shown minimal differences in outcome for mothers or babies. Induction on the due date gives no advantage, while induction at 41 weeks appears to give a small increase in infant survival rates. (This is discussed in more

detail in Chapter 41). On the basis that outcomes are almost as good either way, the decision should be up to the mother.

It's not always an easy decision. While some inductions are simple and straightforward, others become long, drawn-out and difficult procedures (for an example, see the sidebar). Since inductions must be done in hospital, this means that women who have planned a home birth must come to terms with giving birth in hospital. Other women who had planned to have their babies in hospital but hoped to stay home as long as possible may be disappointed about going to the hospital before labour even starts and staying there through the whole process. Some women find this very stressful. Some studies have also found that women describe induced labours as more painful than labours which begin naturally.

Readiness of the Cervix: An Important Factor

The way the cervix feels at the time of starting the induction is the most important factor in how the induction will go. If the cervix is **unripe** (meaning hard, long, and closed), the induction is more likely to fail to start labour at all, labour is more likely to take a long time, and Caesarean section (because of a slow labour) is more likely. If the cervix is **ripe** (meaning soft, thin, and starting to open), the induction is much more likely to go well.

Deciding whether the cervix is ripe or unripe is a subjective thing. A scoring system has been developed to describe the cervix, to try to make the evaluation more objective:

THE NEVER-ENDING STORY: ROBIN'S INDUCTION

Robin's baby was "due" on February 22. That week at her appointment, her doctor examined her and said her cervix was thick and closed. On February 26, she had a biophysical profile, which showed the baby was doing well. On March 3, her doctor examined her again and told her that her cervix still wasn't ripe. She was now nine days overdue (41 weeks and two days) and her doctor told her he liked to induce everyone between 41 and 42 weeks. Robin says, "I didn't think anything of it. I just assumed that it was routine."

She was admitted to hospital that evening and had **prostaglandin gel** put in her cervix to soften it in preparation for labour. The next day an IV with **Pitocin** (a synthetic hormone used to start labour) was started and run all day. This only caused a few contractions, so the Pitocin was stopped at bedtime. She had another dose of prostin gel put in her cervix, and stayed in hospital for the second night. Another day on the Pitocin IV went by, and Robin still wasn't in labour.

That night the prostin gel treatment was repeated, but the next day the labour and delivery department was really busy. Robin says, "The nurse told me that they were too busy to run the IV Pitocin on me; then my doctor came in and told me I might as well go home and come back the next day to be induced again. I was really tired by then—I hadn't slept very well in the hospital. I hadn't had many real meals either, because they kept thinking I was going to be in labour so my meals didn't get ordered. Then they would realize I hadn't had anything to eat and get me a sandwich and juice."

Robin spent a night at home, then "I went back the next day and the doctor said my cervix still wasn't ripe, so I had prostin gel put in every six hours all day long. I stayed overnight again, and the next day I had an IV Pitocin drip again and this time the doctor broke my water. The medication caused what they called **pit contractions** all day, which sure hurt but didn't dilate my cervix very much. By suppertime I was so tired and in pain I asked for an epidural. It worked great for the pain but I still couldn't really sleep because I was shaking and the nurses kept getting me to turn from side to side. Finally, early the next morning I had the baby. Of course, I was excited and happy, but I was so tired I couldn't think straight. It was days before I felt normal again and I think a lot of it was lack of sleep."

Robin wishes she'd asked more questions and been more involved in the decision making. "When I look back, the decision to have the first dose of prostin gel was made so casually, and then things just kept going. It never occurred to me that I could have stopped it by just saying, 'This isn't working—let's stop and wait.' One thing just seemed to automatically lead to another, and I felt like I was on a merry-go-round I couldn't get off."

- **Consistency:** this describes whether the cervix feels hard or soft to the person doing the examination.
- **Effacement:** this measures the length of the cervix. During most of pregnancy, the cervix is about 2 centimetres long. Effacement describes how the cervix becomes shorter and flattens out to become just an opening into the lower part of the uterus. Effacement is measured in per cents—100 per cent effaced means completely flattened out.
- **Position of the cervix:** this refers to whether

the cervix is pointed down towards the mother's backbone or straight forward towards the opening of the vagina. The cervix pointing straight forward into the vagina is the most favourable.

- **Dilation:** this describes how open the cervix is; it is measured in centimetres, between 1 and 10.
- **Position of the presenting part:** this refers to the position of the baby's head (or buttocks if the baby is breech) in the mother's pelvis. The lower the baby's head, the likelier it is the induction will go well.

If the biggest part of the baby's head is lower than the mother's pubic bone, the baby is described as "engaged." For some reason, research has shown that for most white women having a first baby, the baby is engaged during the last few weeks of pregnancy, before labour starts; for later babies or for black women, the baby is usually not engaged until labour is under-way. If your baby is engaged, the induction is likely to be easier.

If the cervix is completely soft and 100 per cent effaced, it is said to be ripe. If it is also in the mid-position in the vagina, the baby's head is very low, and the cervix has started to dilate, these are the perfect conditions to do an induction.

If you are considering induction, it might help in making the decision to know how ripe your cervix is. If it is very ripe, the induction will likely go well. If it is not ripe at all, you can predict that the induction may be more difficult, and you may want to rethink the idea.

Sometimes, induction is chosen even when the cervix is not ripe, so methods to ripen it so that induction will be easier have been developed.

Artificial Ripening of the Cervix

PROSTAGLANDINS TO RIPEN THE CERVIX

Prostaglandins (**prostins**) are drugs that ripen the cervix. A gel or tablet of prostin is placed in the vagina, or the gel squeezed directly into the cervix. Prostaglandin ripening makes it more likely that the induction of labour will succeed. Labours with prostaglandin ripening also tend to be faster. In some cases, prostaglandin causes not just ripening of the cervix but the onset of labour as well.

If oxytocin is going to be used for the induction of labour, it should not be given until six to 12 hours after the prostaglandin ripening is done.

Very strong, frequent contractions and fetal heart rate abnormalities can occur during prostaglandin ripening. Despite this, the rate of Caesarean section and forceps or vacuum deliveries is lower in induced labours in which the cervix has been ripened with prostaglandin first.

Kendra says, "When my doctor told me she wanted to induce me and that she planned to use the oxytocin drip, I asked her about the prostaglandin gel. She said she didn't normally use it, but when I told her what I'd read—that it tends to make induction more successful—she said we could certainly give it a try.

"The plan was to put in the gel in the morning, then start the oxytocin later that day. My doctor inserted the gel, then left for the office, saying she'd come back around noon. Well, my contractions started almost immediately and I had a fast, intense labour. The nurses had to call the doctor back—my baby was born at eleven-thirty! We were very pleased that we had decided to use the gel."

MECHANICAL METHODS OF RIPENING THE CERVIX

The cervix may be ripened by inserting a **balloon catheter** into the cervix and blowing up the balloon. This is left in place, with the other end of the catheter taped to the mother's thigh, for 12 to 24 hours before the induction of labour. The steady pressure of the balloon on the cervix ripens the cervix, possibly by stimulating the release of **natural prostaglandins**. Other mechanical devices have also been used for the same purpose. The disadvantage of these techniques is the pain of the insertion, and a small risk of introducing infection. Research has found this to be less effective in ripening the cervix than the synthetic prostaglandin gel.

OXYTOCIN TO RIPEN THE CERVIX

Oxytocin is a naturally occurring hormone that has been synthesized. While it is most often given to induce labour, it has also been given by intravenous drip over prolonged periods of time to ripen the cervix. Studies have shown that this method of ripening is definitely not helpful.

How Labour Is Induced

Methods used to induce labour include nipple stimulation, sweeping or rupturing the membranes, or giving oxytocin or prostaglandin. Induction of labour is more likely to succeed if the cervix is ripe.

NIPPLE STIMULATION AND SEXUAL ACTIVITY

Women have often been advised to stimulate their nipples, which causes oxytocin release, to start labour. Sex has also been recommended as a way of starting labour; during sexual intercourse prostaglandin is released from the cervix and it is also present in semen. As can be imagined, the data to evaluate these methods come from rather small and uncontrolled studies! However, the research available suggests that nipple stimulation and regular sexual activity in late pregnancy does reduce the number of post-term pregnancies.

Women who are breastfeeding a baby or toddler while pregnant with the next baby are sometimes advised to wean, in case the older baby's suckling causes premature labour. There is no evidence that this is so! Many women nurse through the pregnancy and continue, if they choose, to breastfeed both the older child and the new baby.

Lily became interested in these methods when she reached 41 weeks and her midwife discussed induction with her. "I didn't want to be induced if we could avoid it," Lily says, "and I figured sex and nipple stimulation couldn't hurt and would be fun even if it didn't work. I don't know if that's what did it, but after the third night of sex, I woke up at 3 a.m. in labour."

SWEEPING THE MEMBRANES

Stripping or sweeping the membranes, also called a **stretch-and-sweep**, has been a traditional method of getting labour going. The doctor or midwife inserts a finger through the cervix as far as possible and rotates it in a circle

TWO OPTIONAL INDUCTIONS: CONNIE'S STORY

Connie never imagined she'd want to have labour induced, but in the end she chose induction for both of her children.

"Both of my labours were induced. With my first pregnancy, I was a student. My boyfriend had left me halfway through the pregnancy. My mother, who has always been really close to me, had taken a month's leave of absence from her job so she could fly here and be with me when I had the baby. She came when I was 38 weeks, as my doctor had told me I could go into labour any time after that.

"At almost 42 weeks, we were still waiting! My mother had to fly home to go back to work in five days. We both went to my appointment with my doctor that week. My mother is Dutch and she is really against interfering with pregnancy—she had me at home in Holland—but I couldn't imagine having the baby without her support. At my appointment, we asked about being induced.

"She—my doctor—said that at 42 weeks induction was a very reasonable thing to consider as it was certainly as safe for me and the baby as waiting. Then she suggested feeling my cervix to see if it was ripe. After she examined me, she said my cervix was really favourable and that she was sure the induction would work. By the time we left the office, both my mother and I were comfortable that an induction was what we wanted.

"The next day, I went into the hospital first thing in the morning. My doctor broke the water—I remember how warm it felt. The doctor said that the water was clear and that was a good thing. I walked around for half an hour dripping water and then the contractions started up. I was really glad they started on their own because we had decided that if the contractions didn't start in four hours I would have an IV and Pitocin to start them, something I hoped to avoid. The rest of the labour and birth went fine.

"It was such a help to me to have my mother there—for me that was more important than not being induced.

"With my next pregnancy, I was married. It turned out, though, that I was due right around the time my husband would have to be away on a course for work. When my due date got close, he kept putting off going to the course but finally he was at the point where he had to go. This time I was only 40 weeks and five days. I remember exactly because I was counting!

"My husband really wanted to be here for the birth, and I really wanted him here as well. I talked it over with my doctor, and we agreed that even though this wasn't a medical reason, it was a reason that was important to us as a family.

"The induction went really well. I had hoped that just breaking the water would work again, but this time I only leaked a little bit of water and the contractions didn't start. My husband and I walked and walked all day—still no contractions. In the late afternoon, an IV and Pitocin were started. The contractions kicked in right away; within two hours, the doctor turned the Pitocin off and said my labour was on its own. Two hours later the baby was born.

"I'm really happy with both my inductions, even though I am the type who would have told you that I would never be induced. Both times, the reasons were really important to me."

to separate the membranes from the wall of the lower part of the uterus. There is little good data on this approach, but what there is does suggest that stripping the membranes makes it more likely that the woman will go into labour within the next few days.

This technique is frequently used as an office procedure in post-term pregnancies to avoid formal induction. It is most easily and effectively performed if the cervix is ripe.

Potential concerns are accidental rupture of the membranes, and the introduction of infection.

Eleanor was five days past her due date when her doctor suggested trying a stretch-and-sweep at her regular prenatal appointment. "I was tired of being pregnant, and ready to try just about anything," Eleanor says. "It wasn't comfortable having it done but it wasn't really painful. I went home feeling a bit funny—almost queasy—and by suppertime I was in labour. My doctor said it doesn't usually work that quickly, but I must have been ready to go."

RUPTURING THE MEMBRANES

This is called artificial rupture of the membranes, breaking the water, or **amniotomy**. It is done by putting an **amni-hook** (a long thin plastic stick with a small sharp hook on its end) through the cervix and breaking the membranes with it. The membranes have no nerves so it isn't painful—it just feels wet and warm as the fluid escapes.

Rupturing the membranes to induce labour has traditionally meant that you can't change your mind—once ruptured, there is no turning back. The membranes make a barrier against infection in the uterus, and once they are bro-

ken, it's easier for bacteria to get in. Since something from outside (the amni-hook) has been inserted into the membranes, the risk of infection is probably higher than if the membranes had ruptured on their own.

What if the membranes are ruptured and nothing happens—labour doesn't start? Oxytocin is then administered intravenously to get labour going.

How long should the doctor wait before giving the oxytocin? There are no studies on this. Some doctors will add an oxytocin IV at the same time as they break the water, others will wait for a few hours to see if anything happens.

A rare but very serious complication of rupture of the membranes is the umbilical cord slipping through the cervix (**cord prolapse**). The cord is then between the baby's head and the cervix, and will be compressed when the uterus contracts, cutting off the circulation to the baby. This is an emergency requiring immediate Caesarean section. A cord prolapse is more likely to occur if the membranes are ruptured before the baby's head is well down into the mother's pelvis.

IV OXYTOCIN

Oxytocin is the most widely used method to induce labour. Synthetic oxytocin (Pitocin, hence the name "**pit drip**") is given by IV solution at a carefully regulated rate, which is gradually increased until regular contractions result. Once labour gets going, the rate of oxytocin infusion usually doesn't need to be increased; frequently, the rate of the infusion can actually be reduced or even stopped altogether as active labour "kicks in."

Oxytocin can sometimes induce very strong contractions, causing the baby to be stressed and, rarely, causing rupture of the uterus. There has been a tendency to use continuous electronic fetal monitoring for all labours induced with oxytocin. The research to support this has not been done. In any case, continuous monitoring does not replace careful attention by a bedside nurse. The frequency and strength of contractions can change very quickly with a small change in the dose of oxytocin.

Studies suggest that oxytocin induction without rupture of the membranes will fail to start labour in about one-third of cases. Oxytocin plus artificial rupture of membranes is more likely to establish labour within a few hours of starting induction than oxytocin alone. With this approach, though, traditionally there has been a definite commitment to delivery within 24 to 48 hours, either vaginally or by Caesarean section.

PROSTAGLANDINS

The ability of prostaglandins to ripen the cervix has already been discussed. In some women, prostaglandin used to ripen the cervix also made them go into labour. Prostaglandin gel in the vagina has been investigated as a method of inducing labour. Repeat doses of prostaglandin can be used, usually every six to 12 hours. Prostaglandin is easier to use than oxytocin because no intravenous is required, so women can walk around freely. Prostaglandin can be used whether the membranes are ruptured or not.

How does prostaglandin compare with oxytocin for inducing labour?

Doctors have much more experience with oxytocin, which has been used widely for 40 years, than with prostaglandin, which is a newer drug. Studies comparing the two drugs have only included small numbers of women so far. In the studies that exist, though, the number of women who deliver within 12 hours of induction is the same with both methods. However, after 24 and 48 hours, there are more women who have given birth in the prostaglandin group than in the oxytocin group. Caesarean section rates are very slightly lower in the prostaglandin group, and rates of forceps and vacuum deliveries are significantly lower in the prostaglandin group. There were no significant differences seen in outcomes for the babies.

Are Induced Labours More Painful?

There is a widely held belief that induced labour is more painful than spontaneous labour. Certainly, women who describe their induced labours often comment on the pain, and women who have had both induced and naturally starting labours will often say that the induction was more painful.

Despite this, the incidence of use of epidural anaesthesia is the same in the two groups. This is surprising, given that induced women are in hospital during their whole labour, and that inductions are all carried out during daylight hours: two factors which make anaesthesia very available to the induced women, and might have made it more likely that they would use it.

A different use of oxytocin is to use it to make a slowly progressing labour faster by making the contractions stronger and closer together—this is called **augmenting the labour**. Not surprisingly, women also perceive this as more painful than the labour to that point, and epidural use is more common with augmented labours.

Caesarean Section Rates and Induced Labour

Many people also feel that induction causes a higher Caesarean section rate than spontaneous labour. This is undoubtedly true. However, many inductions are being done because of problems with the mother or baby that make delivery necessary. The induction is being done as an alternative to Caesarean section, not as an alternative to waiting for spontaneous labour. If the induction isn't effective, or doesn't move things along quickly enough, a Caesarean becomes necessary. It is impossible to separate the risk of Caesarean section caused by induction itself, from the risk caused by the *reason* for which induction was being done in the first place.

Talking to Your Doctor about Inducing Labour

If your doctor suggests that you have your labour induced, you will understand the reasons for the induction. If induction is suggested because you are "overdue," for example, you might want to go over the information in Chapter 45. If you have

The Evidence About...
Induction of Labour

Induction of labour is good treatment for complications in which the baby will be better off born than in the uterus.

With an unripe cervix, ripening of the cervix increases the chance that the induction will succeed, that labour will be shorter, and that the baby will be born vaginally. The best method of ripening the cervix is prostaglandin gel applied to the cervix.

Combining oxytocin and rupturing the membranes is more likely to be successful in inducing labour than either alone.

Prostaglandins used to induce labour appear more likely than oxytocin to result in vaginal birth within a reasonable length of time after starting the induction, and to lower the rate of vacuum, forceps, or Caesarean delivery. This information, though, is based on very small studies.

Because induction is easy to attempt does not mean it should be done. If induction is recommended, think about the reasons for doing it first before considering how it will be done.

pregnancy-induced hypertension, see Chapter 33. This will help you make a more informed decision.

Ask your doctor what could happen if you decide not to be induced. If there is not an emergency situation, you could consider trying some of the natural methods of encouraging labour to start first.

-42-
Pre-labour Rupture of the Membranes

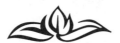

During pregnancy, the developing baby floats inside a bag of fluid known as the **amniotic sac**. The membranes holding the amniotic fluid usually break sometime during labour (although some babies are born with the membranes still intact and in many cultures this has been considered a sign of good luck). Sometimes the membranes break before labour starts. This is called **pre-labour rupture of the membranes**, or PROM.

If your membranes rupture, you might feel or hear a *pop*, or you might not feel anything except the gush or trickle of warm water from your vagina. At first, women often don't realize they are leaking amniotic fluid; they think they've lost control of their bladders. Sometimes the fluid just drips out in small, hardly noticeable amounts; other women have water running down their legs in substantial quantities. There may be an initial gush followed by a slower, steady trickle, or there may be periodic gushes of water once contractions begin.

Alana woke up one morning (a week after her due date) thinking she had heard a noise in the bedroom. When she sat up in bed, she real-ized what that noise had been: her membranes had ruptured and the mattress was now soaked.

Louanne arrived at the hospital when her contractions were five minutes apart. The nurse who examined her asked, "When did your water break? I can't feel any membranes here." Thinking it over, Louanne said it might have happened just before labour started, when she thought she had leaked a little urine. "It was hardly anything," she says, "so I didn't realize that it might have been my water breaking."

In 70 per cent of women, labour will start soon after the membranes rupture and their babies will be born within 24 hours. Ninety per cent of women will give birth within 48 hours of their membranes rupturing. Another 5 to 8 per cent will have their babies within the next couple of days, but 2 to 5 per cent will still be waiting to give birth five days after the membranes rupture.

Why is this wait a concern? Because without the membranes present to act as a barrier, it's easier for germs to get into the uterus and cause an infection which could make the mother and/or the baby ill.

Pre-term Pre-labour Rupture of the Membranes

Christina was just six months pregnant when she noticed a steady trickle of fluid from her vagina. She called her midwife, who suggested she go immediately to the hospital because her baby was so premature. Contractions had started in earnest by the time she arrived, and progressed quickly once in hospital. Baby Emily was born weighing a little less than 3 pounds (1,360 g).

"It took me by surprise," Christina says. "It was pretty frightening to go through, not knowing how the baby would be."

Rupture of the membranes when the baby is premature (before 37 weeks) and labour has not started is called pre-term pre-labour rupture of the membranes.

When pre-labour rupture of the membranes occurs pre-term, the mother is likely going to go into labour, usually right away, and almost always within a week. Research shows that it does not improve the outcome for the baby to use drugs to try to delay the labour, to try to stop it once it starts, or to induce the labour (unless there are signs of infection). Giving the mother antibiotics during the time she is waiting for labour to start can reduce the risk of infection in mother and baby.

Pre-labour Rupture of the Membranes at Term

Christina had extra concerns because her baby was premature. In most cases, though, the membranes rupture when the baby is full term and ready to be born. Labour contractions usually start within a few hours.

Vicky was walking home from the park in the early afternoon with her toddler in the stroller, when she felt a familiar gush of water between her legs. This had happened during her first two pregnancies; right at 40 weeks, her water broke before her contractions started. The previous two times, her doctor had urged her to go to the hospital immediately, even though she wasn't having any contractions. Once at the hospital, she was given oxytocin to induce labour, hooked up to a fetal monitor, and went through many hours of hard contractions before giving birth.

During this pregnancy, just in case it happened again, Vicky had done some research. She had seen studies that suggested the rates of Caesarean section and anaesthetic in labour were higher when women with pre-labour rupture of the membranes were induced. The research found that the rate of infection was no higher if women simply waited to go into labour normally. Some of the research suggested that the risk of infection could be reduced if the woman stayed at home rather than going to the hospital to be examined internally. (Her body would already be resistant to most of the familiar germs at home while the wider variety of germs at the hospital would be more dangerous.)

Vicky decided not to call her doctor this time and simply stayed home, leaking a little fluid throughout the evening. She had a shower rather than a bath, and she changed the sanitary pads she was wearing as soon as they became wet. Shortly after midnight, she began having contractions. At that point, she woke up her husband and they headed to the hospital. Her baby was born four hours later.

"It was my best, easiest labour," Vicky says. "I would do the same thing if it happened again.

I'm not sure exactly how long I would wait, but I definitely would not agree to be induced as soon as my water broke."

Studies found that the total length of time from the moment the membranes ruptured to the moment the baby was born was shorter when labour was induced (an average of 24 hours, compared to 30 hours when labour was allowed to start on its own). But the length of *actual labour* averaged 15 hours with induction, compared to only six hours for the women who waited for labour to begin spontaneously.

The mother who is induced with oxytocin immediately after her water breaks may be facing a harder and longer labour and an increased risk of Caesarean section to deliver her baby, than if she just waits. If an induction is done, the risk of Caesarean section is lower when prostaglandin is used to induce rather than oxytocin.

WILL INDUCING LABOUR REDUCE THE BABY'S CHANCE OF GETTING AN INFECTION?

Concerns about infection have been the main reason for encouraging induction of labour once the membranes have ruptured. However, there is no good research to support this approach. None of the studies examining this question have been well designed or shown clear results. Other factors would need to be included in the design of the study: staying at home versus going to the hospital (where there are more germs); number of vaginal exams, etc. More research is needed in this area.

The Evidence About...
Pre-labour Rupture of the Membranes

Rupture of the membranes before the start of labour at term is a normal event; no good records are available for how often it happens.

Once membranes rupture, 90 per cent of women will deliver within 48 hours spontaneously.

Women with prolonged rupture of the membranes before delivery at term may have a higher risk of infection for themselves and their babies, but it is uncertain whether this risk of infection can be reduced by inducing labour, rather than waiting for labour to start on its own.

Pre-term pre-labour rupture of the membranes almost always leads to premature birth. Administration of antibiotics while waiting for labour and during labour reduces maternal and fetal infections. There is no benefit in trying to stop premature labour once the membranes have ruptured.

Studies were done in the 1960s that compared giving all mothers with pre-labour rupture of the membranes antibiotics versus only giving antibiotics if there were early signs of infection. (These signs include a slight fever in the mother and a rapid heartbeat in the baby.) The studies found no benefits for the babies with routine antibiotics. On the other hand, the mothers who received routine antibiotics did develop fewer infections after this preventive treatment.

-43-
Here Comes the Baby!
The Second (Pushing) Stage

"I have to push."

For many women, the moment when they first feel the baby moving down and their bodies beginning to push the baby out is one of the most exciting moments of labour. Those pushing sensations tell them that the birth of the baby is close and labour is almost over. It can also be a relief to be actively involved, after hours of just trying to cope with contractions.

The **first stage of labour** lasts from the first contraction until the cervix is fully dilated. The **second stage of labour** begins with full dilation of the cervix and ends with the birth of the baby.

Bonnie remembers, "My labour had been a lot more painful than I expected. I had only been in labour five hours and I was groaning and finding it pretty unbearable. I remember saying to my husband 'I can't do this anymore.' He was struggling to find something supportive and comforting to say—actually he looked scared to death every time I groaned—when all of a sudden my water broke and my body pushed.

"I yelled, 'I'm pushing!' He raced out of the room to get the nurse—I think he thought the baby was going to fall right out on the floor.

From then on, the labour was great. The pushing urge was absolutely overwhelming during the contractions—I can't imagine any woman asking if it's time to push. The pushing contractions were really intense, but nothing as painful as the contractions had been up to then.

"In no time at all—my husband says it was about half an hour—I could feel the baby sort of bulging in my vagina. I can't remember if the nurse or my doctor tried to tell me when to push—it wouldn't have mattered what they said, my body just did it. It felt amazing when the baby slid out—it just burned, it really didn't hurt at all."

Maria's memory of her baby's birth is very different but equally happy: "I'd had an epidural when I was 8 centimetres, and promptly went to sleep. I woke up when the nurse came in to do a routine check. She said that I was fully dilated and that the baby's head was right at the opening of the vagina! I couldn't feel a thing—not just the pain was gone, I had no sensation at all.

"The nurse and doctor tried to get me to push when they told me I had a contraction, but all I could do was laugh, I was so excited. They

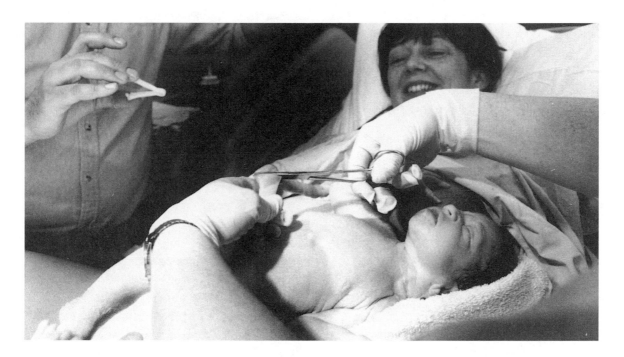

had a mirror so I could see the top of the baby's head—it was unbelievable. The doctor put a plastic thing on Chantelle's head and pulled a bit and out she came, all pink and beautiful. It was all so wonderful because there wasn't a bit of pain. I completely enjoyed the baby's birth."

How will you feel when the second stage begins? The desire to push doesn't always coincide with the moment the cervix finishes dilating. Some mothers feel strong pushing urges before full dilation, and others don't feel pushing urges for some time after the cervix is fully dilated. Sometimes labour seems to slow down at this point, with contractions coming further apart; other women find the contractions are closer together. With epidural anaesthetic, some mothers never feel any pushing urge at all.

There is also a difference between the sensation of "feeling like pushing," which women experience during a contraction, and the actual involuntary "push" that the abdominal muscles give as the baby's head comes down into the pelvis.

Most of the advice you may be given about what to do during the second stage is based on "clinical experience" (meaning the way your physician has always done it) and has not been researched. Nearly all the research that has been done has been very small studies using very few women.

Should Women Be Told How to Push?

Women who are given no directions at all during the pushing stage react to it in very similar ways. Even if they report "feeling like pushing," they seldom make themselves push on purpose. Once the urge to push becomes involuntary, they usually make three to five relatively brief pushes (four to six seconds each) during each contraction. There is usually little holding of the breath—air is released, often with a grunt, during each push.

This is quite different from the way women are often instructed to push. A nurse or other birth attendant may tell you to take a big breath in, hold your breath, and then to push down for a sustained period of time, from 10 to 30 seconds. You might practise this pushing during prenatal classes. Women are often told to push this way as soon as they are fully dilated, whether they have any spontaneous urge to push or not.

Some small studies have been done comparing these two methods of pushing. The coached, holding-your-breath type of pushing results in a slightly shorter second stage, but otherwise has no benefits for mother or baby. Spontaneous (mother-directed) pushing results in better fetal heart rate patterns, higher Apgar scores at birth, and higher pH in the cord blood (all indicative of better fetal well-being).

Interestingly, women with epidural anaesthetic are often encouraged to bear down forcefully as soon as full dilation is diagnosed by a vaginal examination (because of the anaesthetic they often do not feel any pushing urge). If instead you wait until the baby's head appears in the vagina to start pushing, studies show that you are less likely to need forceps to turn the baby's head from a posterior position.

Positions for Pushing

Standing, kneeling, or squatting to give birth are common in most cultures. It has not been common in ours—in hospitals, women have almost universally been encouraged to lie on their backs to deliver, often with their legs up in leg rests or stirrups.

Several (again small) studies have compared being upright for birth with lying down. "Lying down" has meant either the mother lying on her back, or lying on her side. "Upright" in these studies has meant being propped by a backrest or wedge on a bed, or using a specially designed birthing chair. Squatting (with or without support from a low birthing stool) or kneeling has not been researched at all.

The studies found that being upright shortens the length of the second stage. Mothers prefer being upright because they feel less pain and less backache, and a majority of the women said they wanted to use the same upright position for their next birth. Abnormal fetal heart rate patterns and low cord pH (both signs of fetal distress) were slightly less likely with the upright position.

Women who give birth lying on their sides also have infants with better heart rate patterns and better cord pH than those who deliver lying on their backs. It seems that both the upright and the side-lying position avoid the compression of the blood vessels by the uterus that is caused by lying on the back.

Studies did not find any differences in the rate of tears in the vagina depending on position.

Studies have also not so far shown any change in the rates of vacuum, forceps, or Caesarean section between upright posture and lying down for the second stage. However, the studies have been very small, and have included women in the "upright" group who simply had a support or backrest under their head and shoulders while they were on their back in bed with their legs in stirrups.

Birthing chairs have been designed which are just that—a chair in which the woman sits, usually leaning back, to give birth. The use of birthing chairs leads to a higher risk of swollen **perineum** (the opening of the vagina), hemorrhoids and postpartum hemorrhage if the mother sits in the chair for extended periods of time. This seems to be related to the construction of the chair itself, which puts pressure on the thighs and reduces blood flow back from the legs.

Giving birth while lying on your back has not been found to have any benefits to mother or baby.

Vaginal Tears

Delivery of the baby can tear the tissue around the opening of the vagina (the **perineum**). This probably happens in about 50 per cent of births. (We don't really know how many women would tear if they were left alone because so many of them are given episiotomies, a cut made by the doctor in the tissue between the opening of the vagina and the anus, at the time of birth.)

Clearly, in the olden days before **sutures** (stitches) were invented, women had babies, got tears, and most of them healed fine by themselves (although it's also certain that some of the tears didn't heal well and caused the mothers a lot of trouble).

The current assumption is that all tears, except for the tiniest, should be sutured. There is

no research to support this. One study was performed to look at episiotomies that had been repaired with sutures but "broke down." One group of these women were left to heal by themselves, the other group were resutured. The group who were resutured healed faster and had fewer complications. This study supports the already accepted procedure of suturing all *significant* tears. It's not clear, though, that this should apply to smaller tears.

PREVENTING TEARS

There is no evidence from studies to show the best method of preventing the perineum from tearing during delivery. Many techniques have been suggested:

- leaving the perineum strictly alone
- "guarding" the perineum by the caregiver pressing her fingers against it, combined with gentle pressure on the baby's head to prevent rapid delivery
- massaging the perineum with warm oil (either just at birth or for several weeks before the baby is born)
- applying hot compresses to the perineum to help the tissues stretch
- avoiding coached pushing—except at the moment of birth. Then the caregiver encourages the mother to pant or blow steadily out as the baby's head begins to be born. Her uterus will continue to contract and push the baby out but will do it slowly, giving the skin the maximum amount of time to stretch. (This kind of slow birth is sometimes hard to achieve, as some women can't stop pushing.)

None of these methods—all of which have passionate advocates—have been researched to see if they are effective in preventing tears to the vagina. They may be effective, the research has just never been done. This is an example of research which would be of great interest to women.

Some of these techniques at least make the mother feel more comfortable at the time. Marjory remembers, "The hot compresses on my vagina felt so good—they absolutely took away all the pain from pushing. I wouldn't let the midwife stop doing them for one second. I just tore a little when the baby came out. I don't know if the compresses kept it from being any worse, but they sure felt good."

What feels great to one mother may distress another. Elyse says, "Before I had Danny, I had discussed with my doctor not having an episiotomy. She said she massages the perineum with warm oil, and it sounded great. But when I was actually pushing and she started to rub the oil onto me, I couldn't stand it. I actually yelled at her to stop; I was so hypersensitive even that gentle touch felt painful."

Episiotomy

Gary still vividly remembers seeing his wife Lisa being given an episiotomy. After 19 hours of labour, she was finally fully dilated and beginning to push out her baby. She was tired and the doctor and nurse urged her to push harder. Gary held up one of her legs, braced against his shoulder, while the nurse held the other leg. Then the doctor reached over to the green cloth laid out on a metal table and picked up a pair of scissors.

"I'd gotten through labour fine," Gary says, "but when I saw the doctor make that cut, I almost passed out."

Lisa's response was less dramatic. "I think I was feeling so much pain and pressure at that point that I didn't really notice what the doctor was doing. But I noticed it afterwards."

During the birth of Lisa's daughter, the episiotomy that had been cut tore even further. The doctor stitched up both the episiotomy and the tearing. "It took forever," Lisa recalls, and she felt uncomfortable for several months afterwards. When she became pregnant again, Lisa sought out a new doctor who supported her desire to avoid another episiotomy. During her second birth she had only a small tear requiring a few stitches, which was pain-free in about a week.

An episiotomy is a cut made in the perineum to enlarge the opening before the baby's head comes through. Sometimes the cut is done straight down from the bottom of the vagina, and other times it is done at an angle.

While episiotomies were common in the past, the research has clearly shown that:

- Episiotomies to shorten the pushing stage of the labour do not prevent damage to the baby's head and brain. Babies born without episiotomy need no more resuscitation or intensive care than babies born with episiotomy.
- Episiotomy does not protect the mother from "worse tearing." Tearing which damages the muscles around the mother's anus and rectum occurs significantly *more* often—not less—when a midline episiotomy is done, than when a spontaneous tear happens during the delivery.

- The numbers of women who have **stress incontinence** three years after delivery is the same whether they had an episiotomy or not. (Stress incontinence is a fairly common problem in women—when they cough or sneeze or laugh hard, particularly if their bladder is full, they leak some urine.) Episiotomy does not prevent damage to the bladder muscles and other muscles of the pelvic floor.
- There is no evidence that episiotomies heal better than tears. Women who had episiotomies and women who didn't had the same amount of pain at 10 days and at three months postpartum. However, the women who did not have episiotomies started to have sex again sooner than the women who did.

The response to this research has been very positive, as current rates of episiotomy are about 23.9 per cent in Canada and 32.7 per cent in the United States.

RISKS OF EPISIOTOMY

Episiotomy can cause excessive blood loss from the wound edges, particularly if the cut is made well before the delivery of the baby. It can also cause infection and **abscess formation**, injury to the muscles of the anus and rectum, and a hole (called a **fistula**) between the rectum and the vagina.

WHEN IS EPISIOTOMY USEFUL?

There are times when an episiotomy may be helpful:

- If the baby coming through the vagina is in distress and needs to be born quickly, an episiotomy may help speed up the birth.
- If forceps or a vacuum extractor are needed to help the baby emerge, an episiotomy may provide extra room for inserting the instrument to pull the baby out, and in the case of a difficult birth also allows more room for the baby.
- For a breech birth, the smaller body and legs come out first and then the larger head and shoulders have to be born quickly so that the baby can start to breathe. The smaller parts coming first have not stretched the perineum very much, so the head can be a tight fit. Doing an episiotomy when the buttocks reach the perineum may offer some protection to the baby's head and avoid a difficult delivery. This has not been researched, but it is done almost routinely.

Roxanne remembers her episiotomy vividly: "My doctor and I were in agreement that episiotomies were unnecessary. My labour had gone great, I was pushing, the pain wasn't too bad. The nurse had set up a mirror so I could see my baby's head in the vagina with each contraction. The baby's heart rate had been fine—then after one contraction it was really slow. We could all hear it just going *thud...thud...thud*, when before it had been quick.

"My doctor said that sometimes the baby's head gets squeezed at this stage and it doesn't necessarily mean the baby is in distress. I rolled over onto my side and the nurse gave me some oxygen to breathe.

"The baby's heart rate speeded up a little with the next couple of contractions, but it was still a lot slower than it had been. The doctor said she couldn't tell for sure whether the baby was in distress or not, and the quickest way to get the baby born would be to do an episiotomy. I told her to go ahead—I was pretty worried—so she put in some freezing and did an episiotomy with the next contraction.

"The baby's head came out; the cord was around her neck and the doctor had to cut the cord before her shoulders came out. The baby was a bit quiet for a minute, and the doctor rubbed her and gave her some oxygen to breathe. Then she started to cry and everything was fine."

Vacuum Extractors and Forceps

If the mother's efforts to push her baby out don't seem to be working, either forceps or the vacuum extractor can be used to help deliver the baby. The cervix must be fully dilated and the baby's head **engaged**, meaning that the baby's head has moved down under the pubic bone into the pelvis, so that the widest part of the baby's head is in the pelvis. That's usually a good sign that the baby's head will fit through the bones of the pelvis, and that the vacuum or forceps will just be helping to stretch the soft tissues of the perineum.

If the baby's head is *not* engaged, forceps or vacuum are usually not tried because of concerns that the baby simply isn't going to fit through the bony pelvis. If that is the case, pulling on it might damage the baby, without being able to deliver it, and a Caesarean section is probably safer for the baby.

FORCEPS

"I had been pushing for about two and a half hours," says Ann, remembering the birth of her first baby. "I didn't seem to be making any progress at all. My doctor explained that the baby was posterior—face up—and that she'd like to use forceps to turn him."

Ann was feeling tired after a long labour and the time she had spent pushing. "I really felt like the baby wasn't moving at all, so we went for the forceps. I was very disappointed that I had to have an epidural at that point, after going through the whole labour without any drugs. And I had a big episiotomy, too. But a few minutes later, I had my baby in my arms."

Forceps, like the ones Ann's doctor used, are metal instruments that look roughly like salad tongs. They fit around the baby's head, and then the doctor pulls on them to deliver the baby. They can also be used to turn the baby's head from a **posterior position** (with the face looking up) to an **anterior position** (with the face looking down). In an anterior position, the baby's head usually fits through the pelvis better and will deliver more easily.

The safety of forceps for the baby is completely dependent on the physician's training, experience and judgment. Skill is needed to turn the baby's head gently without undue force. When pulling, the baby's head should move down somewhat with each pull; it takes good judgment to decide when a forceps delivery is going to use too much force and that it is safer to do a Caesarean section instead.

Low forceps (a forceps delivery done when the baby's head is at the opening of the vagina) can usually be done with local anaesthetic to freeze the opening of the vagina. **Mid forceps** (a forceps delivery done when the baby is higher in the birth canal) will usually mean the mother needs epidural anaesthesia to handle the pain. Most forceps deliveries that involve rotations of the baby's head from the posterior or transverse position to the anterior position are mid forceps.

VACUUM EXTRACTOR

The vacuum extractor is a soft plastic cup about the size of an egg that is slipped into the vagina and pressed against the baby's head. It has tubing attached that is connected to a pump; the pump creates a vacuum between the cup and the baby's scalp. During contractions, the vacuum is increased and the physician pulls on the extractor to help with delivery. Between contractions, the vacuum is released so that it won't create a pressure sore on the baby's scalp.

The built-in safety of the vacuum extractor is the ease with which the cup "pops off" the baby's scalp. It is difficult to pull hard enough to harm the baby without the vacuum letting go.

The cup often produces a swollen area on the baby's scalp from the vacuum, which is harmless and usually disappears within 48 hours. At times, there can be bleeding into this swollen area, causing a bruise on the baby's head. This takes longer to get better, but causes the baby no lasting harm.

A vacuum extraction can usually be done with just local anaesthetic.

DECIDING TO USE FORCEPS OR VACUUM EXTRACTORS

Marilyn had been fully dilated for about half an hour and was pushing each time the nurse reading the monitor told her a contraction was coming. Because she'd had an epidural, she didn't feel any pushing urge. When her doctor came in to observe, he told her that things were moving slowly.

"I can get this baby out now with a vacuum extractor," he said, "and you won't have to wait any longer to have him in your arms."

What are good reasons for using forceps or the vacuum? The most common ones given are:

Fetal Distress: If your baby is in distress during this pushing stage, forceps or vacuum can help deliver the baby. However, it isn't easy to diagnose fetal distress at this point. There are concerns if the baby's heart rate is very slow and not speeding up between contractions—this is probably a baby in distress.

But what about patterns that are less clearcut? Often during the pushing stage a baby's heartbeat will slow down during contractions then speed up again once the contraction ends. This seems to be normal and is probably caused by the squeezing of the baby's head as it pushes through the birth canal during contractions. However, if the umbilical cord is around the baby's neck, you will see the same pattern of changing heart rate: slow during contractions, faster in between. In the early stages, it's impossible to tell the difference between the normal changes in heart rate and the potentially dangerous cord around the baby's neck. (The baby with a tight cord around its neck will show more serious signs of distress as it moves farther down the birth canal.)

It also gets increasingly difficult to hear the baby's heartbeat as the pushing stage continues. You may notice the nurse or midwife placing the stethoscope on various parts of your belly as she tries to find a good place to listen. If you are moving around, trying to find a comfortable position for pushing, it can get even harder. If you are on your hands and knees, for example, or sitting backwards on the toilet, your caregiver may find it very challenging to listen to your baby.

Long Second Stage: No studies have been performed to determine how long it is safe for the mother to push, or at what point in time the use of vacuum or forceps should be considered. A very long second stage is statistically associated with stillbirths, postpartum hemorrhage, fever in the mother, and seizures in the newborn. However, there is no evidence that it is the length of the second stage itself that causes these complications.

The average length of the second stage for mothers having their first baby is about an hour, and for women having subsequent babies about 30 minutes. That's just an average, though, and there are wide variations. Many doctors use as their definition of an abnormally long second stage two hours for a first birth, and one hour for a second birth; after this they suggest the use of vacuum or forceps.

This arbitrary clock watching is not supported by research. If the mother is not exhausted, the baby's condition is fine (as shown by normal heart rate), and the baby's head is continuing to move down through the birth canal, there is no reason to arbitrarily put a time limit on the second stage.

If you have had an epidural and have no pushing urge, it is reasonable to expect a longer second stage to allow the contractions to move the baby down to the opening of the vagina. Sometimes, the combination of epidural anaesthesia and the reaching of full dilation drastically slows down the frequency of the contractions. In this case, oxytocin might make the contractions more frequent and allow you to give birth without using forceps or vacuum.

This is a situation where you should be involved in making the decision. If you are exhausted and in pain from a long labour and pushing stage, you may want to "get things over with" by having an epidural and forceps or vacuum to deliver the baby. If you are feeling fine and the baby is doing well, however, you can tell your doctor that you would like to continue.

Marilyn chose to wait. "Because of the epidural, I wasn't in any pain, and I knew I'd need an episiotomy if I had the vacuum extractor. It took another 45 minutes before Amy was born, but I only had a small tear, so I was glad we let her arrive at her own speed."

ARE FORCEPS DELIVERIES "SAFE" FOR THE BABY?

There are really two different questions here. If the forceps have been used during a straightforward, normal labour and birth simply to shorten up the second stage, then we want to know if this is safer than a natural, vaginal birth. But if the forceps were used because the mother had been pushing for several hours and the baby was not coming out, we should be asking if the forceps are safer than a Caesarean section, because that would have been the alternative.

Forceps used in a straightforward birth do not seem to cause any harm to the baby, according to the research.

Forceps deliveries can be just as safe as Caesarean sections in more difficult births, provided certain guidelines are followed. The cervix must be fully dilated and the baby's head well down in the mother's pelvis. In this situation, many doctors will try using forceps before suggesting the surgery. If the forceps don't work—the doctor finds he needs to use a lot of force, for example—then the baby will be delivered promptly by Caesarean section instead.

WHICH IS BETTER, FORCEPS OR VACUUM EXTRACTOR?

In North America, forceps have been used much more than the vacuum, while in Europe, the use of the vacuum is more common than forceps.

The Evidence About...
The Pushing Stage

There are many strongly held opinions about the pushing stage of labour but not much research.

Babies are born in better condition when the mother is not coached in how to push, but pushes spontaneously. With this approach, the second stage is only a little longer than when pushing is coached.

Being upright during the second stage is more comfortable for most women, makes the second stage shorter, and slightly improves the condition of the baby when born. For women who prefer to lie down, a side-lying position seems to provide some of the same benefits.

There are many theories, but no proof of the best way (if there is a best way) to prevent tearing at delivery.

There are no benefits from the liberal use of episiotomy. Using episiotomy to avoid a tear is counterproductive, as the risk of tearing is higher when an episiotomy is done.

Research has not established the maximum length of time for the pushing stage that is safe for mother and baby. Setting arbitrary time limits is probably not helpful.

If the baby is not born in a "reasonable" length of time, either vacuum extraction or forceps can be used as long as the cervix is fully dilated and the baby's head is engaged. Vacuum extraction is probably safer for mother and baby, but is not successful as often as forceps.

The vacuum extractor usually requires less pain-relieving medication for the mother. It is less likely to cause tears to the mother's vagina, and causes less pain after the birth. The vacuum extractor frequently causes swelling or bruising of the baby's scalp, while the forceps are more likely to cause cuts or bruises on the baby's face.

As far as getting the baby born quickly, the vacuum extractor and forceps are about the same. It does usually take slightly longer, depending on the hospital, to arrange for an epidural for the mother in order to use forceps. The vacuum extractor is not successful as often as forceps in getting the baby out. However, if the vacuum extractor is tried first, followed by forceps if the vacuum doesn't work, the overall Caesarean section rate is lower.

Since the vacuum extractor causes fewer problems for the mother and requires less med-ication, it is usually the best first choice. However, your doctor's skill and experience with the particular technique is the best guarantee of safety, and will be an important factor in making the choice between vacuum and forceps.

In some hospitals, women are frequently encouraged to have the vacuum extractor used to speed up the births of their babies. Since the vacuum doesn't require an epidural, and is seen as safe for both mother and baby, it has become popular. There is no research to show that this routine use of the vacuum is beneficial, or that it is dangerous.

-44-
Delivery of the Placenta: The Third Stage of Labour

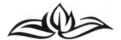

Your baby's born and in your arms. It's over at last, and as you gaze into your baby's eyes you know it was worth it. Then, to your surprise, you feel another contraction...

Well, it's not quite over. Yes, the birth of the baby is what you've been waiting for. But your body has another task to take care of: expelling the no-longer-needed placenta from your uterus. This is called the third stage of labour, and it seems like an anticlimax. Who wants to think about the placenta with a brand new baby to cuddle and admire?

However, your caregiver needs to be alert at this time because there are potential hazards. It's possible for you to bleed heavily at this point, and that can be serious. In fact, it happens in about 8 per cent of births. If the placenta doesn't come out on its own, this is called a **retained placenta** and the doctor may have to remove it by hand (you will usually have anaesthesia if this is necessary). In very rare cases, the uterus can turn inside out and come out of the vagina with the placenta—a very dangerous situation.

The best approach to the third stage will be one that interferes as little as possible with the body's own normal process of delivering the placenta, minimizes the risk of serious complications like hemorrhage and retained placenta, and doesn't disturb the mother's enjoyment of her new baby.

How Is the Placenta Normally Expelled?

After the delivery of the baby, the uterus immediately contracts down to a firm ball about the size of a cantaloupe. The placenta, however, stays the same size as it was and separates from the uterine wall as the uterus contracts. The contracted uterus then pushes the detached placenta down into the lower uterine segment and on into the vagina.

You can often watch your uterus becoming firmer and rounder just above your pelvic bone as the placenta moves down. There is often a sudden gush of blood from the vagina as well. If you have not been given an epidural, and particularly if you are upright, you will probably feel a slight urge to push at this point, and the placenta will slide easily out of your vagina.

THE PLACENTA

Many mothers want to see the placenta once it has been delivered. It is often larger than parents expect, and looks like a generous slab of liver. One side is raw-looking; this is the part that was attached to the uterus. The other side is smooth and shiny and the umbilical cord emerges from the middle of it. This side faced the baby before birth.

Your midwife or doctor will carefully examine the placenta to see that it has come away in one piece. If a piece is left behind in the uterus, it can lead to heavy bleeding and may also interfere with the hormones that make milk by tricking your body into thinking it is still pregnant.

If you are lying down, or have been given anaesthetic so that you don't feel any sensation from the placenta in your vagina, your caregiver may put one hand on your uterus to support it and ask you to push gently. Along with gentle **traction** (pulling) on the umbilical cord, this is usually enough to expel the placenta from the vagina.

Once the placenta is delivered, a nurse or midwife will massage your uterus to make sure it stays firm and contracted and to minimize the amount of bleeding. This can sometimes be quite painful, depending on how vigorously it is done.

Ingrid says, "I hardly noticed the placenta coming out, because I was so absorbed by Jackson. I have vague memories of the doctor telling me to push and somebody showing me what looked like a big hunk of liver in a bowl. Then the nurse kind of grabbed at my belly and started to massage me—and I noticed that!

When she saw my reaction, though, she realized she was doing it too hard, and tried to be a bit more gentle."

Hemorrhage After the Baby Is Born

About 8 per cent of women will bleed heavily after delivery of their baby or the placenta—heavily enough to make their blood pressure fall, feel faint, and need transfusion with intravenous fluid and/or blood. This is called postpartum hemorrhage, and it is slightly more likely in women who:

- have an overstretched uterus, because of a very large baby, twins, or triplets, or a large amount of amniotic fluid
- have very long or very short labours
- have had several previous births
- have had a postpartum hemorrhage with a previous birth.

If this bleeding happens before the placenta is out, the placenta needs to be delivered as quickly as possible. If the placenta has separated from the uterus and is just sitting in the lower uterine segment or in the vagina, your doctor will probably pull on the cord to get it out. You will also be given oxytocin or ergometrine. **Oxytocin** and **ergometrine** are both drugs which make the uterus contract (which is how oxytocin also augments labour). Ergometrine is more likely than oxytocin to cause nausea, vomiting, headache, and temporary elevation of blood pressure.

If the placenta has not separated from the uterus and the mother is bleeding heavily, the doctor may need to manually remove the placenta by putting his or her hand inside the uterus and prying the placenta away. If you have had an epidural, the doctor will be able to do this right away; if not, you will be given a general anaesthetic. You will also have oxytocin given by intravenous. Some research has suggested that injecting oxytocin into the umbilical cord can help the placenta separate and reduce the need to remove the placenta manually.

Priya had an eight-hour labour without any pain medication. "It was very straightforward—the nurses were joking that I'd be great for one of those childbirth videos. I was so thrilled when Sanjay was born, but then the placenta didn't come out. The doctor waited a while, tried massaging my belly, everything we could think of. Then I felt this gush of blood, and the doctor got concerned." Priya was quickly moved to another room and given a general anaesthetic while the placenta was removed. "I felt so groggy when I woke up, but I knew it was necessary. I have to admit it was pretty disappointing to have that happen when the labour and birth went so well, but there are some things you just can't predict."

Prevention of Postpartum Hemorrhage

Prevention is better than treatment. Large studies have been done on giving either oxytocin or ergometrine to women right after birth, and both made a significant difference in the amount of bleeding.

These trials have shown *a reduction of about 60 per cent in incidence of postpartum hemorrhage in women given oxytocin or ergometrine routinely after delivery of the baby.*

Since oxytocin has fewer side effects, it is preferred.

CLAMPING OF THE UMBILICAL CORD

Should the cord be clamped later or earlier?

The usual practice in North America has been to clamp and cut the umbilical cord as soon as the baby is born. However, some have suggested that waiting for a period of time after the baby is born to clamp the cord is better because it allows as much blood as possible to flow into the baby. Different researchers have adopted different definitions of **late clamping**—waiting for 30 seconds after delivery, or until the cord has stopped pulsing completely, or until after the placenta is delivered. The amount of extra blood that the baby gets when the cord is clamped later also depends on positioning—the baby should be level with or slightly below the level of the vaginal opening for the blood to flow downhill.

When the cord is cut right after the baby is born, the baby will have lower blood volume and lower levels of iron. These differences generally disappear by the time the baby is six months old. However, the difference may be significant for premature babies, who may have low iron levels at birth—the cord is often clamped early to facilitate their resuscitation, but they might benefit from the extra blood.

The time of cord clamping does not seem to have anything to do with the risk of hemorrhage. Early cord clamping does reduce the length of time until the placenta delivers. If you would prefer to have the clamping of the cord delayed so that your baby gets the extra blood, be sure to discuss this with your doctor.

CONTROLLED TRACTION ON THE CORD TO DELIVER THE PLACENTA

At many births, the doctor pulls on the umbilical cord to remove the placenta from the vagina. "Controlled" cord traction is such a subjective thing that it is difficult to study meaningfully—there is no way to assess just how hard someone is pulling!

In one study, about 3 per cent of the cords broke while traction was being used. If the cord does break, sometimes the placenta will still deliver spontaneously, but sometimes it means that the placenta has not separated from the uterus, and a manual removal will be required.

How Soon Should the Placenta Be Delivered?

Most placentas will deliver within five to ten minutes of the delivery of the baby.

If there is no unusual bleeding, it is reasonable to wait an hour for spontaneous separation of the placenta and delivery rather than moving immediately to manual removal. Waiting an hour rather than half an hour has greatly reduced the number of manual removals required.

Stella's son Neil was born at home, but the placenta was slow in coming. "The midwives helped me to squat over the basin that they had on the floor, but half an hour went by and nothing seemed to be happening. Then Neil started to fuss, and I put him to my breast. As soon as he began nursing, I felt a couple of sharp contractions and the placenta just plopped out into the basin."

Some physicians routinely remove the placenta manually right after the baby is born if the

SHOULD DAD CUT THE CORD?

Some fathers see cutting the umbilical cord as a symbolic moment, and are eager to take part; others find they are too emotionally caught up in the birth to take on this role. If you are interested, ask your caregiver—you may also need to remind him or her at the time of the birth.

Your doctor or midwife will put clamps on the cord in two places, and you will be handed a pair of scissors to cut through the cord between the two clamps. It is slippery and a bit tough, like a garden hose. Because of the clamps on either side, there will be almost no blood, and neither mother nor baby can feel anything.

mother has an epidural in place for pain relief. There is no research to support this practice.

Researchers have studied the injection of **saline solution** (a mixture of salt and water) or oxytocin into the umbilical cord vein to treat retained placenta, to try to avoid manual removal, but the results have been inconclusive.

Active Management of the Delivery of the Placenta

Some caregivers use "active management" of the third stage. This combines the three components of giving oxytocin as soon as the baby is born, clamping the cord early, and pulling on the cord to remove the placenta. The studies found that these three techniques, used together, produced a lower rate of postpartum hemorrhage and reduced the need for blood transfusions.

However, the studies are a bit confusing and it's not clear that all three steps are helpful. Giving oxytocin is the one element that is clearly associated with decreased risk of postpartum hemorrhage.

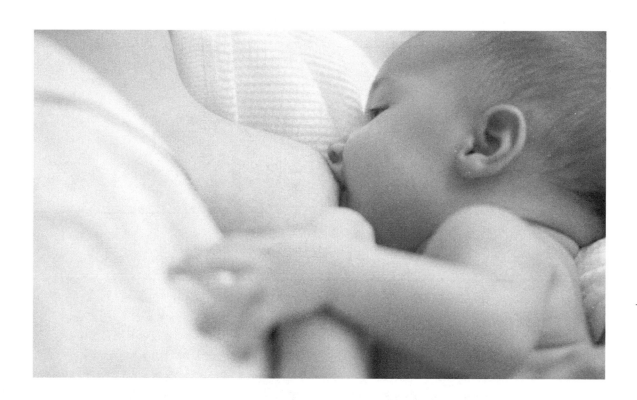

Ten Months
❧ *Birth and Beyond* ❧

Your due date has gone by now, and you might still be waiting for your baby to appear. Read on for more information about what it means to be overdue. And whether your baby arrived at 37 weeks or past 41 weeks, you'll want to know more about what to expect with a new baby and how to get started with breastfeeding.

-45-
"Overdue": Post-term Pregnancy

Lorna felt huge. Her "due date" had gone by two weeks ago, with no sign of a baby appearing. Two nights ago she'd had a dream about giving birth to a watermelon instead of a baby, and she was starting to wonder if labour would ever begin.

"I can't believe I'm actually eager to feel pain," she joked to a friend. "Every time I feel a twinge I keep hoping it will get worse and turn into good hard contractions."

But when Lorna's doctor offered to induce her labour, Lorna surprised herself by saying no, she'd prefer to wait for labour to start on its own. Two days later, her water broke while she was sleeping, and her 9-pound (4,080-g) baby girl was born seven hours later.

Lorna's pregnancy went longer than the average and is described by doctors as **prolonged**, **post-dates**, or **post-term**. Until about 30 years ago, prolonged pregnancy was not considered a problem that anything needed to be done about. People recognized that longer pregnancies led to bigger babies. Gradually, doctors also became aware that there was a slight increase in the rate of babies who died in labour or soon after birth if the pregnancy continued past 40 weeks. At that

time, though, the risks to the baby were considered to be lower than the risks of intervening.

As an example of how recent the concerns about post-term pregnancy are, consider the changes in one medical textbook. *Williams Obstetrics*, a standard text, has had 19 editions since 1903. The 1997 edition was the *first* one to offer an entire chapter devoted to the post-term pregnancy.

Why is there so much concern about post-term pregnancy today?

First, researchers have now done a number of studies to analyze the risks of these longer-than-average pregnancies. Second, doctors now have safer methods of inducing labour, which make it less risky to intervene. Behind these two points, though, is the assumption that recognizing an increased risk means that intervention will be successful in preventing it.

The standard definition of a post-term pregnancy is 42 weeks, or 294 days from the first day of the woman's last menstrual period. This assumes that the baby was conceived two weeks after the day the period began. When the calculation is based on the mother's period, about 10 to 14 per cent of pregnancies will be post-term.

This calculation isn't very reliable for women with irregular periods or longer than average menstrual cycles. When more accurate dating methods, such as ultrasound in early pregnancy, or dating based on the woman's individual ovulation or conception time are used, the number of post-term pregnancies is reduced to 3 to 4 per cent.

There is a definite tendency for some mothers to have more than one post-term pregnancy, and for them to run in families, suggesting that sometimes prolonged pregnancies are genetic.

Julie says, "I went two weeks past my due date with Jason, and when the doctor suggested induction, I agreed. I spent the day on the drip and nothing happened, so I went home and told the doctor I'd changed my mind about being induced. Four days later, labour started and Jason was born. When I went past my due date again with Matthew, I decided to just wait. Sure enough, he was born at 42½ weeks. The funny thing is, my sister Tracey seems to have the same pattern."

What Are the Risks of Post-term Pregnancy?

Put bluntly, slightly more babies will die during labour or shortly after birth when the pregnancy continues past 41 or 42 weeks. Statistically, about 2.5 per 1,000 infants born at 40 weeks will die in labour or shortly after. At 42 weeks, about 4.5 per 1,000 infants die. About 25 per cent of these babies are abnormal, and would not live no matter when they were born. The rest usually die either from a lack of oxygen during labour or from **meconium aspiration**. Meconium is the

THINGS TO CONSIDER IF YOU ARE "OVERDUE"

- Are you certain of the dates of your last menstrual period?
- Are your menstrual cycles normally longer than 28 days, or are they irregular?
- Have you had an ultrasound to confirm the dates? When was it done? (It is only reliable for dating if done early in pregnancy.)
- Has the cervix begun to ripen? This has a big effect on how easy it will be to induce labour (see Chapter 41).
- Have any of your other pregnancies been longer than average but produced a healthy baby? (This may suggest that longer pregnancies are typical for you.)
- What are your "gut" feelings about being induced versus waiting?

dark, tarry substance in the baby's bowels before birth. If the baby has a bowel movement during or before labour, the meconium in the amniotic fluid can be inhaled into the baby's lungs and make the baby ill. This problem seems to be more common in babies born after 42 weeks.

Some research has found that when mothers are having a second or later baby, going past 41 or 42 weeks does not seem to mean an increased risk of death.

Should You Be Induced?

For years, obstetricians have had different opinions on whether or not labour should be induced when a pregnancy becomes post-term. Early studies based on observations without controls

The Evidence About...

Overdue Pregnancy

Prolonged pregnancy is a variation of normal, and in the great majority of cases is associated with a good outcome for mother and baby. It may be part of a particular woman's biology and completely normal for her. However, prolonged pregnancy is also associated with a slightly increased risk to the baby.

Early pregnancy ultrasound gives more accurate due dates and reduces the number of pregnancies that are deemed to be post-term.

Research combining 11 different studies (a meta-analysis) found that induction of labour at 41 weeks (compared to waiting for labour to begin on its own) lowered the perinatal death rate from 2.5 per 1,000 to 0.3 per 1,000.

At 41 weeks it is reasonable, in light of the present evidence, for the mother to make her own decision about whether she wants to be induced or whether she wants to wait for labour to begin on its own.

did not give any conclusive evidence. In the meantime, routine induction of labour at or close to 42 weeks became very common.

More recently, some randomized studies have compared inducing labour at 40 weeks (term) with waiting for labour to start. Large randomized studies have looked at inducing labour at 41 weeks and compared this to waiting. No research has been done on pregnancies after 42 weeks.

What did these studies find?

When the researchers compared inducing labour at 40 weeks to waiting for labour to begin spontaneously, they found no benefit or harm to mother or baby. Both groups had similar numbers of epidurals and Caesarean sections, and the babies had similar Apgar scores.

Induction of labour at 41 weeks versus waiting for labour was compared using a combined analysis of 11 separate studies. This is called a **meta-analysis**—and combining the results of studies in this way can give different results than if one big study is done. The researchers found little difference as far as outcomes for the mothers. For the babies, there was no difference in fetal heart rate abnormalities or in depressed Apgar scores in the two groups. However, there *was* a difference between the two groups in **perinatal** death rates (meaning the number of babies who died during or right after the birth). One baby died in the group of women who had labour induced, versus nine deaths in a similar group of women who waited for the onset of labour.

This is a significant difference, and for this reason many doctors are recommending induction for all women at 41 weeks. However, a meta-analysis such as this should be viewed with caution, as the combined results of several small studies can be less reliable than one big study.

The reviewers on the Cochrane database suggest that induction should be offered to women at 41 weeks—in other words, each mother should make her own decision.

In all these studies, the "waiting for labour" group had some method of observation of the fetus used regularly—either non-stress testing, biophysical profile, or fetal kick counting. These tests may predict pregnancies at higher risk, but there is minimal evidence that this information can be used to improve the outcome for the baby.

The Post-mature Baby

Post-maturity occurs in a small but unknown percentage of both full-term and post-term infants. Post-maturity is abnormal, and the name should not be used as a synonym for post-term pregnancy, which is usually just a variation of normal.

The post-mature infant has a unique and characteristic appearance. This includes wrinkled, patchy, peeling skin, particularly on the palms and soles, a long thin body, and long fingernails. The baby typically is open-eyed and unusually alert, looking worried and "old." These babies are more likely to show signs of stress during labour, have decreased amounts of amniotic fluid, have **meconium** (the baby's first stool) in the amniotic fluid, and are more often stillborn.

Some of these post-mature infants are also post-term, but some are not. It may be that these infants have actually all experienced intrauterine growth restriction at different stages of gestation. There is no research to indicate at the present that even if we could identify these post-mature babies before birth, that their higher risks of stillbirth and lack of oxygen at birth (**birth asphyxia**) could be changed by induction of labour.

-46-
You and Your Newborn Baby

How can you best welcome your newborn baby into the world? Certainly, like any human being, your new baby should be treated with gentleness and respect. The choice of how to demonstrate that loving welcome is up to you.

In his book *Birth without Violence*, French obstetrician Dr. Frederick Leboyer emphasized gentleness in handling the newborn, to reduce the trauma of the baby's sudden separation from his mother into a loud, noisy, bright room. He recommended a dim delivery room, delayed clamping of the cord, silence except for the parents' voices, gentle massage, and a warm bath for the infant. Small studies of all these measures have not shown any specific effect on the newborn's health, good or bad. You should think about what appeals to you and makes sense to you, and ask for those things to be done.

Meeting Your Baby

Most new mothers want to touch and hold their babies as soon as possible. It seems to be a biological process. Petra remembers reaching out for her newborn baby, only to be told that the doctor had to finish stitching her up first. The baby was placed in a bassinet with plastic sides and a radiant heater overhead, and Petra remembers having tears running down her cheeks as she looked longingly at her baby. "I just wanted to touch him," she says.

Fathers may have mixed feelings. Some are eager to hold their newly born babies, others feel suddenly apprehensive. Tarik remembers the nurse wrapping the baby in a towel and saying, "Here you go, Dad." He says, "It was like my arms were paralyzed. I was afraid I might drop him or make him cry or do something wrong. He was so small and I felt so awkward. I'd never even seen a baby that tiny before."

But Rob felt quite differently. When his wife, Sheila, had a Caesarean, "As soon as Miranda was born, the nurse wrapped her up and handed her to me. I held her close to Sheila's face so she could see her, and then unwrapped her a little so we could both check that she had all her fingers and toes. I liked being the first one to hold her."

Norah's midwife urged her to touch her baby's head as it emerged from her vagina, and she reached down to feel the hair. "It felt so weird," she says, "but it made it seem real. As he was born my midwife said, 'Take him, take him,' and I pulled him up onto my chest and it was wonderful." The surge of emotion she felt as she held her wet baby against her skin is still vivid and intense in her memory.

Mothers are sometimes surprised by the intensity of their feelings once the baby is born. Sandra knew her hospital's policy was to keep all babies in the nursery for eight hours after birth for observation, and she thought it sounded like a reasonable idea. Her doctor explained to her that she would be too tired after labour and giving birth to look after the baby, anyway.

But when Sandra's son was born, she found she couldn't bear the thought of being separated from him. When he was taken off to the nursery, she was too restless and anxious to sleep—she wanted him with her. Finally she got out of bed and walked down to the nursery hoping to at least see her baby. When she arrived, she was upset to find that he was crying in his bassinet and nobody was paying any attention.

A nurse escorted her back to her room, where she tossed and turned until her baby was finally brought to her. When Sandra's second baby was born, she let the hospital know in advance that the baby was to stay with her from birth.

Not all mothers feel that way. Cheryl was very tired after a long, hard labour and somewhat groggy from pain medication. She says, "I expected to be all excited once the baby was born. Instead I felt distant. I was just glad it was over, and I wanted to go to sleep."

Anne says, "I remember looking at my daughter and saying, 'Hello, stranger.' I knew she was my baby, but I didn't feel any connection to her. It took me a while to get to know her and fall in love with her."

If the mother is tired or experiencing the side effects of pain medication, the hospital staff may suggest taking the baby to the nursery. The baby's father might choose to hold the baby and keep the new family together, or he might follow the baby to the nursery and supervise the process of weighing, examining, and bathing the baby.

Keeping mother and baby together after birth is important, not just because mothers prefer it, but because it produces better outcomes for mothers and babies. One well-conducted study found that the risk of child abuse and neglect was lower when mothers and babies "roomed-in" together from birth, compared to mothers and babies who were separated for most of their hospital stay.

Other studies have noted more affectionate behaviour and more self-confidence when mothers kept their babies with them. Mothers who have kept their babies with them are also more likely to succeed at breastfeeding, and to breastfeed longer than three months.

Researchers have observed typical ways in which many mothers greet and examine their new babies. A mother will often study her baby's face without saying much until the baby opens his eyes, and then she will speak softly to the baby, saying "hello" or "there you are" or calling the baby by name. She will touch the baby first with the tips of her fingers and then with her whole hand, and will usually undress the baby (if she has been wrapped in a blanket or gown) and examine the baby's entire body. The freedom to go through this process in her own way, and at her own speed, seems to be important for the new mother as she builds a connection with her baby.

All the above does not mean that mothers and babies who miss that immediate "bonding" time because of hospital routines, illness, or other complications will have problems relating or will never fall in love with each other. They will! But the early hours after birth do seem to be a sensitive time, when both mother and baby are primed to make that connection. Caregivers and hospitals should promote this time together, and not infringe on it with unnecessary routines.

Studies on fathers and new babies have not been done in the same way mothers and babies have been researched.

The risk of the baby catching an infection while in the hospital is significant, and any infection can be serious in a newborn infant. At least one study found lower rates of infection in babies who roomed-in with their mothers when compared to babies who stayed in the nursery. Hospital routines to prevent infection, including using gowns and restricting visitors, have not been demonstrated to reduce infection rates.

Routine Treatments of the Newborn

Will keeping the mother and baby together interfere with the care the baby receives? What immediate care do healthy newborns need?

The doctor, nurse, or midwife will usually suction the baby's mouth and nose as soon as it is born. This hasn't been studied even though it is so frequently done. It is intended to clear any mucus or fluid from the baby's airway so that he can breathe more easily. There are some risks: if it is done too vigorously, the baby can bleed from its mouth or nose, or the catheter can cause spasms in the baby's throat and abnormal heartbeats.

If the baby has passed meconium before birth, suctioning of the nose, mouth, and throat as soon as the baby's head emerges may help prevent the baby inhaling any meconium into his lungs. This procedure is safe enough to be recommended, although its benefit has also never been demonstrated in clinical trials.

"I wish somebody had told me beforehand that they always suction babies," Mieke says. "When the doctor yelled at the nurse, 'Okay, suction here,' I panicked. I thought something must be wrong. And the baby made this horrible gurgling and gagging noise that scared me even more. But the doctor and nurse were completely calm and unconcerned, so I realized everything was okay. Then Theo started to cry, and it was the most beautiful sound I ever heard."

The other concern is to keep the baby warm. Even healthy newborns can lose a lot of heat in a cold room (and many hospital delivery rooms are air-conditioned), and infants cool down even more because they are wet at birth. The best way to keep your baby warm is to gently dry her with a warm towel, then settle her, tummy down, against your bare chest. The two of you can then be covered with a pre-warmed blanket, or a heater could be set up near you if necessary. The newborn examination can be done while the baby is in your arms or lying beside you (roll over onto your side so that you can see her better).

If the mother is unable to hold the baby, the baby can be wrapped well and given to the father to hold, or the baby can be placed in a bassinet with a heater overhead for warmth. The father could also remove his shirt and have the baby against his bare skin with a blanket around the two of them.

If the baby requires some resuscitation, a pre-warmed area must be available so that the baby does not get cold. As much as possible should be done where the parents can still see their baby.

When Margaret's son was born, he didn't breathe well at first. The nurse moved him quickly to a heated bassinet and continued to suction him. James followed, and from his position beside the bassinet described to Margaret what was going on: "He's opened his eyes now and he's looking at me. He probably thinks I'm the one sticking that tube in his mouth. Oh—did you hear that? He sneezed. And now he's crying. His little face is all red." His running commentary was incredibly reassuring to Margaret.

Another routine treatment is swabbing the umbilical cord stump with either **neomycin** or **triple dye**. This has been shown to reduce the incidence of certain skin infections.

An injection of vitamin K has been given routinely to newborns to prevent **hemorrhagic disease of the newborn**, a rare condition in which the baby's clotting mechanism is deficient because of lack of vitamin K. The incidence of this disease is probably 1 in 200 to 1 in 400 or less, and significant complications from the disease are much less than that.

The studies on hemorrhagic disease were done when first feedings of babies were often delayed 12 or even 24 hours, and breastfed infants were routinely supplemented so that the infant did not get much of the **colostrum** (the early breast milk), which is high in vitamin K. It is probable that the risk of this disease for breastfed babies is even lower than the statistics suggest.

However, giving these routine injections of vitamin K makes the risk even lower, and there do not seem to be any harmful effects. Vitamin K can also be given by mouth. However, new studies showing that the oral dose is not as well absorbed by the body as the injected form have prompted the Canadian Paediatric Society (CPS) to release new guidelines for the administration of vitamin K to newborns.

The CPS recommends that all newborns receive vitamin K by injection within six hours of birth. If parents choose an oral dose, the CPS recommends giving this at the first feeding, with follow-up doses during the first six to eight weeks of life. CPS cautions that parents should be aware that the oral dose is still not as effective in preventing the disease as the injected dose.

This is something you could discuss with your doctor if you would prefer that your baby not have the injection.

In many countries, the law requires that all newborn babies have their eyes treated to prevent gonorrhea. Silver nitrate, once the mandated treatment in North America, should not be used, as it is irritating to the eyes and is ineffective against infection with chlamydia. Either **tetracycline** or **erythromycin** antibiotic ointment is a better choice.

The ointment may blur the baby's vision temporarily, so the baby may not look so alertly at her parents. There is no urgency to put the ointment in the baby's eyes; the ointment can be delayed until you and your baby have had a long visit, a chance to breastfeed, and to get to know each other a little.

No matter what the normal routines are at the hospital where your baby is born, understand that you have the right to refuse any treatment or

SAFE SLEEP

A safe sleep environment reduces the risk to your baby of **SIDS** (sudden infant death syndrome) or suffocation hazards. The following precautions are recommended:

Baby in a Crib	Baby Sharing Parents' Bed
Crib should meet current safety standards with a mattress that fits snugly	Bed should have a firm, standard mattress (not a waterbed).
No bumper pads, fluffy duvets, pillows, or large stuffed animals	Parents sleeping with baby should be non-smokers and avoid consuming alcohol, medications, or drugs that cause drowsiness, and extreme exhaustion
Position crib away from blind cords, lights, and other hazards	Keep duvets and pillows well away from baby's face
Be sure mattress is at lowest setting and sides are all the way up once baby can sit up	Don't leave baby alone in an adult bed
Crib should be in parents' room for the first year, unless the parents smoke	Don't sleep on a couch, chair, or recliner with the baby
Baby should sleep on her back	Baby should sleep on her back
Breastfeed your baby	Breastfeed your baby

procedure, including the ointment. You can insist on keeping your newborn with you, insist on feeding your baby whenever you (and the baby) wish, leave earlier than the hospital's normal discharge time, and ask that the baby wear clothes you have brought from home rather than the hospital's gowns.

Establishing family-centred maternity care is a goal of most hospitals and is encouraged by guidelines published by both the Canadian and American colleges of obstetricians and gynaecologists. Institutes in both countries work to encourage hospitals to become sensitive to the needs of families. You can help this trend by letting the hospital know before you deliver what kind of care you would like. After you go home, take a minute to write the hospital and tell them all the things you liked (or didn't like) about your stay. It makes a difference!

-47-
Postpartum Depression

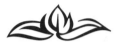

"The birth went well," says Kelly. "Really, everything worked out the way I had hoped. And Evan was perfect—a beautiful, healthy baby boy. I was so happy for a week or so. Then I just gradually started to feel really sad and black. It was more than just being tired, though I was exhausted. I thought that I was an awful mother who didn't deserve to have this beautiful baby. Every week I felt worse. Luckily my midwife was still making regular visits and she could see how terrible I was feeling. She talked to my husband and they pushed me to talk to my doctor about what was happening."

Postpartum depression usually starts in the month or so after the baby is born, though it may arise at any time in the first year. Unhappy thoughts and feelings come and stay most of the day. The unhappiness is strong enough that often the mother cannot enjoy her baby, and sometimes cannot even take care of her baby or herself.

SYMPTOMS OF POSTPARTUM DEPRESSION CAN INCLUDE:

- feeling sad, anxious, or panicky most of the time
- feeling hopeless, that things will never get better
- loss of interest and pleasure in most usual activities
- feeling vaguely guilty, worthless, and angry
- feeling that everything is too much effort (this is on top of the usual new mother fatigue)
- either worrying about the baby, or feeling indifferent towards the baby
- feeling your baby would be better off without you, or having scary thoughts about harming the baby or yourself
- sleeping too much or not at all, having headaches or stomach aches, or having a big appetite change—either eating all the time or less than usual

POSTPARTUM PSYCHOSIS

Postpartum psychosis is a rare and serious illness affecting 1 to 2 per 1,000 women. This illness puts women out of touch with reality. They often have delusions that something is wrong with the baby or someone is trying to harm the baby. They often have persistent thoughts (which they sometimes act on) about harming themselves and the baby. Women with postpartum psychosis need immediate medical help.

"Baby Blues"

Postpartum depression is quite different from the "baby blues," which are *short* periods of sadness, irritability, or crying. Many women have these feelings in the first few days after having a baby. The blues clear up within a week or so with no treatment.

Diagnosing Postpartum Depression

It can be very hard for a woman to tell that she is having a postpartum depression. Often she does not realize that the feelings she is having are not normal. She imagines that everyone feels this way after they have a baby. Feelings of vague guilt are made worse if she is also having feelings of indifference to the baby, or excessive worry about the baby. She may be afraid to tell anyone about these thoughts. Depressed women may also believe that they will never feel any better. Kelly says, "When I was depressed, I felt so hopeless. I knew I would never feel any different. I

didn't have the energy to think about talking to a therapist. My husband and midwife really had to push me, and convince me that how I was feeling wasn't normal."

Friends and family (and occasionally professionals) often unintentionally make the woman feel worse by saying, "What do you have to be depressed about?" or by suggesting that she "snap out of it" or "get it together." Women in a depression *can't* just make themselves feel better. They already feel angry at themselves because they don't understand why they feel so awful. Women need their friends and family to recognize their distress, and they need their midwife, physician, or any other professional they are in contact with to be alert for the symptoms they are showing.

What Causes Postpartum Depression?

We don't know why some women experience postpartum depression. Hormonal changes in the body, heredity, and life circumstances are all probably involved. Any woman who has a baby can get a postpartum depression, even women who planned and wanted their babies and are living otherwise happy lives.

However, women who have already had a depression, either after another pregnancy or at some other time in their life, and women who have a mother or sister who has been depressed, are more likely to experience postpartum depression. Women who have severe premenstrual symptoms are more likely to become depressed postpartum. And women in troublesome life circumstances, or with a difficult relationship with their family or partner, are more likely to be depressed postpartum.

Getting Better: Help for Postpartum Depression

Like most illnesses, postpartum depression can range from mild to severe. Some women with postpartum depression will recover without any treatment. But it can take six months to a year to feel completely better, and during this time they will suffer. Because they cannot interact happily with their babies and partners or families, everyone suffers. Most women do recover faster with treatment.

In many cases, help is provided by a professional counsellor or therapist who will listen to the woman talk, and not tell her how she "should" feel. A therapist can reassure the woman that this is an illness, it is not her fault, it will get better, and she is not alone. The therapist will help the woman see that many of her distressing thoughts (that she is a bad mother, that she is guilty, that she will never feel better) are caused by the depression. A support group of other women dealing with postpartum depression can reinforce the knowledge that she is not the only person to suffer from this condition.

Antidepressants can be useful in the treatment of postpartum depression. They work in the body to correct depression, just as penicillin treats pneumonia or insulin treats diabetes. They are not "uppers" or "downers" and they are not addictive. Antidepressants can be used safely during breastfeeding. They do take two to three weeks to work, and are usually fully effective in six weeks. The improvement is gradual and brings a return to feeling normal, not a feeling of being drugged or high. Kelly says, "At first, the appointments with the therapist were kind of useless—I would either just cry or not be able to talk. Then my doctor put me on an antidepressant and after a couple of weeks I could actually feel the black feeling lifting off my body. Then I could talk to the therapist about how I was feeling. After that, I really started to feel better. I didn't want to take drugs, particularly because I was breastfeeding Evan, but I know they helped me get better."

Like many health issues, postpartum depression is easier to treat and gets better faster the earlier treatment is started. Although it can be very difficult to ask for help when you are depressed, it is the first step to feeling better. Depression is an illness. You can't make yourself snap out of it any more than you can will yourself to heal a broken leg. It is important to tell your caregivers how you are feeling. Women deserve to be able to enjoy their babies and to enjoy the experience of being a mother.

Getting Started with Breastfeeding

Annette says, "I decided to breastfeed because of the allergies in both my family and my husband's family. I've really suffered with mine, and I wanted to prevent them if I could."

Noor says, "Breastfeeding just seemed like the normal thing to do. You know—human milk for human babies, cow's milk for calves..."

Rena says, "Sharla will be in daycare soon, and I think that because I'm breastfeeding her she won't be sick as often. That means not only is she happier and healthier, but I have less time off from work."

Celine says, "When I started really looking at reasons to breastfeed, I was amazed. It really does make a difference in so many areas—baby's health, development, even intelligence."

The reasons to breastfeed have been solidly demonstrated and ongoing research continues to come up with new ones.

Knowing this, the vast majority of mothers want to breastfeed their babies; unfortunately, many of them will give up or wean early because they run into problems and don't get the help they need. What happens during labour, birth, and the first few feedings can

SOME IMPORTANT REASONS TO BREASTFEED

Babies who are not breastfed have an increased risk of:

- respiratory infections and ear infections
- gastrointestinal infections, diarrhea, or constipation
- allergies, including food allergies, eczema, and asthma
- iron-deficiency anemia
- problems with jaw and dental development that may require braces or other orthodontic work
- illnesses serious enough to require admission to hospital
- **SIDS** (sudden infant death syndrome)
- diabetes
- obesity
- some childhood cancers
- lower scores on intelligence and achievement tests

have a lot to do with the success or failure of breastfeeding.

Glenda's labour went very slowly at first then quickly at the end. "I had been given Demerol in labour because they thought it would be several hours before the baby was born," she says. "Then suddenly things went fast and Gordon was born an hour later. Because of the Demerol, we were both pretty sleepy. I tried to nurse him but honestly, I could barely hold him and he was out of it, too."

Glenda fell asleep, and woke up six hours later. "I asked the nurse to bring Gordon to me and she did. He had a pacifier in his mouth because they said he'd been crying a lot. I tried to nurse him then and it was pretty awkward, I don't think he really got any milk."

The next time Glenda tried to feed her son, she couldn't get him to nurse at all. She tried repeatedly to push his head towards her breast, as the nurse showed her, but to no avail. "I was in tears, and Gordon was screaming. The nurse said we'd better get some food into him, and brought me a bottle of formula. He drank it right down. I guess he was starving."

Four hours later, Glenda tried again and finally got the baby to nurse. "I was so relieved. It really hurt, though, and I hadn't expected that. The nurse said some pain was normal until my nipples got toughened up."

Glenda went home with her baby boy and the hospital's "new mother gift pack" that included a sample can of formula. When her nipples became even more painful a day later, she decided to give the baby another bottle of formula from the free sample, to give her nipples a break from feeding. But they hurt even more by the next day, so she gave another bottle and

within a couple of weeks, Gordon was completely formula-fed.

Glenda was very disappointed that breastfeeding hadn't worked out for her, but she didn't realize that some of the problems she encountered were due to some not-very-helpful routines and policies at the hospital where her baby was born.

The Best Start

What will help breastfeeding mothers and babies get off to the best start?

The Baby-Friendly Hospital Initiative is a worldwide program sponsored by UNICEF and the World Health Organization (WHO), aimed at creating in-hospital birth environments that will facilitate breastfeeding. To earn this designation, hospitals have to follow certain guidelines (such as not accepting free formula from formula manufacturers) and be inspected to show that all the steps are being followed. The 10 steps of the program are well-supported by research and, where they have been applied, have led to more mothers breastfeeding and longer breastfeeding duration.

While these recommendations apply to hospitals, they let you, as a parent and consumer, know what things you should be looking for to help you and your baby get off to a good start.

To support infant health, hospitals should follow these guidelines:

1. **Have a written breastfeeding policy that is routinely communicated to all health care staff.** This is important because mothers are often frustrated when they are given different

information and advice by different people on staff. For example, when Elaine's son was born prematurely, the midwife who attended the birth encouraged her to begin expressing her milk immediately for him, even though he was not yet mature enough to actually breastfeed. When she went to the nursery to see her son, however, the nurse there discouraged her from pumping until the baby was bigger, saying she wouldn't get much milk at this stage anyway. Elaine was already concerned about her very tiny baby and didn't know what was right. Having all staff given consistent, accurate information can prevent situations like this. Fortunately, Elaine did begin pumping because this was important in establishing and maintaining a good milk supply for her baby.

2. **Train all health care staff in the skills necessary to implement this policy.** Policy isn't helpful unless people have the knowledge to assist mothers in solving breastfeeding challenges. For example, mothers may need to know how to hand-express milk, how to deal with inverted nipples, how to deal with engorgement of the breasts, how to deal with oversupply, how to recognize the baby's feeding cues, and many other practical aspects of breastfeeding.

3. **Inform all pregnant women about the benefits and management of breastfeeding.** If the hospital where you are planning to give birth does not have a Baby-Friendly designation, you may not be automatically given this information—but this is something you could do for yourself. Look for books about breastfeeding that are up to date and written by people with breastfeeding expertise, or videos that are produced by breastfeeding experts, not formula manufacturers. (Research has shown that when mothers are given breastfeeding information created by formula companies, they are less likely to breastfeed and wean earlier if they do breastfeed than the mothers who receive information prepared by breastfeeding experts.) If at all possible, attend La Leche League meetings while you are pregnant, so that you will be prepared to get breastfeeding off to a good start once your baby is born. At the meetings you will be able to see other mothers with their babies and discover the various positions for latching the baby on, for example. If you do have problems, you will probably feel more comfortable about phoning the La Leche League leader for help because she'll be familiar to you. (Of course, you can also call even if you haven't attended any meetings.)

4. **Help mothers initiate breastfeeding within one half-hour of birth.** Your hospital may not do this routinely, but you can discuss this with your caregiver and ask to have it written into your birth plan. To help initiate breastfeeding successfully, you may also want to take the step of minimizing medication during labour and birth. All medications, including epidurals, do affect the baby's ability to suck effectively. With good help, many mothers and babies are able to overcome this difficult start to breastfeeding. But where other problems are also present, the baby's uncoordinated sucking in the first days may lead to the mother weaning early.

The medication itself is not the only factor. When a labouring woman has an epidural anaesthetic, for example, she will also be given intravenous fluids, and after the baby is born, this extra fluid can cause **edema** (swelling) and **breast engorgement**. This engorgement—caused not by too much milk in the breasts, but by too much fluid—often makes latching the baby on very difficult, even if the baby had managed to breastfeed before the engorgement set in. Women are often then advised to pump to relieve the pain, only to find that pumping simply pulls more fluid into the breasts and makes the situation worse.

Keeping mothers and babies together after birth and encouraging immediate breastfeeding is very helpful. When babies nurse in the first two hours after birth, they are less likely to be weaned early than babies who didn't nurse until four or more hours after they are born. This doesn't mean that the baby who needs special care (or is not able to nurse for some other reason) is doomed to breastfeeding failure, but it does point out that these babies and mothers may need some extra help in getting nursing established.

What if your baby doesn't latch on and start to nurse even after an hour or two? The skin-to-skin contact you are both enjoying is still very valuable—it helps to stabilize your baby's temperature and blood sugar.

What if your baby was born by Caesarean? The Baby-Friendly guidelines suggest that your baby should still be given the opportunity to breastfeed in that first half hour. With a knowledgeable person to help you, your baby can latch on even while the surgical incision is still being closed.

5. **Show mothers how to breastfeed and maintain lactation even if they should be separated from their infants.** Perhaps your baby is too premature or ill to feed at the breast. In that situation, it is important to establish and maintain milk production. The **colostrum**—the milk that mothers make in fairly small quantities during the first couple of days after a baby is born—is very valuable for a premature or ill baby because it contains high levels of antibodies and other protective factors. Frequent pumping or hand-expressing will signal the breasts to produce more milk and help to make sure you have plenty of milk once your baby is ready to go to the breast.

6. **Give newborn infants no food or drink other than breast milk unless medically indicated.** The research is very clear that when babies are given supplements in the first few days, they are much more likely to be weaned early than babies who are not supplemented. Supplements can interfere with the mother's milk production. In addition, studies also show that these early supplements increase the baby's risk of allergies, infection, and other health problems. Medical indications for early supplementation are rare. Jennifer's baby was 9 pounds, 12 ounces (4,422 g) at birth and seemed hungry right from the start. He latched on eagerly and breastfed about once an hour for the first two days. One of the nurses suggested that her colostrum was just not enough to meet this larger-than-average baby's needs and that she should supplement with formula. But while Jennifer was still trying to make up her mind about that, she noticed that her breasts were

SELF-ATTACHMENT

Increasingly, research is showing that babies know more about how to breastfeed than people used to believe. Sometimes if the baby is held to the breast after birth it will nuzzle or lick at the nipple and not be interested in nursing. But many babies will actively seek out the breast and begin to suckle. One researcher filmed a number of newborns who were simply placed, tummy down, on their mother's abdomens after they were born. The babies soon began to crawl on their stomachs towards the nearest breast. They found the nipple, then attached themselves and began sucking well without any assistance. The study involved only a small number of babies, but others have reported observing a similar self-attachment process with newborns, and in some places (such as Sweden) this has become incorporated into hospital routine.

This ability to self-attach at the breast lasts beyond the newborn period, and sometimes mothers who have had difficulty getting their babies to breastfeed effectively find it helps to go back to basics and let the baby latch on his own way. American pediatrician Dr. Christina Smillie has developed an approach to baby-led latching for babies past the immediate newborn stage. The mother sits comfortably in a chair or on the bed and holds the baby skin-to-skin (baby in just a dia-per, mother not wearing a blouse or bra) in an upright, vertical position. The baby will typically move so that he can see the mother's face, and this helps him orient himself. If he is hungry and ready to nurse, he will shortly begin to bounce to one side or the other, seeking the breast. These movements can be surprisingly strong. The mother supports the baby's shoulders and bottom and follows him as he moves. When he finds the breast, he may bob his head a few times as he positions himself, and then will latch on.

Once the baby has learned to breastfeed effectively, it isn't necessary to start in a vertical position every time. However, this approach can be very helpful with a baby who hasn't latched at all, who resists being held in a nursing position, or who tends to keep coming off the breast.

Patience is essential in this self-attachment process. In studies where newborns are allowed to crawl to the breast, the researchers found that many took over an hour to complete the process and begin nursing. The baby can be checked over while it is lying on the mother's tummy and other routines (such as weighing and bathing) can wait until breastfeeding has gotten started. It seems to be helpful not to wash the baby or the mother before allowing him to search for the breast.

feeling much fuller. Her baby's frequent nursing had brought in the "mature milk" more quickly than usual, and there was no need to supplement.

7. **Practice rooming in—that is, allow mothers and infants to remain together 24 hours a day.** Many breastfeeding problems can be prevented or solved simply by keeping mothers and babies together, especially if the mothers are encouraged to have the baby in skin-to-skin contact with them as much as possible. It's not true that mothers will become exhausted and won't get enough rest if their babies are in the same room. If the mother is shown how to breastfeed lying down, she'll get plenty of rest.

8. **Encourage breastfeeding on demand.** Some breastfeeding experts feel the phrase "on demand" sounds as though the parents should wait until the baby is crying hard and insisting on being fed, and they prefer to talk about feeding "on cue." The basic idea is that parents pay attention to the baby's signals, rather than watching the clock and feeding the baby on a schedule. The early cues may be fairly subtle—the baby may smack his lips or make sucking movements; he may put his hands up to his mouth; if he's being held, he may turn towards the breast or try to move down his mother's body to find the breast. Waiting until the baby is actually crying means you've missed the early cues, and a crying baby may be too upset to nurse well, or may have swallowed a lot of air, causing intestinal pain later.

How often will your baby want to eat if he's fed on cue? There are great variations between babies. Some feed very frequently, others less often. The average is between 8 and 12 times in 24 hours, but that doesn't mean there is a problem if your baby nurses 13 or 15 or 20 times in 24 hours. Research in tribal societies in Africa, for example, found that the babies nurse an average of every 15 minutes, for a few minutes at a time. It *can* be a concern if your baby is nursing fewer than 8 times in 24 hours, though, and you may need to keep a close eye on his diaper output and weight gain.

How long should the baby breastfeed at each feeding? Again, there should be no set limits. When mothers time feedings, they are much more likely to wean early. It is important to know when the baby is actually drinking milk at the breast, as some babies who are not latched on well may suck on the nipple but not be getting much milk. Those babies can nurse for an hour or more at a time and still not be satisfied.

Pediatrician Dr. Jack Newman, an internationally known expert on breastfeeding who runs a breastfeeding clinic in Toronto, Ontario, has described an easy way for mothers to tell if the baby is actually getting milk. When a baby sucks slowly and rhythmically, and pauses with his mouth wide open at the height of each suck, he is getting mouthfuls of milk.

9. **Give no artificial nipples (i.e., bottles) or pacifiers to breastfeeding babies.** Babies who are given bottles of sugar-water, formula, or even expressed breast milk are more likely to be weaned early. Babies who are given pacifiers are also more likely to be weaned early. Why? It may be **nipple confusion**. A baby sucks quite differently on a bottle than at the breast, and a baby who has become used to the bottle method may find it difficult to suck correctly at the breast—and may make his mother's nipples very sore in the process. It may also have more to do with the flow of milk than the nipple. Milk comes very quickly out of a bottle nipple (especially if the hole is large) but the baby has to work harder to get milk from the breast. A baby who has become accustomed to the fast, effortless flow of milk from the bottle might be frustrated by the slower flow of milk from the breast. While the baby doesn't get milk from a pacifier, he does learn an incorrect sucking technique that can interfere with effective nursing at the breast. If the baby does need to

be supplemented there are many other ways to provide the supplement—cup-feeding, spoon-feeding, using a tube at the breast or on a parent's finger, using a syringe, etc.

10. **Foster the establishment of breastfeeding support groups and refer mothers to them.** This is directed at medical staff, but you can take a big step on your own by seeking out and joining a group for breastfeeding mothers such as La Leche League. This is an international organization which has been providing mother-to-mother breastfeeding support for more than 50 years. Other organizations may be available in your community as well. The ideal time to start attending meetings is before your baby is even born, so that you can learn the tips that will help get you off to a good start.

Here are some comments from mothers who attended La Leche League meetings in Canada, taken from a 2005 survey:

"I enjoy coming to the meetings for many reasons...to meet other moms, to get out, to get answers to questions. I feel I could ask anything without feeling shy or embarrassed. La Leche League has been a wonderful experience for me!"

"I like the relaxed atmosphere at LLL meetings. I feel comfortable sharing experiences with other moms and learning from other moms. A great source of support and encouragement."

"LLL has been my lifeline through all my children. During my first breastfeeding experience I learned lots of valuable information

and certainly continued to breastfeed longer than I expected."

"Book info is great, but what you can learn from other mothers' experience is invaluable."

"LLL has taught me to trust my instinct—I have felt so confident in my mothering skills since I have attended LLL."

Each support group—and each meeting—will be a little different, depending on the mothers who show up. If you feel that the first one you attend doesn't really suit you, don't give up. Look for another group or perhaps try a couple more meetings and see if it can work for you.

Breastfeeding Techniques

When the baby shows interest in nursing—which can be right after birth or not for several hours, especially if the mother's had medication during labour—you may want to start by encouraging your baby to self-attach. Sit upright with your back well-supported and place the baby vertically and skin-to-skin against your chest (remove any clothes and your bra). This position is usually very calming for the baby as well. If your baby is ready to feed, he'll begin to bob his head and usually will move back so that he can see your face. Then he'll begin to move down to one side or the other, usually in a series of "bounces." Sometimes the baby will move quite vigorously and you may feel like he is throwing himself sideways. Support him with one hand behind his shoulders and the other behind his

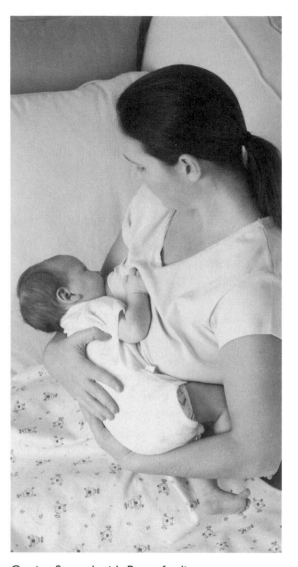 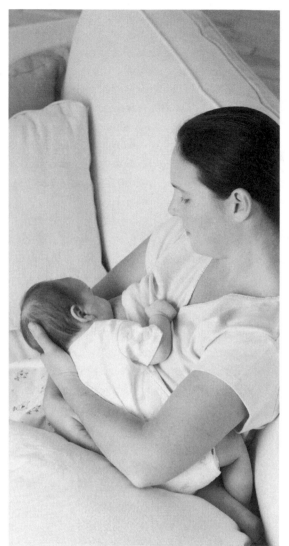

Getting Started with Breastfeeding

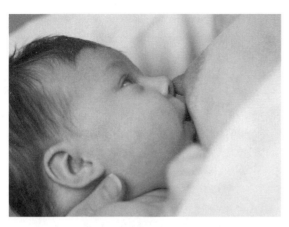

You may need to support your breast with one hand, keeping a finger or your thumb on top and your other fingers well back from the nipple. With your baby in a secure and comfortable position, aim your nipple at his nose.

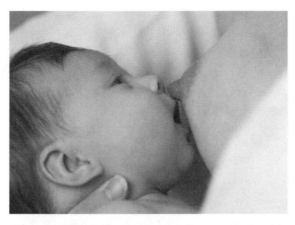

The curve of the breast below the nipple should naturally rub against the baby's mouth. This will encourage the baby to open his mouth wide. Be patient and wait for that wide-open mouth.

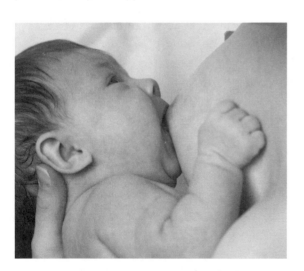

As he opens his mouth and takes in the breast, you can use your finger or thumb to help tuck the nipple under his top lip and jaw if necessary. This approach will help him get a large mouthful of breast and will position the nipple at the back of his mouth. As he latches, pull his body in close and allow his head to stay tipped back with his chin buried in your breast and his nose clear.

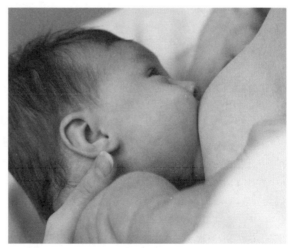

You'll see that more of the breast is covered by his bottom lip and jaw than by his top lip and jaw. It is the action of the baby's tongue and jaw that extracts milk from the breast. This asymmetrical position helps the baby feel the nipple in his mouth, which stimulates him to suck, and also makes it easier for him to extract milk from the breast.

hips and bottom as he moves down. When his face is close to your breast, he'll begin bobbing his head again as he searches for the nipple. As he finds it, he'll get his chin buried into the breast and his nose away from it, and be well-latched on.

If there is any pain as he latches on and begins to nurse, that's a sign that the latch isn't as good as it should be. Pediatrician Dr. Christina Smillie, who has studied this baby-led latching approach, recommends "wiggling around" to make it better. In other words, adjust the baby's position and your own position until you find something that is more comfortable. It often only takes a small adjustment to make a big difference in how the latch feels and works.

If you are feeling that you need to give your baby more help in latching, you can try this approach. Position the baby on your lap with his stomach against yours or with his body slightly rolled away from you. Hold him with your hand behind his shoulders and neck and his weight on your forearm, his bottom near your elbow. He should be very close to you, ideally skin-to-skin. Tuck the baby's bottom arm around your waist; use your elbow to tuck his bottom in. Let his head tip back so that his chin can be pressed into your breast as he latches on. Use your other hand to support your breast, with your thumb on top and the rest of your fingers under the breast. His nose should be level with the nipple.

There are different approaches suggested to get the baby to open his mouth wide. Some experts like to use the nipple to stroke the baby's lips from side-to-side, others stroke the top lip then the bottom lip. Another approach recommends starting with the nipple at baby's nose, then stroking down the grooved area between nose and mouth and onto the top lip. Whichever method she chooses, the mother should "aim" her nipple towards the top of his mouth, to help get the baby's lower lip onto the breast well below the nipple. As the baby opens his mouth wide, she can pull him in closer with a little pressure on his shoulders and hips, allowing his head to tip back. He will take a large mouthful of breast, covering more of the breast with his bottom lip and jaw than with the top lip and jaw, and the nipple will go right to the back of baby's mouth.

If this is done properly, it won't hurt. When the mother feels an initial painful tugging sensation on the nipple it means that the baby is trying to pull the nipple into position. She probably needs to either wait until the baby opens his mouth wider, or pull the baby in closer when he takes the nipple. (Taking the baby off and re-latching repeatedly tends to cause more damage to the nipple, though, so you may want to try to adjust your position while the baby is still at the breast—perhaps by tucking baby's bottom and shoulders in a bit more.)

As the baby nurses, the mother should see and hear a changing pattern. It may begin with a series of rapid sucks, as the baby stimulates the milk to **let down** (move from the ducts further back in the breast, where it is made, to the ducts right behind the nipple so the baby can drink it). Then the mother should notice a suck-suck-pause-suck-pause or similar pattern, with the baby's mouth open wide during each pause—he is swallowing a mouthful of milk at each pause. If the baby continues with the fast suck-suck-suck pattern, with no pauses or noticeable swallowing, he is probably not latched on correctly. The mother should slide her finger in the baby's mouth to break the suction and start over.

"This 'latching-on' thing isn't always easy," says Roberta. "When Germaine was born, he had such a tiny mouth and my nipple looked so big. I was so happy at the first couple of feedings when he started to suck, even though it hurt.

"But then the hospital lactation consultant came by to see how we were doing, and she said he wasn't on right. He was only getting a little of the milk, and my nipples were sore." Roberta learned to wait until Germaine opened his mouth really wide—"and that took some persistence because by this point he thought it was okay to nurse just on the end of my nipple"—and to make sure he was taking in part of the breast as well. "I knew when we got it right because it stopped hurting, and Germaine started to suck differently—I could tell he was getting a real mouthful of milk."

Engorgement

"I felt like I had two large rocks on my chest," says Linda, remembering her experience with engorgement three days after her baby was born. "I couldn't bear to take a shower, it was so painful to have the water hit my breasts. And feedings were incredibly difficult."

The first milk the breasts produce, called **colostrum**, is made in small quantities and the mother's breasts remain soft for the first 48 hours or so after the baby is born. Then the "true milk" begins to arrive, and if milk production is over-enthusiastic ("I think my breasts thought I'd had twins," Linda says) and the milk is not

removed, engorgement can be the result. The breasts become painfully swollen, but the swelling is not only from increased milk production. The spaces between the milk ducts also fill up with extra fluid, both from pregnancy and from any intravenous fluids the mother may have been given during labour.

The best prevention and treatment for engorgement is avoiding interventions in labour that require IV fluids (such as epidurals), and unrestricted breastfeeding: letting the baby nurse as often as he wants, for as long as he wants. This allows milk production to be adjusted to meet the baby's needs.

If engorgement does become a problem, some research has found that hand-expression of milk gives some relief to the mother. Pumping is not helpful, as the vacuum of the pump tends to pull more fluid into the breast and make the engorgement worse. Some research has shown that applying well-washed cabbage leaves to the breast will reduce engorgement. Other treatments, including ice packs or moist heat applications, may be helpful but have not been formally researched. Another approach which has, again, not been formally researched, is described by American lactation consultant Jean Cotterman as "reverse pressure softening." This involves using the fingertips to firmly press the engorged tissue around the nipple back towards the mother's ribcage. The idea is to create a circle of softened tissue where the fluid has been pushed back into the breast. If this is done right before nursing, it will be easier for the baby to latch on well and get more milk, reducing the engorgement.

The Sleepy Baby

Some babies—especially those who have had a difficult birth, or who have **jaundice**—may be sleepier than usual. Bronwyn says, "My friends were envious because Talia slept so much, but it was a real problem. My breasts were so hard and full, and at every feeding I'd struggle to wake her up, somehow get her on the breast, and then she'd fall asleep again after about three sucks. I was so worried that she wouldn't get enough milk."

Bronwyn called a La Leche League leader who gave her some suggestions about getting the sleepy baby to nurse. "It helped to keep her close to me all the time, for two reasons. I could be alert to any signs of her starting to stir or wake up so that I could try feeding her. If I didn't pick her up when she started to make those little noises, often she'd go back to sleep again. Secondly, just me moving her from room to room and all our normal household noises kept her from going into such a deep sleep."

Bronwyn also learned some tips on keeping Talia awake during feedings. She undressed her—both to keep her a little bit cool and provide more skin-to-skin contact—and changed her diaper before each feeding. If Talia dozed off at the breast, she would stroke under Talia's chin with her finger to encourage her to keep sucking. Rubbing the baby's feet also helped at times. Switching sides frequently—after every couple of minutes—was another method of keeping Talia awake and interested.

"It didn't take long before Talia was more wakeful and a better nurser," Bronwyn says, "and pretty soon there were days when I wished she was my sleepy baby again!"

The Fussy Baby

Jennifer's baby was the opposite of Talia. Michael slept very little and mostly took short catnaps, even during the first day after his birth, and he seemed to want to nurse 24 hours a day.

"And if he wasn't sleeping or nursing, he was crying," Jennifer says. "The first time I tried to feed him, he was screaming and it just seemed impossible to nurse him. I'd push my nipple into his mouth—it was open wide because he was crying so hard—and he didn't seem to notice it was there. He just kept screaming. After a couple of tries I started crying, too."

Jennifer's midwife showed her how to touch her little finger against the top of Michael's mouth. That would start him sucking, and help him to calm down. Holding him vertically, skin-to-skin, against her chest was also very helpful in calming him down. Once he was calm, he often began to move towards the breast, and Jennifer would help him get into position. If he didn't take the nipple readily, she would try touching either his lips or the corner of his mouth with the nipple. That would often encourage him to root for the nipple, and make it easier to feed him.

Do I Have Enough Milk?

Frightening stories in newspapers and on TV about breastfed babies who became seriously dehydrated have made new mothers even more anxious than usual about their milk supply. Most women who give up breastfeeding early say they didn't have enough milk. How common is this problem, and what can be done to make sure the baby is getting enough?

The Evidence About...
Breastfeeding

Breast milk is the biologically appropriate food for babies. When babies are not breastfed, they are at higher risk of a number of illnesses and developmental difficulties in both the short and long term. Breastfeeding is most easily established when the mother and baby are kept together from birth and the baby is nursed as often as he wants for as long as he wants. Supplementation with either formula or water and the use of pacifiers should be avoided.

Despite the strong evidence about the value of breastfeeding, our society makes it difficult for mothers to nurse their babies. Breastfeeding in public is often discouraged, and mothers may have a hard time finding a private place for feedings. Our whole society would benefit from the lower medical costs and reduced strain on the environment if breastfeeding was truly supported.

Finding support and practical help with breastfeeding is often the key to success.

HOW LONG CAN I BREASTFEED?

The World Health Organization (and both the Canadian and American organizations of pediatricians) recommends that breastfeeding be exclusive for the first six months, that solid foods may be added at that point but are only supplementary to breast milk, and that breastfeeding should continue for two years or longer. Yes, even with teeth. Babies breastfeed quite easily (and usually quite painlessly, although occasionally babies do bite), even with a mouthful of teeth. Once it's an ingrained habit, they don't forget how to breastfeed, even if they are given occasional bottles or drinks from a cup. Many women continue breastfeeding well beyond the minimum two years recommended—the American Academy of Pediatrics specifically notes that there is no upper limit for breastfeeding. Women will continue to produce milk as long as the child is breastfeeding.

It's hard to tell what percentage of mothers are actually physically incapable of making enough milk for their babies, because many of the common routines (restricting the length and frequency of feedings, giving supplements, and using pacifiers for babies) have the effect of reducing milk supply. Often when mothers who think they don't have enough milk learn to position their babies correctly and begin feeding on cue they find their milk production increases dramatically.

Other women become concerned about their milk supply because their babies nurse more frequently and sleep less than they had expected. "I

didn't know that breastfeeding a new baby could be a full-time job!" says Lorraine. "Somewhere I had the idea that babies nurse for about 20 minutes every four hours or so, and you have the rest of the day to do what you want while they sleep. I had a whole list of projects I expected to take care of during the first month while my baby napped. When Matthew wanted to nurse every hour-and-a-half, naturally I thought there must be something wrong with my milk. It helped to talk to some other mothers and find out that he was perfectly normal."

Some physicians have tried **test weighings** of babies to see if they are getting enough milk.

This involves weighing the baby before and after a feeding and then calculating how much milk the baby has consumed. This is very inaccurate and not very helpful, because the amount of milk the baby takes at each feeding can vary quite dramatically. Research shows that when babies are routinely weighed before and after feedings, mothers are more likely to give up breastfeeding.

A better way to decide if the baby is getting enough milk is to observe the baby. Is he clearly swallowing milk as he feeds? Is he alert and active? In the first few weeks, expect to see at least two or three substantial bowel movements every day. Regular weight checks by your midwife or other caregiver can also reassure you that the baby is gaining properly.

-Conclusion-
Making Decisions: Applying the Best Evidence

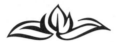

The experience of growing and giving birth to a baby is in some ways a simple process that, most of the time, works beautifully without any intervention at all. It is also a very complex process, with potential complications and challenging dilemmas. In Western society, pregnancy and birth can be made more complex by the medical system which has been designed to deal with those challenges—but which can, at times, get in the way of the simple and straightforward parts of pregnancy and birth.

A considerable amount of research has been done on pregnancy and birth, but it hasn't always produced clear answers. In some cases, the research has demonstrated that once-common routines are not helpful—as with electronic fetal monitors, episiotomies, and shaving the mother's pubic hair. Some research has discovered life-saving treatments—such as gammaglobulin for Rh-negative mothers and corticosteroids for premature babies. Other research has only confirmed what women have always believed—that walking and moving around is helpful in labour, that having a support person present is valuable, and that

women do know how and when to push their babies out.

The research, though, is only a foundation. It's up to you to decide how to apply the results of that research to your individual situation. This is your baby, your body, your family, and you are the ones who will live with the consequences of the decisions you make. You know what things are important to you, and can make the best choices for your pregnancy, with the research results as only one factor (although certainly an important one) in the decision-making.

Discussing Decisions with Your Caregiver

Florence was expecting her second baby. She'd had trouble breastfeeding her first, and was determined to get off to a better start this time. After seeing a video of newborns who were allowed to "self-attach" at the breast, she decided to ask her doctor to let her baby begin breast-feeding that way. She brought a copy of the research study to show the doctor.

"Well, there's a lot we have to do when the baby is first born, Florence," her doctor said. "The baby has to be suctioned, we have to check everything over, the baby has to have eye ointment. We can't just leave him or her lying on your stomach until he nurses—if that ever happens."

"In the video, they said the longest it ever took was one hour. Couldn't the eye ointment wait until after that?" Florence asked. "And couldn't you examine him while he's lying on me?"

"I guess so. I'll want to suction him first, and then I could put him on your abdomen. Really, though, I'm most concerned about the baby getting cold."

Florence thought back to the research she'd seen. "I think they used the heater that usually goes over the baby's incubator over both mother and baby. Could we do that?"

"I don't know if the equipment we have moves that way. I've never tried it." Her doctor sounded doubtful.

"Okay," said Florence. "I'll call labour and delivery and see what I can find out about getting a heater over me and the baby. I'll let you know what they say. And maybe after you've read this research, I'll lend you the video."

Florence was able to arrange for a heater to keep her and her newborn daughter warm. The baby lay on her abdomen for about ten minutes after birth, and then begin to move towards her mother's breast. Before long, she had found the nipple and latched on beautifully. Florence was very pleased with the results of her decision.

Not all caregivers are as easy to talk to. Some simply have a more intimidating way about them, and some are not interested in discussion.

Julie was less than pleased with the care her labour and delivery nurse provided. The nurse seemed impatient with Julie's slowly progressing labour and repeatedly told her to be quiet when she moaned during contractions. When Julie finally felt like pushing, the nurse seemed eager to get things over with.

Julie pushed as she felt the urge. She made a low moaning sound—almost a grunt—then took another breath.

"No, you're doing it wrong," the nurse said. "You have to hold your breath as long as you can and push as hard as you can, through the whole contraction. I want to see your face turn purple and your veins pop out." Julie was puzzled. This wasn't what she'd learned in prenatal classes or in the book she'd read.

"You've read that you shouldn't hold your breath too long, haven't you?" asked the nurse, noticing the expression on Julie's face. "Well, the books are wrong. I've been delivering babies for a long time, and the way to get them out is to hold your breath and push, push, push."

Julie thought back to what she'd read, and made a quick decision. She decided to ignore the nurse's instructions, and listen to what her body was telling her. When she felt the urge to push, and to hold her breath, she did. When she wanted to let the air out and take another breath, she did—even though the nurse was instructing her to keep holding her breath and push harder. It was clearly not a time to try to discuss it, so she simply kept her focus on the messages she was getting from her own body.

What can help you in discussing your options and your decisions with your doctor?

- Approach your doctor as a partner. He or she certainly has information and training that will be helpful in making decisions, and the two of you (or the three of you, since your partner may also be included) should work together to find the best choices for your situation.

- Ask lots of questions, but understand that your doctor won't always have the answers. Many aspects of pregnancy and childbirth have not been researched; in other cases the research has produced unclear or contradictory results.

- If your doctor recommends a certain course of action, ask why. Ask if he or she can direct you to any research studies or other sources of information. If your doctor seems offended or taken aback by your questions, explain that this is a significant decision for you and you want to know more about it.

- You can look up research yourself—either in books such as this one, in medical journals, or through the Internet—and bring it in to the doctor to discuss.

- If your doctor is not supportive of your decisions, you can change doctors. This is not always easy to do, but may be your best option if you are really not compatible. You can also ask for a second opinion if a planned Caesarean or other major intervention is being recommended.

Liam's Birth: Decision-making in Action

How does this decision-making process work out in real life? Each birth has its own challenges and each family has its own priorities.

Lenore has had five children, and a wide range of birth experiences—from a Caesarean section for a transverse lie, to a planned home birth. You might think that by the fifth baby, there would be few surprises or issues left to deal with. Not so! Lenore's last labour and delivery—Liam's birth—involved perhaps more unexpected setbacks and decisions than any of his siblings'. Here is Liam's birth story, which illustrates how women can play an active role in decision-making—in partnership with their caregivers—even when labour doesn't go according to plan.

Lenore had planned a home birth. At her midwife's appointment just before her due date, she commented on how big the baby seemed to be getting, and the midwife suggested she do an internal examination since that can sometimes trigger labour. It worked. Lenore's water broke as she walked in the front door of her home.

"Labour started normally," Lenore said, "but as it continued, I kept feeling that the contractions weren't hard enough, weren't painful enough. It's hard to believe, but I was wanting to feel more pain because I knew from experience that the contractions had to be more painful to get the baby born."

As the night went on, the midwives became concerned about Lenore's lack of progress. They encouraged her to walk, to sit on the toilet, to sit in the Jacuzzi, but she was still not dilating very quickly. They begin to talk to Lenore about moving to the hospital.

"I didn't want to go, but I did understand their concerns," Lenore said. "Finally, at six in the morning, I agreed that we should go. It was just a gut feeling that something was not right."

When they arrived at the hospital, the midwives asked the obstetrician on call to examine Lenore. "The obstetrician said it was a big baby, I'd probably need a Caesarean, and we might as well do it now. I said absolutely not. I'd had big babies before, and I wasn't ready to just give up on a vaginal birth. So she said I should have an IV with oxytocin to stimulate my labour and an epidural. If the baby wasn't out by noon, she wanted to do a Caesarean. I thanked her as politely as I could, and said we would like to talk things over alone."

Lenore discussed her options with her midwives and support people. "I decided I could take things one step at a time, that I didn't have to buy 'the whole package' right away." She decided she would have an IV and oxytocin, to see if stronger contractions would help.

But when the oxytocin was started, the baby's heart rate dropped drastically in response. "We had it turned off right away," Lenore says. Her contractions then stopped altogether—she thinks from the stress of the situation. Lenore knew she had to do something, so she asked to have the IV (with fluids, since she was a little dehydrated, but no oxytocin) put on a moveable pole, and she headed into the shower—where she spent the next two or three hours.

"I felt safe in there. I could relax better. My contractions started again and then got quite strong. When I came out, my friend who was supporting me went around making the room as home-like as she could. She took down all the signs about epidurals, and she set out the blankets and sleepers we had brought for the baby. That really helped."

As the morning wore on, the midwife checked Lenore and found she was fully dilated, but the baby's head was very high. Lenore lay on her side and began to rock her pelvis back and forth, with her support people helping by pushing against her hip.

At noon, the obstetrician returned. She asked Lenore to move onto her back, and as she did, she felt the baby move down. "Then I pushed him out," Lenore says, "and it was a wonderful feeling. I lifted him up to my chest as he was born and didn't want to let go, I was just so glad he was born and everything was okay." The obstetrician was quite surprised, and said so. Liam weighed 10 pounds, 1 ounce (4,564 g) and was home meeting his brothers and sisters an hour later.

Liam's story has an interesting sequel. Lenore explains, "We found out later that Liam had a serious heart defect, and he had to have major heart surgery when he was seven months old. I suspect that's why his heart rate dropped so dramatically when I was given oxytocin. I think, too, that this might have been just the right kind of labour for Liam—slow and easy—given his heart problem. I guess I'll always wonder about that."

"I used to be quite a shy, quiet person, but I've become much stronger, much more assertive, in part through my experiences giving birth," muses Lenore. "With each one, there were decisions and choices to be made. Some of the decisions I could make in advance, but you have to be prepared to deal with things as they come up." In a similar situation, you might make different choices than Lenore did—and those choices would be right for you.

Just the Beginning

When you decided to pick up this book and read it, you were taking responsibility for your own care, and for the health and well-being of your baby, during your pregnancy and birth.

This is, however, just the beginning. As a parent, you will be responsible not only for decisions about your own life, but for your child as well. The decisions you make about how to care for and raise your child can affect that child for the rest of his life. All parents worry about making the right decisions for their children, and you will too.

You will have choices to make about how your baby is fed, who will take care of your baby if you go out to work, what kind of diapers you will use, where your baby will sleep, how you will teach or discipline your child. You will have decisions to make about your child's medical care and education. It's a big—and sometimes overwhelming—responsibility. How do you know the right thing to do? Just as with pregnancy and childbirth, you will work out the right choices for you, your baby, and your family. These decisions may or may not be in step with the routines of your community. Any skills you can develop to help you be assertive in promoting your child's well-being will be tremendously helpful.

Your willingness to speak up and make decisions will benefit both other women having babies and the medical community. Women need to keep questioning whether medical procedures produce better outcomes, to keep asking why, to keep looking for better ways. Most of the changes—and many of them have been quite dramatic and substantial—in the way women are cared for during labour and birth have happened because women were determined to make their own decisions. The acceptance of vaginal births after Caesareans is a one good example, and policies allowing fathers, doulas, and other support people to be present for births is another.

Most of these women had no thought of changing hospital policies—they just wanted to have the kind of birth experience that was important to them. But along the way they initiated changes that have benefited hundreds of other women—perhaps including you!

We hope that the memories of your pregnancy and your baby's birth will be positive ones, and that you will feel satisfaction in having made decisions that were right for you and your family. And as the arrival of your child leads you into the unique adventure of parenthood, we hope that your baby brings you as much joy and pleasure as our own children have given us.

Northern Babies: Difficult Choices

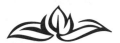

Women who live in northern Canada or Alaska, far from hospitals, have to make decisions about childbirth which have never been researched by studies and which can be very difficult.

Jana, for example, recently had her sixth child. She hired a nanny to care for her older children while her husband was working so that she could travel to a southern city to give birth. "I went into labour the day I was to fly to Victoria. I had to leave at 6:30 a.m. to catch a ferry to the airport (and it was a two-hour drive to the ferry). My plane left at 10:20 a.m. I arrived in Vancouver at noon, then changed planes and flew to Victoria around 1 p.m. My first words to my sister were, 'I'm in labour!' to which she replied, 'Well, I guess dinner's off.' My healthy baby girl was born at 7 p.m."

Lois was also living in a remote northern town when she discovered she was pregnant with twins. "I was strongly advised to deliver in a large city as facilities here would not accommodate twins. I flew to Calgary on March 1, leaving my two-year-old behind with my husband. My due date was April 1, and on March 31 I finally went into labour." Her twin boys were born later that day, and her husband drove 14 hours in snowy weather to pick her up. After just four days in hospital, Lois headed home with her husband and babies—a two-day trip.

Kim says her greatest fear during her pregnancy was that her baby would be born on the boat on the way into town. "We live in a remote community with no road access and our closest hospital is 22 nautical miles away. Fortunately, I had gone to town on our local freight and passenger boat on the Thursday, so that I would be there for a doctor's appointment the next morning. I confidently told the crew on the boat, when they kidded me about going into labour on the trip, that I had two weeks to go." But Kim's baby had decided differently. When she went into labour during the night, she had to call neighbours on an Autotel and ask them to please contact her husband. One hopped in his boat and travelled a mile further down the island to wake her husband and start him travelling into town. After her son was born, Kim had to wait three days until the passenger boat sailed again to make the trip home.

Some parents decide not to make the trip into a larger community when they give birth. Daria had her baby in the tiny community hospital of her small town in northern Saskatchewan. It was a quick, unmedicated birth, and Daria commented, "Darby was born on September 18, and she was the New Year's Baby for 1996 at our hospital!"

Rebecca says, "You must trust your own instincts and do what feels right for you, no matter what everyone else says." In her small community, she could choose either the local hospital, or a hospital in the city nearly an hour away. "We decided to opt for the rural hospital, hoping we would have more individualized care. Everyone thought we were crazy. No one seemed to understand why we wouldn't want to be where the latest technology was. I am so glad we chose not to listen to those people."

Rebecca describes her birth experience as "wonderful." Theirs was the only family in the hospital's small maternity wing, so they had lots of privacy and excellent care. "I felt it was the closest thing to giving birth at home."

Kim decided to have her third baby at home after the small community hospital only 45 minutes from her home closed its maternity ward. Rather than make the long trip into a larger city to give birth, she arranged to have a midwife attend her and describes her labour this way: "My labour was a mixture of hard work and fun; I used the warm bath for a while but it was so relaxing my contractions began to get irregular. So I went up to our bedroom and spent the rest of my labour beside our bed, on my knees, holding onto Bruce for support. Being in our own home made me so much more comfortable and relaxed that I occasionally laughed with the joy of it all between contractions." After her daughter was born, Kim says, "It was heavenly to cuddle into our own bed afterwards to rest and recuperate.... In the days and weeks following the birth, whenever I rested or was alone with my thoughts, happy memories of the experience made me feel all warm."

Laurie also felt it was important to trust her feelings about where to give birth. She says: "During a perfectly normal pregnancy, I had reservations about giving birth in our small hospital in northern Ontario. My gut feeling said that this was not the place to be. So three weeks before my due date I packed a few bags, grabbed all our savings, and headed to Sault Ste. Marie (four hours south) to wait for our daughter to be born."

Miranda was born five weeks later—but she arrived blue and not breathing, and had to be placed on a ventilator. A few days later she was transferred to the Hospital for Sick Children in Toronto where she had open heart surgery. At three weeks, Miranda had a second operation for a rare liver problem, and spent another two months in the hospital recovering from that surgery before her parents were able to bring her home. Laurie is convinced that some inner mother's wisdom told her that Miranda would need this special help at birth.

Sometimes plans to head south for the birth are changed when baby decides to make an early arrival. Tracey had planned to leave her small community in northern Ontario and have her baby in Toronto, where she had relatives. However, three weeks before her expected due date, Tracey's water broke. She headed for her community hospital, only to find her family doctor was away on holidays and the only other doctor in town who delivered babies was off on a shopping trip. Tracey was having contractions at this point, and the doctor decided to send her, strapped onto a stretcher, by helicopter to Thunder Bay, the closest city.

Tracey remembers, "My husband was not allowed on the helicopter and had to drive the four-hour trip to Thunder Bay. Fortunately, he made the trip safely and I delivered a healthy baby girl that evening. All we faced now was getting her home in the middle of winter..."

Families in the more remote communities of northern Canada have a number of decisions to make that families in other parts of Canada may never consider. If they decide to travel south before the expected arrival time of the baby, the expenses of staying in the city can quickly mount up, especially if there are no friends or family with a handy spare room.

Inducing labour looks far more appealing when every day you wait for labour to begin means more money paid out for food and hotel bills, as well as another day separated from your older children and your partner. Some mothers have described feeling depressed and lonely as they waited out their pregnancies "in the company of strangers." Those who had family to stay with were more positive about the experience, but it was still difficult to be away from their partners.

If the mother decides to stay in her home community to give birth, she may have a very positive experience. However, if she or the baby need extra care it may mean a sudden traumatic trip by plane or helicopter to a larger hospital.

There is no right decision in these situations. Each family has to weigh the resources available in their own community and their own feelings to make a plan that is right for them.

Understanding Research Methods

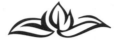

Every pregnant woman is guaranteed to receive plenty of information and advice. Some of it is "old wives' tales"—stories that have been around for years. (One such tale, for example, advises pregnant women not to lift their arms over their heads, because that action might make the umbilical cord wrap around the baby's neck. Mothers who've heard that are usually relieved to find out that this is simply physically impossible.)

Other advice is based on the experience of the person sharing the information—or on something heard from "a friend of a friend." Other people's experiences are interesting, but they may not mean much for you and your pregnancy.

Finally, there is information about pregnancy and birth that has been demonstrated or discovered through research.

Most of the studies talked about in this book have been reviewed by the Cochrane database and only included if the reviewers considered it to be good, valid research.

What makes "good" research? How do you know when the results or conclusions from a particular study are likely to be meaningful?

The best, most reliable medical research includes:

- large numbers of people in the study, to reduce the risk that any benefits seen are simply chance or coincidence. This also allows for any rare or uncommon effects to be seen.
- a "control" group to be compared to the "treatment" or "intervention" group. The two groups need to be as similar as possible (except, of course, for the one aspect of medical care being treated). One way to achieve this is to assign the people coming into the study randomly to the two groups.
- a plan to eliminate bias as much as possible. The best way to do this is the **randomized, double-blind** study. In this kind of study, people are assigned randomly to either the control group or the intervention group, and neither the doctors caring for the people or the researchers know who is in each group.

It isn't always possible to have all these elements in a study, and that is especially true when it comes to pregnancy and childbirth. The ran-

TWO NON-RANDOMIZED STUDIES

One study sought to compare home birth with hospital birth to determine which was safer. However, it included in the home birth group women who had their babies at home unattended, because they were too mentally ill or developmentally delayed to realize that they were pregnant or to get medical care. The hospital group all had prenatal care. Because these two groups were not comparable, the study was not meaningful.

Another non-randomized study compared two groups of women who had already had a Caesarean section. Some chose a repeat C-section for their next baby, while others chose to have a vaginal birth (VBAC). Because the two groups were otherwise very similar, the researchers were able to show that VBAC is just as safe for the baby, and is safer for the mother, than a repeat Caesarean.

TWO "RANDOMIZED" STUDIES: NOT RELIABLE

Researchers wanted to find out if giving breast-fed babies one bottle a day would lead to early weaning. They assigned the breastfeeding mothers they were studying to either the "one-bottle-a-day" or the "no-bottles" group, and found that the babies in both groups weaned at about the same time. The problem with this study was that mothers who wanted to exclusively breastfeed refused to be part of the study, because they didn't want to risk being assigned to the "one-bottle-a-day" group. In fact, the researchers found that the women in the "no-bottles" group were giving their babies as many bottles as the other group, and no conclusions could be made.

In another study, researchers wanted to compare two approaches to handling babies who woke up and cried at night. Parents in one group were told to leave the baby to cry herself back to sleep; parents in the other group would go to the baby at night and offer comfort or feeding. After a few weeks, the researchers found the "cry it out" babies were sleeping longer than the "comforted" babies. However, a high percentage of the parents in the "cry it out" group dropped out of the study—possibly those whose babies were sleeping less (and crying more). This makes it impossible to draw any meaningful conclusions.

domized, double-blind type of study is most easily designed to research drugs. It's impossible to research something like the use of electronic fetal monitors during labour this way, because it will be quite obvious to everyone who is attached to a monitor and who isn't.

In evaluating research, it helps to be aware of some of the limitations of different approaches. For example, some studies compare the past to the present: before Caesarean sections could be safely done, almost all pregnant women with the placenta placed over the cervix (**placenta previa**) would die, along with their babies, when they went into labour. When these babies are delivered by Caesarean section, almost all the

mothers and babies are fine. This is a clear example of a new treatment that worked and could easily be compared to past practice.

But comparisons between past and present are risky. Too many other things may have

> The results of research studies do not set up rules for the treatment of pregnant women. These studies give doctors a direction for giving women advice, and they give women a foundation for making decisions. It is your right and your responsibility to make your own decisions about your care during pregnancy, birth and beyond.

changed, as well as what is being studied, so that the "present" group is now very different from the "past" group of women.

Sometimes it is difficult to arrange for randomized studies. The people who are potential candidates may refuse to be randomly assigned to one group or the other—they want to make their own choices. Some studies simply look at

---

The Evidence About...
Research

The best research method is the randomized controlled study, but this kind of study is often difficult to do for pregnancy and childbirth.

When studying pregnancy and childbirth issues, studies of women who have chosen different treatments, approaches, or interventions are more frequently used. In these it is especially important to be sure we are comparing women who are as similar as possible in all ways, except in regards to the issue being studied.

A lot of pregnancy and childbirth studies have only included small numbers of women. These results are less meaningful than studies with larger groups. Meta-analyses, which combine several smaller studies, have often been used, but these may not be reliable.

---

the results when people make these choices, and try to ensure that the groups being studied are as similar as possible.

Even when researchers try to set up randomized studies, there can be problems. People who are asked to be part of the study but choose not to be can affect the results—their absence may mean that an important group is being left out. People may also drop out part way through the study, and this can affect the results, making them less reliable.

Why is it important to know about these factors? You may read or hear about research results, but only when you know how the study was designed and carried out will you know if it is truly valid.

Meta-analysis: Combining Research Studies

When large studies have not been performed, sometimes the results of several smaller, but well-designed, studies are combined. Combining several studies in this way is called a meta-analysis. Meta-analyses are often used in medical research; however with a meta-analysis one can never be sure that the results would be the same if a very large trial were actually done. A meta-analysis combines all the possible errors in each small study as well as their results.

What Gets Researched?

Decisions about what to research are not primarily based on what pregnant women would like to know. There has been very little research on many areas of great concern and interest to pregnant women—nutrition during pregnancy, for example. Researchers are more likely to do studies on topics that are easy to study or that can readily find sponsors—drug companies, for example, sponsor lots of research on drugs.

How to Deliver a Baby: Just in Case

Heather's first labour lasted 12 hours. A few days after her due date with baby number two, she felt a couple of contractions. They were fairly strong, so she called her husband, Steve, at work and said, "I think labour is starting, but I've only had a couple of contractions so there's no rush." Next, she called her midwife to let her know. As soon as she put the phone down, the contractions started coming fast and furious. She realized that things were moving much more quickly than she'd expected. Suddenly, after one huge contraction, she felt like pushing.

Wanting to protect the carpet in her living room, Heather struggled into the bathroom and spread towels out on the tile floor. With her three-year-old daughter encouraging her from just outside the door, she gave birth to a baby boy a few minutes later.

When Steve arrived home half an hour later, he was stunned to find Heather in bed and the midwife checking the baby. "You said there was no rush!" he exclaimed.

Sometimes babies arrive very quickly! It's helpful to be prepared, just in case. The good news is that a quick birth usually proceeds without difficulties—it's the long, slow labours that are more likely to be complicated.

Here's what to do in these rapid situations:

If You Are Helping the Mother

1. Remember, you are not going to deliver the baby, the mother is. Your role is to try to provide a safe, calm environment for that to happen.
2. If you're in a car, pull over, and in cool weather turn the car heater on high. If you're at home or outdoors, try to get the mother to a safe and comfortable place.
3. Call your midwife, doctor, hospital, or 911, if you can do so without leaving the mother.
4. Help the mother lie down on her side and get the bottom half of her clothes off. Prepare a nice, soft landing spot for the baby. Put towels, blankets, clothes, cushions, or whatever you have between the mother's legs. Try to get some dry cloth (your own shirt will do nicely if there is nothing else) ready to dry the baby off.

5. Use your hands to support the baby's head and body as it emerges. Remember that the baby will be slippery, wet, and may arrive in a big hurry!

6. You need to keep the baby as dry and warm as possible. Lift him onto the mother's belly and dry him off. Then cover both mother and baby with dry towels or blankets. Leaving him covered and skin-to-skin on the mother's belly will help to keep him warm. If you have lots of towels, toss the damp ones away and cover mother and baby with the dry ones.

7. Usually the baby will start crying right away. If the baby does not breathe right away, keep rubbing him with a towel or blanket or even your hands to encourage him to breathe. Keep it up until he is crying loudly.

8. Don't cut the cord—just leave it be. The placenta probably won't come out for a while.

9. When the placenta does come out, just wrap it in a cloth or put it in a bowl and keep it close to the baby (so that the cord doesn't get pulled). If the mother can put the baby to her breast, this will help to reduce bleeding.

If You Are Having a Baby Alone

1. These quick births, especially if you are alone, can be scary. Remember that your body knows how to give birth. It will happen with very little deliberate effort on your part.

2. Call for help from anyone—even if it's just a next-door neighbour who can then make the call to your midwife, doctor, or 911.

3. Get your clothes off—at least the bottom half. Either lie down on your side or on your back with your back propped up against something. Choose a place that will be safe for the baby to land. Try to get some blankets or towels under you, and to have some dry things—your own clothes if necessary—to dry the baby off after she is born.

4. Reach down and support the baby as she is born. You can lift her up onto your belly. Remember, she will be slippery.

5. You need to keep the baby as dry and warm as possible. Dry her off then cover yourself and the baby with dry towels or blankets. Leaving her covered and skin-to-skin on your belly will help to keep her warm. If you have lots of towels, toss the damp ones away and cover yourselves with dry ones.

6. Usually she will start crying right away. If the baby does not breathe right away, rub her with a towel or blanket or even your own hands to encourage her to breathe. Keep it up until she is crying loudly.

7. Don't worry about cutting the cord. After a while, you will feel more contractions and the placenta will slide out. If you can do it easily, wrap it in a towel and move it beside you so you can bring your baby up to your breast. Breastfeeding right away will help reduce the amount of bleeding.

8. If you weren't able to call for help before, do so now. You may feel weak and shaky at this point; keeping warm will help.

Resources

Midwifery

Midwives Alliance of North America
www.mana.org

American College of Nurse-Midwives
www.acnm.org

Canadian Association of Midwives
www.canadianmidwives.org

Obstetrics

American College of Obstetricians and
Gynecologists
www.acog.org

Society of Obstetricians and Gynaecologists of
Canada
www.sogc.org

Doulas

DONA International
www.dona.org
Toll-free: 1-888-788-3662

Drugs, Medication, and HIV/AIDS during Pregnancy

Motherisk
www.motherisk.org
In Toronto, Ontario: 416-813-6780
Alcohol and substance: 1-877-327-4636
Nausea and vomiting: 1-800-436-8477
HIV/AIDS: 1-888-246-5840

Multiple Births

National Organization of Mothers of Twins
Clubs (U.S.)
www.nomotc.org

Multiple Births of Canada
www.multiplebirthscanada.org

Premature Babies

Prematurity
www.prematurity.org

Kangaroo Mother Care Promotions
www.kangaroomothercare.com

Postpartum Depression

Postpartum Support International (PSI)
www.postpartum.net

Diaper-free Babies

Diaper Free
www.natural-wisdom.com

Breastfeeding Help

La Leche League International
www.llli.org

La Leche League Canada
www.lllc.ca
Toll-free: 1-800-665-4324

Dr. Jack Newman
www.drjacknewman.com

International Lactation Consultant Association
www.ilca.org
In Raleigh, North Carolina: 919-861-5577

Canadian Lactation Consultants Association
www.clca-accl.ca

Academy of Breastfeeding Medicine
www.bfmed.org

Index

abdominal decompression, 99
abortion, 72–73, 86, 92, 93, 94, 96–97
acupressure, 63, 216
acupuncture, 216
acute cystitis, 116
African-Americans, 71, 80, 245
AIDS, 144–45
alcohol, 33–35, 85, 187
allergies, 53, 285, 288
American Academy of Pediatrics, 297
American College of Nurse-Midwives, 23
American College of Obstetricians and Gynecologists, 136, 280
American Institute of Medicine, 78
amni-hook, 248
amnio-infusion, 192, 209
amniocentesis, 58, 73, 93, 95, 102
amnioscope, 209
amniotic fluid, 14, 86, 96, 93, 96, 101, 120, 121: problems with, 208–10, 232
amniotic sac, 14–15, 120, 251
amniotomy, 204, 248
anaesthetic gas, 219–20
anaesthetists, 220
anemia, 52, 76. 80
anencephaly, 51, 95, 96
antacids, 150, 155
anterior position, 173
antibiotic eye ointment, 145, 146

antibiotics, 35, 42, 70, 116, 117, 126, 132, 133, 146, 167, 168–70, 190, 242; overuse of, 169–70
anticonvulsants, 183–84
anti-D antibodies, 72–74
anti-D gammaglobulin, 72, 74
antidepressants, 283
antihistamines, 63, 64
antihypertensives, 183
antinauseants, 219
anxiety, 92, 112, 162, 170, 199, 201
aorta, 231
Apgar score, 15, 59, 156, 209, 219, 221, 229, 232, 256
apnea, 186
appetite, 78
aspiration pneumonia, 131, 156, 209, 210, 226
assertiveness, 27–29, 299–303
asthma, 33
asymptomatic bacteriuria, 115

babies: large, 79, 80, 97, 98, 129, 159–60, 161, 242–43; small (See small for dates); measurement of, 57, 58, 97–99; post-mature, 275; premature, 186–87, 193–95; sharing parents' bed, 280; supplementation, 195, 288; test weighing of, 297–98; vision of, 145, 146, 279 (See also under fetal; newborns)
baby blues, 282

baby equipment, 122–24, 199, 280
Baby-Friendly Hospital Initiative, 286: guidelines, 186–91
back labour, 214
bacteria, 166–70
balloon catheter, 246
bed rest, 87, 99, 113, 151, 183
Benedictin, 63, 64
betamimetics, 99, 189, 191
beta strep. See Group B strep
bikini cut (Caesarean), 130
bilirubin, 73
birth. See childbirth
birth asphyxia, 275
birth defects, 34, 35, 54, 63, 94, 187
birth plan, 25–27
birth supplies (home birth), 44
birth weight. See low birth-weight; weight, baby
Birth without Violence (Leboyer), 276
birthing centres, 24, 39, 41–42
Birthing from Within, 107
birthing positions, 154, 155, 156, 158, 214, 256–57
birthing stool, 257
bladder infections, 116, 126, 168, 224
bleeding: into brain, 181, 189, 192; during pregnancy, 58, 73, 85; after sex, 67; in third trimester, 164–65
blighted ovum, 86
blindness, 70, 145, 146

blood clots, 80, 86, 126
blood clotting, 48, 81, 164, 181, 279
blood patch, 226
blood pressure: high. See hypertension; cuff, 76; normal, 180
blood sugar, 85, 155, 160, 161, 162, 163 (See also diabetes; gestational diabetes)
blood tests, 12, 74, 76, 86
blood transfusions, 42, 74, 145, 164, 268
blood type, 71–72, 73, 76
bloody show, 15, 164
BMI (body mass index), 79
body temperature, 34, 278–79
bonding, 276–78
bowel movement, infant, 298 (See also meconium)
Bradley Method, 107
brain: baby, 95, 192, 199; damage, 73, 178; hemorrhage, 181, 183; maternal, 181, 189
breast: changes, 66; edema, 224; engorgement, 288, 295; infections, 124; shape, 110; surgery, 110
breast milk, 110, 124, 194, 289, 295: supply, 296–98
breast pump, 124, 295
breastfeeding: Baby-Friendly guidelines, 286–91; Caesarean and, 132; classes, 107; duration of, 297; epidurals and, 221, 224; equipment, 124, 295; fre-

quency of, 290; fussy baby, 296; HIV and, 144–45; hospitals and, 286–91; on demand, 290, 295; pacifiers and, 123; positions, 132, 289, 291–95; premature baby, 194–95; in public, 297; self-attachment and, 289, 291, 294, 299–300; session, duration of, 290; readiness for, steps, 109; sleepy baby, 296; special situations, 110; supplementation and, 53; surgery and, 110; vaccination and, 69; value of, 285, 297; and weight loss, 79–80 (See also La Leche League)
breathing patterns, labour, 104, 105, 213
breathing problems: baby, 126, 136, 186, 189, 210, 219, 221, 226 (See also respiratory distress syndrome)
breech presentation, 70, 73, 114, 126, 129, 138, 175–77, 191, 259; Caesarean vs. vaginal delivery and, 178–79; exercises, 176; turning baby, 176–77
brow presentation, 174–75
bulking agents, 64

Caesarean section, 8, 12, 21, 42, 48, 58, 60: anaesthesia and, 130–31, 226; complications of, 126, 136; and continuous monitoring, 229, 230; elective, 133; epidurals and, 221, 224, 225; exercise and, 81; incisions, 126, 130, 135, 137; infection and, 132, 133; and labour induction, 242, 249, 250; lawsuits and, 129–30; morbidity rate, 136–37; planned, 129; rates of, 125, 133; reasons for, 80, 111, 114, 125, 143–44, 161, 164, 165, 174, 175, 177, 178, 79, 185, 192, 203, 232, 248; recovery from, 132, 133; repeat, 126, 127, 129, 134–36; step-by-step description of, 131–33; trial of labour after, 135, 136; unnecessary, 126–30; vaginal birth after, See VBAC; vs. forceps delivery, 263; vs. vaginal birth,

126, 133, 192; vs. vaginal breech delivery, 178–79
caffeine, 34
calcium, 53, 54, 55
calcium channel blockers, 99
Canadian College of Obstetricians and Gynecologists, 280
Canadian Pediatric Society (CPS), 279
cancer, 34, 88, 142, 242
caregiver, choosing, 20–29
car seats, 122–23
cat feces, 70
catheters, 131, 132
cephalic presentation, 172–73
cerebral palsy, 113, 129, 229
cervical cerclage, 188
cervix, 15: artificial ripening of, 245–46; placenta covering. See placenta previa; progression of labour and, 201, 203; readiness of, 243–45
charley horse, 150–51
cheeses, pregnancy risk, 34
chemicals, toxic, 34
child[birth]: attitude towards, 105; husband-coached. See Bradley Method; ideal settings, 37; in remote communities, 305–7; practices, changes in, 8, 108; quick, 312–13; resources, 106; resuscitation at, 25, 221, 279 (See also fetal positions; labour; labour induction; prenatal classes; specific types of delivery)
Children's Aid Society, 32
chlamydia pneumonia, 146
chlamydia trachomatis, 146, 279
chorion, 93
chorionic villae, 14
chorionic villus biopsy, 58, 73, 92–94
chorioretinitis, 70
chromosomal abnormalities, testing for, 92–97
cirrhosis, 142
clothing, baby, 123
cocaine, 32, 35
Cochrane Collaboration, 10
cold sore, 142, 144
colostrum, 288, 295, 279
compound presentation, 175

conception, determining date of, 57
corticosteroids, 183
congenital rubella syndrome, 68
constipation, 64, 151, 152
continuous epidural, 220
continuity of care, 24–25
contraction stress testing, 100
contractions: exercise and; frequency of, 201
cord prolapse, 178, 190, 248
corticosteroids, 189, 190, 192
counterpressure, 215
cribs, 123, 280

D&C (dilation and curettage), 57, 84, 86, 87
death: infant, 42, 126, 136–37, 161, 167, 185, 186, 189, 209, 272; maternal, 42, 126, 130, 136–37, 144, 178, 181, 185 (See also perinatal death; SIDS)
decision-making, 299–303
dehydration, 63, 156
Demerol, 42, 218–19, 231, 286
depression, 81, 218, 221 (See also postpartum depression)
DES (diethylstilboestrol), 87–88
diabetes, 21, 26, 47, 48, 81, 85, 161, 163, 181, 187, 189, 190 (See also gestational diabetes)
diapers, 122
diastolic blood pressure, 180
Diclectin, 63–64
diet, 50–55: diabetes and, 81, 159, 162; in early labour, 237; heartburn and, 150; pre-eclampsia and, 182; to prevent allergies, 53; morning sickness and, 63 (See also supplementation; names of supplements)
dilation, 15, 201, 203, 245
doctor–patient relationship, 250–51, 299–301
DONA (Doulas of North America), 157
Doppler ultrasound, 101, 102
doulas, 21, 48, 126, 157–58, 215
Down's syndrome, 46, 48, 93, 94, 95, 96, 97
doxylamine, 63
dreaming (fetus), 120
drugs: illegal, 32, 35; injectable,

42; intravenous use of, 141, 145; over-the-counter, 35–36; prescription, 35–36; recreational, 32, 85, 187 (See also medications)
due date, 15: calculating, 30–31; and ultrasound, 57
dura, 224, 225
dystocia, 127, 133, 204

ear infections, 123
eating disorders, 55
eclampsia, 181 (See also pre-eclampsia)
ectopic pregnancy. See tubal pregnancy
edema, 151, 180, 181–82, 224, 288
effacement, 15, 201, 244
effective care, 10–11
elective pre-term delivery, 190
electronic fetal monitors (EFM), 38, 100, 126, 128, 129, 139, 140, 154, 155, 156, 214, 228–29, 249: 20-minute strip, 230 (See also fetal heart/heart rate; heart rate monitoring)
embryo, 14, 88
endocrinologists, 25
engaged (head), 245, 260
epidural anaesthesia, 24, 42, 105, 126, 127, 129, 130, 131, 139, 156, 174, 192, 220–21, 224–25, 231, 249, 256
epidural space, 220
enema, 104, 154
epilepsy, 48 (See also seizures)
episiotomy, 10, 24, 155, 192, 257, 258–60
ergomtrine, 266, 267
erythomycin, 146, 279
ethical medical care, 97
exercises: Kegal, 152; to turn breech babies, 176; value of, 81–82; and weight loss, 80
external version, 125, 126: of breech babies, 176–77; timing for, 177–78
eye infections, 70, 145–46 (See also blindness)
eyebrows/eyelids, fetus, 120

face presentation, 174–75
factor D, 71
failure to progress, 127, 128, 204, 205

Fallopian tubes, 14, 88
false negatives, 95, 96
false positives, 95, 96
family-centred maternity care, 38, 41, 104
family doctors, 22
fast foods, 50
fasting blood sugar, 160
fathers: and blood type, 71; cutting cord, 268; fraternal twins and, 112; as labour partner, 105, 107, 157, 158, 215, 236–40; miscarriage and, 90; –newborn relationship, 276, 278–79; ultrasound and, 60
"feeling pregnant," 86
fertility treatments, 89, 112
fetal alcohol effect, 33–34
fetal alcohol syndrome (FAS), 33, 34
fetal assessment test, 91–101
fetal biophysical profile, 101, 102
fetal distress, 128, 134, 256: forceps vs. vacuum delivery and , 261–64; management of, 231–33; monitoring for, 227–31
fetal growth, 58, 76, 92, 97–101, 181, 242–43: milestones, 120–21
fetal heart/heart rate, 57, 76, 87, 100, 120, 128, 177, 192, 208, 210, 221, 227–31, 256 (See also electronic fetal monitors; fetal distress)
fetal movement, 101, 119, 120, 171: counting, 99–100
fetal positions, 60, 171, 172–79
fetal sac, 86, 87
fetal scalp sampling, 230–31
fetal size, 58, 97–99, 120
fetal weight, 58
fetus, 14
fingers, fetus, 120
fish, 34
fluid retention, 151, 180, 181
folic acid, 51, 53–54
food cravings, 52
food myths, 52
footwear, 151
forceps deliveries, 21, 24, 81, 129, 155, 192, 203, 221, 225, 229, 230, 232, 249, 259, 260–61: vs. vacuum, 261–64; safety of, 263

formula, 109, 144, 286, 287
fortified foods, 52
fraternal twins, 112
full-term pregnancy, 15, 30–31
fundal height, 97–98

general anaesthetic, 131, 155, 156, 226
general practitioners, 22
genetic abnormalities, testing for, 92–97
genetic counselling, 97
genetics: miscarriage and, 84; post-term pregnancy and, 273
genital herpes, 142, 143–44
German measles. See rubella
gestational age, 14, 58
gestational diabetes, 10, 12, 159–62
ginger, 63
glucometer, 160
glucose intolerance, 160
glucose tolerance test, 159, 160–61
glue-sniffing, 32
gonococcus, 145
gonorrhea, 145–46
grief, 89–90
Group B strep, 46, 117, 166–69
guilt, 33, 107

hand washing, 70, 144, 167
head-down position (birth), 172–73
Health Disciplines Act (Alberta), 23
health insurance plans, 8, 23, 24
Health Protection Branch (Canada), 64
heart disease, 48, 81
heart rate, fetal. See electronic heart monitors; fetal heart/heart rate; heart rate monitoring
heart rate monitoring, 227–30 (See also electronic heart monitors)
heartburn, 150
HELLP syndrome, 183, 185
hemoglobin, 52
hemolytic disease of the newborn, 72, 73, 74
hemophilia, 93
hemorrhage, 126 (See also postpartum hemorrhage)
hemorrhagic disease of the

newborn, 279
hemorrhoids, 151–52, 257
hepatitis, 74
hepatitis B, 141–42: immune globulin, 142
herbal: remedies, 35; supplements, 53
heroin, 35
herpes simplex, 142–44
high blood pressure. See hypertension
high-risk pregnancy, 46–48, 92, 94, 96
HIV, 48, 74, 139, 144–45
home birth, 8, 22, 26, 39, 40: choosing, 43–45; safety concerns, 42–43; siblings at, 43; supplies, 44; VBAC and, 139, 140
hormone therapy, 87–88
hospital births, 37–38, 40, 43: choosing, 38, 49, 49
Hospital for Sick Children (Toronto), 36, 306
hospital tours, 105, 153
hospitalization, 113, 117, 183, 185
hospitals: admissions procedure, 153–54; breastfeeding and, 286–91; family-centred care, 280; high-risk, 139; length of stay in, 145; in remote communities, 305–7; routines, 153–56; teaching, 24, 139, 154
hot tubs, 34
hyperemesis, 63
hypertension, 21, 26, 80, 101, 113, 180, 187, 189, 190, 250
hypno-birthing, 107
hypnosis, 216

identical twins, 112
imidazole, 65
incubator, 193
infertility, 88
informed consent, 97
inhaled painkillers, 219–20
insulin, 155, 160, 161, 162
International Childbirth Education Association, 107
Internet, 106, 139
intramuscular injections, 89
intrauterine transfusion, 73, 74
intrauterine growth restriction, 98–99, 101, 181, 183, 187, 189

inverted-T (Caesarean) incision, 135, 136
iron, 51–52, 54, 64
IUDs, 85, 88
IV fluids, 38, 104, 107, 132, 133, 139, 140, 155, 168, 170, 214, 231, 232, 248–49, 266, 295

jaundice, 73, 296

Kangaroo Care, 193
Kegel exercises, 152
kidneys, 116–17, 125, 181, 183, 242

labour, 211–12: abnormal, 201; active, 15, 127; anatomy of, 15, 16–18; assessing baby during, 227–33; attitude toward, 105, 212, 217–18, 222–23; augmenting, 204–6, 249–50; and breathing patterns, 104, 105, 213; comfort technique, 237, 240; exercise and, 81; failure to progress, 127, 128, 204–5; false, 188, 204; food/drink and, 155–56; hospital routines for, 155–56; freedom of movement during, 107, 126, 127, 154, 156, 205, 206, 214–15; latent, 127, 128, 129; long, latent, 203–4; music during, 217; pain management and, 8, 10–11, 38, 39, 41, 42, 104, 107, 213–26; progression of, 201–3; prolonged, 204–6; positions during, 156, 231, 237; precipitate, 206–7; premature, 112–14, 166, 167, 168; signs of, 200–1; stages, 15, 202, 254–64; VBAC, 139 (See also epidural; fathers, as labour partner; spinal anaesthesia; trial of labour)
labour induction, 8, 10, 31, 73, 99, 100, 126, 128–29, 139, 161–62, 184–85, 190, 241–50:discussing with doctor, 250–51; and infection (newborn), 253; methods, 246–50; pain of, 249–50; and post-term pregnancy, 273–74; reasons for, 241–43; vs. waiting, 243
labour support people, 21, 107, 126, 157, 240 (See also

doulas; fathers; midwives)
lactation consultant, 110, 132
(*See also* La Leche League)
lactose intolerance, 55
La Leche League, 26, 77, 109, 287, 291, 296
Lamaze Method, 107
laparoscope, 89
late clamping, 267
lawsuits, 129–30
laxatives, 64
legs, 150–51
libido, 66, 196 (*See also* sex)
lifestyle risks, 32–36
light for dates, 98
lips/mouth, fetus, 120
listeria bacteria, 34
liver, 70, 96, 141–42, 147, 181, 183, 185
low birthweight, 79, 99, 113, 115 (*See also* small for dates)
low forceps, 260–61
low umbilical artery pH, 209, 221
lungs, 32, 33, 189, 190, 191, 199, 210, 273, 278 (*See also* respiratory distress syndrome)

magnesium, 52–53, 54, 183; citrate, 151; lactate, 151; sulphate, 183
malnutrition, 50, 54, 81, 99, 243
massage, 104, 150, 152, 215, 237, 257
mastitis, 124
maternal herpes Type 2, 143–44
maternal mortality. *See* death, mothers
maternal serum screening (MSS), 59, 94–95, 102
maternal weight, 48, 50, 63, 77, 78–81
meat, 34, 70
meconium, 208–9, 221, 273, 275
medical training, 11–12
medicalization (pregnancy), 8, 9–10, 11–12, 91–92
medications: breastfeeding and, 287–88; fetal distress, 233; hypertension, 35, 47, 48, 51; intrauterine growth restriction, 99; labour pain, 8, 10–11, 38, 39, 41, 42, 104,

107, 218–26; nausea/vomiting, 35, 63–64; postpartum depression, 283; pre-eclampsia, 182, 183–84; pre-labour rupture, membranes, 190; premature labour, 113–14, 189, 191; respiratory distress syndrome, 189, 193
membranes: rupturing, 248; sweeping, 246, 248 (*See also* PROM)
menstrual cycle, 14, 30, 57, 59
mental retardation, 95, 309
mercury, 34
meta-analyses, 274, 310
methotrexate, 89
mid forceps delivery, 261
midwifery, 8, 10, 22–24, 76–77, 240
Midwifery Act (SK), 23
Midwives Alliance of North America, 23
milk: allergies, 53; fortified, 52 (*See also* breast milk; lactose intolerance)
milk of magnesia, 151
miscarriage, 32, 34, 57, 66, 68, 72–73, 81, 83–90, 95, 112
morning sickness, 62–67, 75
mother:–baby relationship, 170, 193, 194, 224, 276–80, 288; -directed pushing, 256; illness of, 242; older, 47, 48, 85, 93, 96, 112; young, 47, 50, 79, 105, 107, 187 (*See also under* maternal)
Motherisk, 36
mucous plug, 15, 201
multiple pregnancy, 21, 57, 106, 111–14, 181, 187
multivitamins, 51, 54
music (during labour), 217

narcotics, 218–19, 231
natural birth, 107
natural prostaglandins, 246
nausea/vomiting, 35, 63–64 (*See also* morning sickness)
navel, baby, 14 (*See also* umbilical cord)
neomycin, 279
neonatologists, 191
neural tube defects, 51, 54, 95–96, 97
newborn: hemolytic disease of, 72, 73, 74; intensive care, 187, 191; meeting, 276–78; rou-

tine treatments of, 278–80; supplementation, 288
nipples, 110, 196, 246, 286, 290–91
nitrous oxide, 219
non-stress testing, 100
normal flora, 166
normal show, 164
northern communities, 23, 305–7
nuchal translucency screening, 94
nursing pillows, 124
nystatin, 65

obesity, 48, 54, 78, 79, 80–81, 133, 152, 161
obstetricians, 21–22
old wives' tales, 52, 308
olgohydramnos, 208, 232
oral sex, 67
organs, fetus, 120, 121
orgasm, 66, 196
outcome, 11
ovaries, 14, 88, 89
overdue pregnancy. *See* post-term pregnancy
overweight mothers, 78, 79, 80–81, 152, 159, 161
ovulation, 30, 57
ovum, 14, 88
oxytocin, 100, 127, 129, 139, 184, 204–6, 221, 231, 232, 245, 246, 248–49, 253, 262, 266, 267, 268, 269

pacifiers, 123, 290
pancreas, 161
pediatricians, 131
pelvic infections, 88
penicillin, 147
perinatal death, 34, 57, 59, 73, 112, 113, 147, 181, 274, 275
perineum, 257
peritoneum, 131, 132
pesticides, 34
pH, 209, 221, 230, 256
phenobarbital, 192
piracetam, 233
pit contractions, 244
pit drip, 248
pitocin, 128, 129, 244
placenta, 14, 266: abruption of, 58, 73; active management of delivery, 268–69; blood flow to, 98–99; and blood type, 72; delivery of,

265–69; manual removal of, 267, 268; retained, 265, 268; separation of, 32, 58, 131–32, 136, 181, 187, 190
placenta previa, 58, 130, 165, 177, 196, 309–10
platelets, low, 185
polyhydramnios, 208
polyp, 85
posterior position (birth), 173–74
post-mature baby, 275
postpartum depression, 281–84
postpartum hemorrhage, 43, 208, 257, 262, 266–69
postpartum psychosis, 282
post-term pregnancy, 15, 57, 59, 272–75
practice vs. research, 11–12, 31
poverty, 80, 187, 188
pre-eclampsia, 53–54, 80, 151, 112–13, 136, 151, 180–85, 242 (*See also* HELLP syndrome)
pre-existing health problems, 25, 26, 47, 48
pregnancy hormone, 86
pregnancy-induced hypertension (PIH), 180
pregnancy test kits, 30
premature birth, 15, 48, 55–53, 74, 81, 113, 115, 116, 120, 191–95
premature labour, 187–93
prenatal checkup, 24, 76–77
prenatal classes, 77, 104–8, 152, 153, 213, 214
presentation, 172 (*See also* fetal positions)
presenting part, 172, 245
pre-term pre-labour rupture of membranes, 252 (*See also* PROM)
progesterone, 88
prolapse: umbilical cord, 178, 190, 248; vagina, 130
prolonged pregnancy, 15, 243, 272 (*See also* post-term pregnancy)
PROM (pre-labour rupture of the membranes), 190–91, 242, 251–53
prostaglandin (prostins), 139, 242, 244, 245, 249, 253
protein, 54
proteinuria, 180, 181, 182, 183, 185

pubic hair, shaving, 104, 131, 154
pushing stage, 155, 254–64
pyelonephritis. See kidney
pyridoxine, 63, 233

quadruplets, 111–12

randomized (double blind) studies, 42, 308–10
red measles. See rubella
regional anaesthesia, 130–31, 132
remote communities, 305–7
research methods, 308–10
respiratory distress syndrome (RDS), 126, 136, 186, 189, 190, 193
resting up, 214
Rh gammaglobulin, 71
Rh incompatibility, 71–72
Rh-negative, 71–74, 177
Rh-positive, 71-72, 74
ripe cervix, 243–245
ritodrine, 176, 189
rooming in, 289
rubella, 68–69, 76, 85, 98
rubeola, 69
running, 81–82

sacrum, 216
safety: anti-D gammaglobulin, 74; cribs, 123; exercise, 82; forceps delivery, 263; home/hospital birth, 42–43; sleep environment, 280; ultrasound, 59, 60, 61
saline solution, 268
saunas, 34
second-hand smoke, 33
sedatives, 218
seizures: maternal, 181, 183–84; newborn, 70, 231, 262
self-attachment, 289, 293, 294, 299–300
septuplets, 111
serum AFP (alpha-fetal protein), 96
sex, 66–67, 196–97, 246, 259
sexual positions, 66, 196
sexually transmitted diseases (STDs), 76, 141–48
siblings, 43
sickle cell anemia, 93
SIDS (sudden infant death syndrome), 32, 33, 280, 285

silver nitrate eye drops, 145, 146, 279
single mothers, 105, 106, 107, 158
skin-to-skin contact. See touch
sleep, 81, 120, 218
slings, 123
small for dates, 98–99, 243
small for gestational age, 98, 113
smoking, 32–33, 79, 85, 98–99, 187
social interventions, 188 (See also poverty)
Society of Obstetricians and Gynecologists of Canada (SOGC), 127, 133, 143, 154, 230
sound: during labour, 217; monitoring fetus, 231
spina bifida, 51, 54, 95, 96
spinal anaesthesia, 130, 131, 225–26, 231
spinal cord: baby, 95; maternal, 220
spinal headache, 226
spotting, 57, 67
steristrips, 132
stethoscope, 227, 262
stillbirth, 51, 262, 275
stool softeners, 64
strep. See Group B strep
stress, 33, 48, 79, 81, 82, 92, 162, 204, 243
stress incontinence, 152, 259
stretch marks, 152
stretch-and-sweep, 246, 248
strollers, 124
sun exposure, 52
sunny-side up (birth), 173
supplementation, 51–53, 63, 195, 288
Supreme Court of Canada, 32
surfactant, 193
sutures, 257
swelling, 151, 180, 181–82
swimming, 82
swings, mechanical, 124
syphilis, 85, 146–47
systolic blood pressure, 180

tastebuds, fetus, 120–21
tears, vaginal, 257 (See also episiotomy)
teeth buds, 120
TENS (transcutaneous electrical nerve stimulation), 217

teratogenicity, 35, 68
terbutaline, 189, 233
test weighing, 297–98
tetracycline, 146, 279
thalidomide, 35
therapeutic abortion, 92, 93, 94, 96–97
threatening to miscarry, 85–86
thrush, 65
thyroid disease, 242
tobacco, 32–33
toes, fetus, 120
touch, 193, 194, 215, 231, 237, 288
toxemia. See pre-eclampsia
toxoplasmosis, 70, 98
trachea, 210
tranquilizers, 218
transient tachypnoea of the newborn, 126
transverse (Caesarean) incision, 130, 135
transverse lie, 60, 125, 126, 137, 179
transverse lower uterine segment incision, 135–36
trial of labour, 135, 136, 137
triple dye, 279
triplets, 21, 47, 111, 114, 187, 193
tubal ligation, 88
tubal pregnancy, 88–89
twins, 57, 58, 111, 112, 113, 114, 187
Type 1 diabetes, 47, 161
Type 2 diabetes, 47, 161, 162

ultrasound, 28, 30, 56–61, 84, 87, 98
umblicial artery, 101
umbilical cord, 14, 101, 190, 209, 221, 266–68, 279
underweight mother, 79
UNICEF, 286
unripe cervix, 243–44
urinary tract infections (UTIs), 115–17
U.S. Center for Disease Control, 144
uterus, 14, 88: incision on, 130; measuring, 76; placenta across bottom. See placenta previa; rupture of, 135–36, 137, 139

vaccination, 68

vacuum delivery, 24, 155, 221, 225, 229, 230, 232, 249, 259, 261: vs. forceps, 261–64
vagina, 14, 15: prolapsed, 130; tears, 256, 257; yeast infections, 65
vaginal birth, 81, 114: and premature birth, 192–93; vs. Caesarean, 126, 133, 178–79, 192
vaginal breech delivery, 178–79
vaginal cancer, 88
vaginal examination, 154, 165, 167, 231, 253, 256
varicose veins, 151
VBAC (vaginal birth after Caesarean), 104, 106, 107, 133, 134–40
vegetarianism, 54–55
vena cava, 231
ventilator, 189, 193
vertex presentation (birth), 172–78
videos, 105, 106, 109
visualization, 213
vitamin B6, 52, 63, 233
vitamin D, 52, 53, 54
vitamin K, 192, 279

walking, 82, 107, 126, 127, 154, 156, 204, 205, 206, 214, 221
water, breaking. See under membranes
water: immersion in (labour), 215–16; drinking, 64, 116, 231; sterile, 216
weaning, 287, 288, 290, 309
weight: baby, 32, 51, 52, 53, 54, 58, 79, 80, 81, 98, 121; gain, 79, 80, 81; loss, 79–80, 81; maternal, 48, 50, 63, 78–81
William Obstetrics, 217–18, 272
windpipe, suctioning, 210, 278
witch hazel, 151
World Health Organization (WHO), 144–45, 286, 297

X-rays, 34

yeast infections, 65, 170
yeast vaginitis, 65
young mothers, 47, 50, 79, 187

zidovudine, 144